Recent Advances in PEDIATRICS
(Special Volume–28)
Child Nutrition in Practice

The most up-to-date compendium of peer-reviewed, evidence-based and state-of-the-art topical issues of special relevance and applicability to the Indian subcontinent and other resource-limited countries, especially in the South-East Asian Region (SEAR)

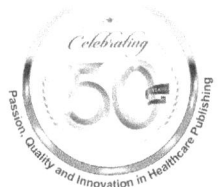

Academic Editor
Suraj Gupte

Executive Editors
Shamma-Bakshi Gupte
Manu Gupte

Excerpts from Reviews in Journals

"...provides a wealth of much-sought information... An indispensable series for modern pediatricians of resource-poor nations..."
—*Asian Journal of Tropical Pediatrics, Kuala Lumpur, Malaysia*

"A remarkable blend of excellence and state-of-the-art information in child health with special reference to the Indian subcontinent..."
—*European Bulletin of Child Health, Edinburgh, UK*

"...series of extraordinary merit... a boon for pediatric scholars in India and other developing countries."
—*Journal of Pediatrics and Child Health, Victoria, Australia*

"An essential reading for pediatric postgraduates, scholars and practitioners looking for state-of-the-art information."
—*Indian Practitioner, Mumbai, Maharashtra, India*

"Strongly recommended...an extraordinary, meritorious series."
—*Academy Today (Bulletin, Indian Academy of Pediatrics), Mumbai, Maharashtra, India*

"A commendable work... a must for pediatric scholars."
—*Journal of the Indian Medical Association, Kolkata, West Bengal, India*

"An immensely valuable series, combining much-sought-after information and its clinical applicability."
—*Current Pediatric Practice, Bhavnagar, Gujarat, India*

"A highly recommended desktop reference series... with excellent format."
—*Asian Medical News, Hong Kong, China*

"An excellent series with tremendous potentials...an essential reading for pediatric scholars having thirst for updates providing latest developments and projections for the future."
—*Asian Journal of Maternal and Child Health, Manila, Philippines*

Jaypee's Other Titles by Professor (Dr) Suraj Gupte

- *Recent Advances in Pediatrics (RAP): Hot Topics (General/Miscellaneous Pediatrics)*
  Vol 26 (2018), Vol 25 (2017), Vol 24 (2016), Vol 23 (2015), Vol 22 (2014), Vol 21 (2013), Vol 20 (2011), Vol 19 (2010), Vol 18 (2009), Vol 17 (2007), Vol 16 (2006), Vol 15 (2005), Vol 14 (2004), Vol 13 (2003), Vol 12 (2002), Vol 11 (2001), Vol 10 (2000), Vol 9 (1999), Vol 8 (1998), Vol 7 (1997), Vol 6 (1996), Vol 5 (1995), Vol 4 (1994), Vol 3 (1993), Vol 2 (1992), Vol 1 (1991)

- *Recent Advances in Pediatrics (RAP): Special Volumes*
  RAP Special Vol 27: Infectious Diseases-II/Book 2
  RAP Special Vol 26: Infectious Diseases-I/Book 1
  RAP Special Vol 25: Perspectives in Neonatology
  RAP Special Vol 24: Respiratory Diseases
  RAP Special Vol 23 : Pediatric Gastroenterology, Hepatology and Nutrition
  RAP Special Vol 22 : Immunology, Infections and Immunization
  RAP Special Vol 21 : Neonatal and Pediatric Intensive Care
  RAP Special Vol 20 : Nutrition, Growth and Development
  RAP Special Vol 19 : Developmental and Behavioral Pediatrics
  RAP Special Vol 18 : Pediatric Neurology
  RAP Special Vol 17 : Adolescence
  RAP Special Vol 16 : Pediatric Cardiology
  RAP Special Vol 15 : Nephrology
  RAP Special Vol 14 : Critical Care Pediatrics
  RAP Special Vol 13 : Pediatric Endocrinology
  RAP Special Vol 12 : Neonatal Emergencies
  RAP Special Vol 11 : Community Pediatrics
  RAP Special Vol 10 : Pulmonology
  RAP Special Vol 09 : Neurology
  RAP Special Vol 08 : Emergency Pediatrics
  RAP Special Vol 07 : Hematology
  RAP Special Vol 06 : Gastroenterology, Hepatology and Nutrition
  RAP Special Vol 05 : Neonatology-2
  RAP Special Vol 04 : Neonatology
  RAP Special Vol 03 : Tropical Pediatrics-2
  RAP Special Vol 02 : Tropical Pediatrics
  RAP Special Vol 01 : Nutrition, Growth and Development

- *Recent Advances in Pediatrics (RAP) Volumes in Pipeline*
  RAP Special Vol 29: Emergencies and Intensive/Critical Care
  RAP 27 Hot Topics: General/Miscellaneous Pediatrics
  RAP Special Vol 30: Child Neurology and Developmental Pediatrics

Other Jaypee Books by Prof (Dr) Suraj Gupte
- The Short Textbook of Pediatrics, 13th edition, 2020
- Case-based Reviews in Pediatric Emergencies, 2017
- Pediatric Drug Directory, 9th edition, 2018
- Differential Diagnosis in Pediatrics, 6th edition, 2020
- Instructive Case Studies in Pediatrics, 5th edition, 2011

Recent Advances in PEDIATRICS
(Special Volume–28)

Child Nutrition in Practice

Academic Editor

Suraj Gupte MD FIAP FSAMS (Sweden) FRSTMH (London)
Professor and Head (Emeritus)
Postgraduate Department of Pediatrics
Mamata Medical College and Mamata General and Superspecialty Hospitals
Khammam, Telangana, India
drsurajgupte@gmail.com
www.drsurajgupte.com

Editor: The Short Textbook of Pediatrics; Recent Advances in Pediatrics (Series); Textbook of Pediatric Emergencies, Neonatal Emergencies, Pediatric Nutrition, and Pediatric Gastroenterology, Hepatology and Nutrition; Pediatric Infectious Diseases; Influenza: Complete Spectrum; Case-based Reviews in Pediatric Emergencies; Clinical Problem Solving in Neonatal Emergencies and Intensive Care, etc.

Author: Differential Diagnosis in Pediatrics, Pediatric Drug Directory, Instructive Case Studies in Pediatrics, Influenza, Perspectives in Influenza, Nutrition in Neonatal ICU, Speaking of Child Care, etc.

Chief Editor (Gastroenterology Section): International Journal of Gastroenterology, Hepatology, Transplant and Nutrition (Jaipur, India)

Co-editor: Asian Journal of Maternity and Child Health (Manila, Philippines).

Section and Guest Editor: Pediatric Today (New Delhi).

Editorial Advisor: Asian Journal of Pediatric Practice (New Delhi).

Editorial Advisory Board Member/Reviewer: EC Pediatrics (London), Indian Journal of Pediatrics (New Delhi, India) Pediatrics (New Delhi), Indian Journal Child Health (Gwalior), Synopsis (Detroit, USA), Maternal and Child Nutrition (Preston, UK), Journal of Infectious Diseases (Turkey), EC Pediatrics (London), Journal of Clinical Pediatrics (Patna), etc.

Examiner: Several Universities, including National Board of Examinations (NBE) for DNB, New Delhi; All India Institute of Medical Sciences (AIIMS), New Delhi; Postgraduate Institute of Medical Education and Research (PGIMER), Chandigarh; Sher-I-Kashmir Institute of Medical Sciences (SKIMS), Srinagar; Indira Gandhi Open University (IGNOU), New Delhi.

Pediatric Faculty Selection Expert: All India Institute of Medical Sciences (AIIMS), Punjab Public Service Commission, Jammu and Kashmir Public Service Commission, Union Public Service Commission.

Executive Editors
Shamma-Bakshi Gupte
Manu Gupte

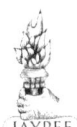

JAYPEE BROTHERS MEDICAL PUBLISHERS
The Health Sciences Publisher
New Delhi | London

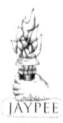 **Jaypee Brothers Medical Publishers (P) Ltd.**

Headquarters
Jaypee Brothers Medical Publishers (P) Ltd
4838/24, Ansari Road, Daryaganj
New Delhi 110 002, India
Phone: +91-11-43574357
Fax: +91-11-43574314
Email: jaypee@jaypeebrothers.com

Overseas Office
J.P. Medical Ltd
83 Victoria Street, London
SW1H 0HW (UK)
Phone: +44 20 3170 8910
Fax: +44 (0)20 3008 6180
Email: info@jpmedpub.com

Website: www.jaypeebrothers.com
Website: www.jaypeedigital.com

© 2020, Shamma-Bakshi Gupte, Manu Gupte (Executive Editors)

The views and opinions expressed in this book are solely those of the original contributor(s)/author(s) and do not necessarily represent those of editor(s) of the book.

All rights reserved. No part of this publication may be reproduced, stored or transmitted in any form or by any means, electronic, mechanical, photocopying, recording or otherwise, without the prior permission in writing of the publishers/editors.

All brand names and product names used in this book are trade names, service marks, trademarks or registered trademarks of their respective owners. The publisher is not associated with any product or vendor mentioned in this book.

Medical knowledge and practice change constantly. This book is designed to provide accurate, authoritative information about the subject matter in question. However, readers are advised to check the most current information available on procedures included and check information from the manufacturer of each product to be administered, to verify the recommended dose, formula, method and duration of administration, adverse effects and contraindications. It is the responsibility of the practitioner to take all appropriate safety precautions. Neither the publisher nor the author(s)/editor(s) assume any liability for any injury and/or damage to persons or property arising from or related to use of material in this book.

This book is sold on the understanding that the publisher is not engaged in providing professional medical services. If such advice or services are required, the services of a competent medical professional should be sought.

Every effort has been made where necessary to contact holders of copyright to obtain permission to reproduce copyright material. If any have been inadvertently over-looked, the publisher will be pleased to make the necessary arrangements at the first opportunity. The **CD/DVD-ROM** (if any) provided in the sealed envelope with this book is complimentary and free of cost. **Not meant for sale.**

Inquiries for bulk sales may be solicited at: jaypee@jaypeebrothers.com

Recent Advances in Pediatrics (Special Volume–28): Child Nutrition in Practice

First Edition: **2020**

ISBN: 978-93-5270-476-7

Printed at

Dedicated to

My dear Parents
whose inspiration, motivation, blessings
and moral support continue to contribute a great
deal to our academic endeavors
and
Everybody striving to contribute to child health
and welfare for a brighter future globally

Contributors

Anuradha Bansal
Assistant Professor
Department of Pediatrics
Punjab Institute of Medical Sciences
Jalandhar, Punjab, India
Ch 23: Handling Nutrtional Problems in Office Practice

Aruna Chandra
Senior Fellow in Nutrition
Institute of Child and Adolescent Health
London, United Kingdom
Ch 1: Nutritional Needs in Children

Ashish Simalti
Assistant Professor
Department of Pediatrics
Army Hospital R and R
New Delhi, India
Ch 18: Immunology of Malnutrition

Anita Singh
Assistant Professor,
Department of Neonatology
Sanjay Gandhi Postgraduate
Institute of Medical Sciences
Lucknow, Uttar Pradesh, India
Ch 21: Feeding Low Birth Weight Babies

Anup Thakur
Consultant Neonatologist, Sir Ganga
Ram Hospital, New Delhi, India
Ch 21: Feeding Low Birth Weight Babies

Aditi
DM Senior Resident
Pediatric Gastroenterology
Department of Gastroenterology
Postgraduate Institute of Medical
Education and Research (PGIMER)
Chandigarh, India
Ch 30: Diet in Chronic Liver Disease

Bhavana B Lakhkar
Professor of Pediatrics
Shri BM Patil Medical college
BLDE University
Vijayapur, Karnataka, India
Ch 13: Infant and Young Child Feeding

Dhiren R Patel
Assistant Professor, Department of
Pediatrics, Division of Gastroenterology,
Hepatology and Nutrition
Saint Louis University School of
Medicine, Saint Louis, Missouri, USA
Ch 27: Nutrition in Cystic Fibrosis

Edwin Dias
Professor and Head, Department of
Pediatrics, Srinivas Institute of Medical
Sciences and Research Center
Mangaluru, Karnataka, India
Ch 32: Food Intolerance and Allergy

EW Kawasaki
Associate Professor, Gasatroenterology,
Hepatology and Nutrition, University of
Tokyo Hosptal, Tokyo, Japan
Ch 7: Vitamin D Deficiency Rickets and Other Rickets

E William
Senior Consultant in Nutrition
Institute of Child and Adolescent Health
London, United Kingdom
Ch 1: Nutrtional Needs in Children

GS Latha
Professor of Pediatrics
SS Institute of Medical Sciences and
Research Center (SSIMS and RC)
Mangaluru, Karnataka, India
Ch 2: Antioxdants

Harmesh S Bains
Professor and Head, Department of
Pediatrics, Punjab Institute of Medical
Sciences, Jalandhar, Punjab, India
Ch 6: Vitamin D Deficiency
Ch 11: Zinc in Childhood Malnutrition
Ch 16: Severe Acute Malnutriton
Ch 17: Refeeding Syndrome
Ch 22: Pedatric Obesity
Ch 23: Handling Nutrtional Problems in Office Practce
Ch 26: Nutrtional Management of Diarrhea

Isobel Tanapong
Chairman, Human Nutrition Division
Bangkok Christian Hospital
Bangkok, Thailand
Ch 5: Vitamin A Deficiency

Jeffrey H Teckman
Chief of Gastroenterology and Professor
of Pediatrics, Department of Pediatrics
and Department of Biochemistry and
Molecular Biology, Saint Louis University
School of Medicine, Saint Louis,
Missouri, USA
Ch 27: Nutrition in Cystic Fibrosis

Jatinder Singh
Associate Professor
Department of Pediatrics
Punjab Institute of Medical Sciences
Jalandhar, Punjab, India
Ch 26: Nutritional Management of Diarrhea

Kareena Naidu
Research Fellow in Human Nutrition
Bangkok Christian Hospital
Bangkok, Thailand
Ch 5: Vitamin A Deficiency

Manu Sharma Sareen
Assistant Professor
Department of Pediatrics
Punjab Institute of Medical Sciences
Jalandhar, Punjab, India
Ch 16: Severe Acute Malnutrition

Novy Gupte
Drug Regulatory Consultant
Clinical Development Service Agency
(CDSA)
Department of Pharmacology
All India Institute of Medical Sciences
New Delhi, India
Ch 4: Vitamins: Essentials and Therapeutics in a Nutshell
Ch 8: Micronutrients and Macrominerals

Noopur Singhal Sud
Assistant Professor, Department of
Pediatrics, Punjab Institute of Medical
Sciences, Jalandhar, Punjab, India
Ch 22: Pediatric Obesity

Nithya Thuruthiyath
Senior Resident, Department of
Pediatrics, Government Medical College
Thrissur, Kerala, India
Ch 19: Malnutrition and the Nervous System

Pushwinder Kaur
Assistant Professor
Department of Pediatrics
Punjab Institute of Medical Sciences
Jalandhar, Punjab, India
Ch 17: Refeeding Syndrome
Ch 20: Prevention of Childhood Malnutrition

Pushpendra Magon
Professor, Department of Pediatrics
Punjab Institute of Medical Sciences
Jalandhar, Punjab, India
Ch 11: Zinc in Child Nutrition
Ch 20: Preventon of Childhood Malnutrition

Piyush Upadhyay
Assistant Professor of Pediatrics
Dr Ram Manohar Lohia (RML) Institute
of Medical Sciences
Lucknow, Uttar Pradesh, India.
Ch 9: Iron Deficiency Anemia
Ch 34: Sports Nutrition
Ch 35: Nutritional Supplements

Contributors ix

Pankaj C Vaidya
Additional Professor
Department of Pediatrics
Advanced Pediatrics Centre (APC)
Postgraduate Institute of Medical
Education and Research (PGIMER)
Chandigarh, India
Ch 30: Diet in Chronic Liver Disease

Rashmi Dwivedi
Professor and Head, Department of
Pediatrics, Gandhi Medical College
Bhopal, Madhya Pradesh, India
*Ch 12: Antenatal Nutrition: Effect on
Fetal and Neonatal Outcome*
Ch 14: Adolescent Nutrition

Rakhi Jain
Lecturer in Pediatrics
GSVM Medical College
Kanpur, Uttar Pradesh, India
Ch 9: Iron Deficiency Anemia
Ch 34: Sports Nutrition
Ch 35: Nutritional Supplements

Rajiv Sinha
Associate Professor and Head
Division of Pediatric Nephrology
Institute of Child Health
Consultant Pediatric Nephrologist
AMR and Fortis Hospitals
Kolkata, West Bengal, India
Ch 31: Nutrition in Acute Kidney Injury

Sheikh Minhaj Ahmed
Full-time Pediatric Intensivist
Lilavati Hospital and Research Centre
Mumbai, Maharashtra, India
Ch 18: Immunology of Malnutrition
Ch 33: Drug-Nutrient Interaction

Sandeep Dhingra
Assistant Professor, Department of
Pediatrics, Armed Forces Medical
College, Pune, Maharashtra, India
Ch 33: Drug-Nutrient Interaction

Suraj Gupte
Professor and Head (Emeritus)
MMC and General and Superspecialty
Hospital, Khammam, Telangana, India

Ch 1: Nutrtional Needs in Children
Ch 3: Assessment of Nutritional Status
*Ch 4: Vitamins: Essentials and
Therapeutics in a Nutshell*
Ch 5: Vitamn A Deficiency
*CH 7: Vitamin D Deficiency Rickets and
Other Rickets*
Ch 8: Micronutrients and Macrominerals
*Ch 15: Protein-Energy Malnutrition:
Overview*

Shaveta Kundra
Head, Department of Pediatrics
ESIC Model Hospital
Ludhiana, Punjab, India
Ch 24: Nutrtion in Diabetes
Ch 28: Nutrition in Celiac Disease

Sumantra Kumar Raut
DM PGT in Pediatric Nephrology
All India Institute of Medical Sciences
(AIIMS), New Delhi, India
Ch 31: Nutrition in Acute Kidney Injury

TM Ananda Kesavan
Additional Professor in Pediatrics
Government Medical College
Thrissur, Kerala, India
*Ch 10: Neuropsychiatric Dysfunctons in
Iron Deficiency Anemia*
*Ch 19: Malnutrition and the Nervous
System*

Thomas L Ratchford
Fellow, Division of Gastroenterology
Hepatology and Nutrition
Department of Pediatrics
Saint Louis University School of
Medicine, Saint Louis, Missouri, USA
Ch 27: Nutrition in Cystic Fibrosis

Utpal Kant Singh
Professor, Department of Pediatrics
Nalanda Medical College
Patna, Bihar, India
Ch 3: Assessment of Nutritional Status
*Ch 4: Vitamins: Essentials and
Therapeutics in a Nutshell*
Ch 8: Micronutrients and Macrominerals
*Ch 15: Protein-Energy Malnutrition:
Overview*

VN Tripathi
Senior Professor of Pediatrics
Government Medical College
Kanpur, Uttar Pradesh, India
Ch 9: Iron Deficiency Anemia
Ch 34: Sports Nutrition
Ch 35: Nutritional Supplements

Vibhor V Borkar
Consultant Pediatric Hepatologist and
Gastroenterologist, Department of
Hepatology and Liver Transplantation
Global Hospital; Consultant Paediatric
Gastroenterologist and Hepatologist
SRCC Children's Hospital, Haji Ali
Visiting Pediatric Gastroenterologist
Lokmanya Tilak Medical College
Mumbai, Maharashtra, India
Ch 30: Diet in Chronic Liver Disease

Waheeda Shaik
Senior Fellow, Gastroenterology,
Hepatology and Nutrition, University of
Tokyo Hospital, Tokyo, Japan
Ch 7: Vitamin D Deficiency Rickets and Other Rickets

Yogesh Waikar
Consultant Gastroenterologist
Superspeciality GI Kids Clinics and
Imaging, Nagpur, Maharashtra, India
Ch 25: Nutrition in Pediatric Irritable Bowel Syndrome

Preface

Balanced nutrition is the lifeline of child's optimal growth and development, and cognition. Not just that! Nutrition impacts the health and well-being across the entire lifespan, i.e. from the earliest stages of fetal development, at birth, and through infancy, childhood, adolescence and adulthood. Appropriate feeding practices stimulate bonding with the caregiver and psychosocial development. They lead to improved nutrition and physical growth, reduced susceptibility to common childhood illnesses and better resistance to cope with them. Improved health outcomes in young children have long-lasting health benefits throughout the life-span, including increased performance and productivity, and reduced risk of certain noncommunicable diseases.

Erratic nutrition — more often related to erroneous knowledge, beliefs and attitude rather than food deficiency — leads to nutritional problems, such as undernutrition (including micronutrient deficiencies), overweight and obesity. In the Indian subcontinent, we have abundance of undernutrition in one or the other form. But, along with that, there exists growing problem of overweight and obesity especially during adolescence in prosperous populations. This double burden of undernutrition and obesity is a matter of considerable concern.

With this background, *RAP Special Vol 28* presents up-to-date information on topical issues in child nutrition and nutrition-related disorders in order to promote health for children including those who have special needs, based on the recent and current medical and scientific concepts and breakthroughs.

In keeping with the mission and the policy of the RAP series ever since its inception and first appearance in 1990-91, the volume presents 35 chapters developed by 40 experts drawn from India and abroad focusing on the contemporary concepts, concerns, and controversies with emphasis on new and evolving concepts in child nutrition as relevant in India and other South-East Asian countries. Each and every chapter is outstanding by its excellence, providing a stimulating, mature, informed, state-of-the-art and, at places, even provocative update.

The startup Part 1, a spotlight on the fundamentals of child nutrition presents a grid of 3 well-written chapters. Unwinding with the first chapter on nutritional needs of infants and children, it provides information on basics of nutrition that is crucial for normal growth and development. Next comes the chapter on antioxidants that are critical in neutralizing the harmful free radicals and eliminating them. The third chapter emphasizes the importance of clinical parameters, especially the anthropometry, in the assessment of nutritional status.

Part 2 deals with vitamins and Part 3 with micronutrients and macrominerals (that are essential for balanced nutrition) as also their deficiencies and excesses. They play important roles in child's development and well-being including the regulation of metabolism, cellular pH, and bone density. Their significance should never be downplayed in clinical nutrition.

Three fine chapters of Part 4 provide information on nutrition in different age groups. The impact of maternal nutrition on the growing fetus and the newborn and, in subsequent life is aptly made out. The importance of enhanced nutrition needs in adolescence — the period of rapid growth stands duly emphasized.

Part 5 dwells on the paradoxically dual burden of undernutrition and obesity. Undoubtedly, undernutrition continues to remain extraordinarily high in the poorer populations of India. But, paradoxically, overweight and obesity too are heading for endemic levels in prosperous segments of population.

A somewhat off-beat Chapter 6 puts forward a workable approach of tackling nutritional problems of infants and children in office practice in Part 6. This should be of considerable interest and utility for the busy practitioner.

Part 7 deals with nutrition in such systemic diseases as pediatric diabetes, diarrhea, irritable bowel syndrome (IBS), cystic fibrosis, and celiac disease.

Part 8 are incorporated excellent chapters on somewhat neglected though very important areas, i.e. food intolerance and allergy, drug-nutritive interaction and sports nutrition.

Finally, we have miscellaneous topics in Part 8 that provides in-depth descriptions on food intolerance and allergy, drug-nutrient interaction — an area that has remained neglected until recently, and sports nutrition. The chapter on sports nutrition rightly sets out to dependable information for promoting nutrition practices that enhance fitness and sports performance.

Notably, a multidisciplinary approach with an eye on future, a well-tested and well appreciated conviction with the RAP series, continues to occupy pride of place in the present volume too. Such an approach is known to be befitting when the goal is not only to inform but also to motivate discussion, interaction, research and innovation.

The volume is intended to be used by pediatric scholars, practitioners and health providers working in preventive and curative services around the world including both high- and low-income settings.

We are confident that the *RAP Special Vol 28: Child Nutrition in Practice* shall provide the potential readers an enjoyable, fruitful and productive source of much-sought-after information in child nutrition.

Suraj Gupte
Academic Editor

Acknowledgments

Grateful acknowledgments are made to:
- The contributing authors, both from India and abroad, for providing excellent state-of-the-art chapters on various topical issues. They were gracious enough to repose confidence in our editorship.
- The Advisory Editorial Board for providing inputs and advice in various matters.
- The peer-reviewers, for critically reviewing the contributions, thereby providing us the benefit of their expertise.
- Dr Gagan Hans, Assistant Professor (Psychiatry), All India Institute of Medical Sciences, New Delhi, for voluntarily helping us in several ways.
- Dr Novy Gupte, for voluntarily helping us in various ways in taking the project to its logical conclusion.
- Shivani-Mahendru Gupte, Project Officer, TCS, Jammu and Kashmir, for considerable help.
- Various journals and periodicals for editorial and critical reviews of RAP volumes and for permission to use their references in the state-of-the-art chapters.
- The readers who provide us the feedback to maintain and enhance the excellence of the series.

Finally, M/s Jaypee Brothers Medical Publishers (P) Ltd, New Delhi, India, and their dedicated staff deserve our appreciation for the skillful and commendable production qualities of the book.

Contents

PART 1: PRINCIPLES OF CHILD NUTRITION

1. **Nutritional Needs in Children** — 1
   Suraj Gupte, Aruna Chandra, E William

2. **Antioxidants** — 20
   GS Latha

3. **Assessment of Nutritional Status** — 32
   Suraj Gupte, Utpal Kant Singh

PART 2: VITAMINS

4. **Vitamins: Essentials and Therapeutics in a Nutshell** — 40
   Novy Gupte, Suraj Gupte, Utpal Kant Singh

5. **Vitamin A Deficiency** — 64
   Suraj Gupte, Kareena Naidu, Isobel Tanapong

6. **Vitamin D Deficiency** — 72
   Harmesh S Bains

7. **Vitamin D Deficiency Rickets and Other Rickets** — 78
   Suraj Gupte, Waheeda Shaik, EW Kawasaki

PART 3: MINERALS

8. **Micronutrients and Macrominerals** — 95
   Novy Gupte, Suraj Gupte, Utpal Kant Singh

9. **Iron Deficiency Anemia** — 109
   VN Tripathi, Piyush Upadhyay, Rakhi Jain

10. **Neuropsychiatric Dysfunctions in Iron Deficiency Anemia** — 116
    TM Ananda Kesavan

11. **Zinc in Child Nutrition** — 126
    Pushpendra Magon, Harmesh S Bains

PART 4: NUTRITION IN DIFFERENT PEDIATRIC AGE GROUPS

12. **Antenatal Nutrition: Effect on Fetal and Neonatal Outcome** — 133
    Rashmi Dwivedi

13. Infant and Young Child Feeding ... 147
    Bhavana B Lakhkar

14. Adolescent Nutrition ... 169
    Rashmi Dwivedi

PART 5: UNDERNUTRITION AND OBESITY

15. Protein-Energy Malnutrition: Overview ... 184
    Suraj Gupte, Utpal Kant Singh

16. Severe Acute Malnutrition ... 227
    Harmesh S Bains, Manu Sharma Sareen

17. Refeeding Syndrome ... 235
    Pushwinder Kaur, Harmesh S Bains

18. Immunology of Malnutrition ... 242
    Ashish Simalti, Sheikh Minhaj Ahmed, Uday Bodhankar

19. Malnutrition and the Nervous System ... 254
    TM Ananda Kesavan, Nithya Thuruthiyath

20. Prevention of Childhood Malnutrition ... 261
    Pushwinder Kaur, Pushpendra Magon

21. Feeding of Low Birth Weight Babies ... 270
    Anita Singh, Anup Thakur

22. Pediatric Obesity ... 286
    Noopur Singhal Sud, Harmesh S Bains

PART 6: PEDIATRIC PRACTITONER AND NUTRITION

23. Handling Nutritional Problems in Office Practice ... 303
    Anuradha Bansal, Harmesh S Bains

PART 7: NUTRITION IN SYSTEMIC DISEASES

24. Nutrition in Diabetes ... 317
    Shaveta Kundra

25. Nutrition in Pediatric Irritable Bowel Syndrome ... 330
    Yogesh Waikar

26. Nutritional Management of Diarrhea ... 335
    Jatinder Singh, Harmesh S Bains, Vaneeta Bhardwar

27. Nutrition in Cystic Fibrosis ... 342
    Thomas L Ratchford, Jeffrey H Teckman, Dhiren R Patel

28. **Nutrition in Celiac Disease** — 356
   Shaveta Kundra

29. **Diet in Inflammatory Bowel Disease** — 369
   Pankaj C Vaidya

30. **Diet in Chronic Liver Disease** — 379
   Aditi, Pankaj C Vaidya, Vibhor V Borkar

31. **Nutrition in Acute Kidney Injury** — 386
   Sumantra Kumar Raut, Rajiv Sinha

PART 8: MISCELLANEOUS

32. **Food Intolerance and Allergy** — 401
   Edwin Dias

33. **Drug-Nutrient Interaction** — 409
   Uday Bodhankar, Sandeep Dhingra, Sheikh Minhaj Ahmed

34. **Sports Nutrition** — 420
   VN Tripathi, Rakhi Jain, Piyush Upadhyay

35. **Nutritional Supplements** — 426
   VN Tripathi, Piyush Upadhyay, Rakhi Jain

Index — 433

PART 1: PRINCIPLES OF CHILD NUTRITION

1 Nutritional Needs in Children

Suraj Gupte, Aruna Chandra, E William

ABSTRACT
An understanding of the nutritional requirements of infants, children and adolescents is important not only in relation to macronutrients (carbohydrates, fats, proteins) but also minerals, including macrominerals and microminerals (micronutrients or trace elements) in health and disease. Also, it needs to be appreciated that nutrition needs are at peak in the first 3 years of life because of the rapid growth and adolescence when the growth spurt occurs. To counter the free radicals, defenses are provided in the form of antioxidants which are defined as substances in food that significantly decrease the adverse effects of free radicals. Examples of antioxidants are superoxide dismutase, transferrin, glutathione peroxidase, vitamin C (ascorbic acid), vitamin E (tocopherol), β-carotene, selenium, zinc, iron, manganese, nicotinamide, riboflavin and lycopene. Immunonutrition has bright prospects and potentials for cutting down morbidity and mortality in critically ill children with the above indications. Nevertheless, more work is warranted to establish their efficacy and safety in children.
Keywords: Antioxidants, Carbohydrates, Fats, Immunonutrients, Microminerals, Macronutrients, Micronutrients, Minerals, Nutritional requirements, Protein, Trace elements.

INTRODUCTION

Adequate nutrition is of paramount importance during childhood, especially in the first three years of life, when growth is most rapid and the child is, by and large, totally dependent on caretaker(s), usually the parents.[1-5] Suboptimal nutrition leads to poor weight gain and growth failure.[5-8] Naturally, a basic knowledge of nutritional requirements at various ages as also sources of vitamins and other micronutrients and minerals is mandatory.[1]

NUTRIENTS

The term, *energy requirement* or *needs*, denotes the amount of dietary energy required to balance energy expanded and deposited in new tissues (growth). Table 1 gives the break-up of energy expenditure.

Table 1: Break-up of energy expenditure.

Growth	12%
Physical activity	25%
Basal metabolism	50%
Fecal loss	8%

In order to meet the growth needs in first three years and during adolescence, a higher energy dense diet (less complex carbohydrates and larger quantity of fat) is needed. Seven principle classes of nutrients are—carbohydrates, fats, proteins, fiber, mineral, vitamins and water. Leaving aside fiber, the remaining six are the chief constituents of food. These six factors form the human body in the following way:

- **Water:** 63%
- **Proteins:** 17%
- **Fats:** 12%
- **Carbohydrates:** 1%
- **Vitamins and minerals:** 7%.

The term, **macronutrients**, refers to carbohydrates, fats and proteins—the building blocks of the body that are needed in large amounts (g).

The term, **micronutrients**, denotes vitamins and minerals that are needed in only very small amounts (µg, mg). Their role in enhancing immunity and in various metabolic pathways as cofactors is indispensable.

The term, **macrominerals,** is used for such elements as calcium, sodium, potassium, magnesium, etc. that are needed in grams rather than mcg or mg.

The term, **microminerals**, is synonymous with micronutrients.

The term, **recommended dietary allowance**, refers to recommended daily levels of nutrients estimated to be sufficiently high to meet the physiologic needs of nearly all healthy individuals in a particular age and gender group. Alternative terms used include **daily requirement, safe intake of nutrients** and **recommended daily amounts of nutrients**.

WATER

It is second only to oxygen as a must for survival. Compared to adults, infants require much larger amount of water per unit of body weight. Its requirements at different ages are given in Table 2.

CARBOHYDRATES

Carbohydrates, the major source of energy (4 kcal/g), add up to the bulk (55–60%), taste and texture of the diet. Two types are known:

1. **Simple:** Monosaccharide, disaccharides, e.g. glucose, fructose (sucrose in sugar, lactose in milk), fruits, vegetables.
2. **Complex:** Oligosaccharides, polysaccharides, e.g. starch, pulses, millets, roots.

Table 2: Daily requirement for water.

Age range	Water requirement (mL/kg)
First 3 days	80–100
3–10 days	125–150
15 days–3 months	140–160
3–12 months	150
1–3 years	125
4–6 years	100
7–9 years	75
10–12 years (and thereafter)	50

Table 3: Daily calorie requirement of infants.

Age range (months)	Requirement (cal/kg)
0–3 months	120
3–6 months	115
6–9 months	110
9–12 months	105

Table 4: Daily requirement for calories.

Age range (years)	Requirement (Kcal/kg)
Under 1 (average)	110
1–3	100
4–6	90
7–9	80
10–12	70
13–15	60
16–19	50
Adult	40

With the exception of fiber, all carbohydrates are converted to glucose which is either employed as a fuel by the brain and muscles or stored in liver and muscles as glycogen. Carbohydrates consumed in excess are converted to fat.

Glucose from starch and sugar in diet constitute the main source of energy. The cells use glucose as a fuel. The liver and muscles convert it to glycogen. Excess carbohydrates are converted to fat.

Calorie or energy requirement varies from age to age as is shown in Tables 3 and 4. On an average, 50% of calories should come from carbohydrates, 35% from fats and 15% from protein.

It is worth remembering that daily requirement is 100-120 kcal/kg for the first year of life. During the subsequent period, it decreases by around 10 kcal/kg for each succeeding three year duration.

Table 5: Absolute daily requirement for calories during first year.

Age (months)	Calorie requirement
1	500
2	600
4	700
5	800
9	900
10	1,000

Table 6: Holliday and Seger formula for daily calorie and fluid calculations.

Weight range	Calories	Fluids
3–10 kg	100 kcal/kg/day	100 mL/kg/day
10–20 kg	1,000 + 50 kcal/kg/day for each kg >10 kg	1,000 + 50 mL/kg/day for each kg >10 kg
20 kg	1500 + 20 kcal/kg/day for each kg >20 kg	1,500 mL/kg/day for each kg >20 kg

Box 1: Break-up of energy requirement.

- Maintenance of basal metabolism: 50%
- Specific dynamic action: 5%
- Growth: 12%
- Physical activity: 25%
- Losses in stools, etc.: 8%

Table 5 presents the total daily calorie requirement during the first year of life. An infant of 1 year of age needs about 1,000 kcal. A rough rule is to add 100 calories per each year of age up to a maximum of 1,500 kcal. About adolescence; when the growth spurt occurs, calorie needs are much higher. According to this rule, a child of 5 years of age needs 1,000 + 400 = 1,400 kcal. Calculations according to another widely-employed formula (Holliday and Seger formula) are given in Table 6. Box 1 gives the break-up of energy requirement.

PROTEINS

Proteins of animal origin are termed ***biologically complete proteins*** since these provide a good deal of essential amino acids, namely—lysine, leucine, isoleucine, tryptophan, valine, methionine, phenylalanine, threonine and histidine. On the contrary, proteins of vegetable origin are usually ***biologically incomplete*** since they lack one or more of the essential amino acids. However, when different vegetable sources of protein are combined, result is a product that is likely to provide all the essential amino acids. Higher amounts of vegetable proteins are needed to make allowance for low biological value (Table 7).

Table 7: Daily requirement for proteins.

Age range (years)	Protein requirement (g/kg)
Under 1	2.6–3.5
1–3	2.0–2.5
4–6	3.0
7–9	2.8
10–12	2.0
13–15	1.7
16–19	1.5
Adult	1.0

Box 2: Protein quality indices.

- Biologic value (BV)
- True digestibility (TD)
- Net protein utilization (NPU)

Box 3: Nutritive value of an average-size hen's egg.

• Fat (6 g)	54 kcal
• Proteins (6 g)	24 kcal
• Carbohydrates	Negligible
• Total calories	78 kcal
• Cholesterol	200 mg
• Sodium	65 mg

Biologic value (BV) is defined as the fraction of absorbed nitrogen retained in the body for growth or maintenance. It is 100 for egg protein which is regarded as the ***reference protein***, 75 for milk and fish and 67 for rice. Energy value of protein is four kcal/g. Protein quality is judged by biologic value, true digestibility and net protein utilization (NPU) (Box 2).

Egg protein is considered a ***reference protein*** on account of its highest BV and NPU (Box 3 and Fig. 1). Since egg protein BV is taken as 100%, other foods are expressed in relation to this value. As a rough rule, animal proteins possess higher BV than plant protein.

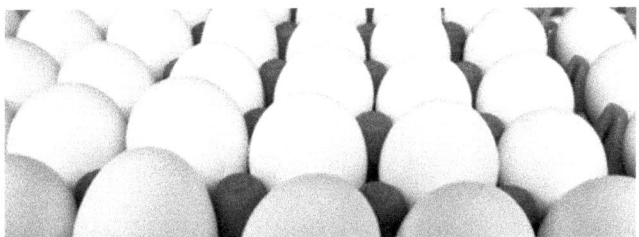

Fig. 1: Egg protein, a standard reference protein, is known for the highest biological value. On an average, one hen's egg provides 6 g protein (24 kcal), 6 g fat (54 kcal) and a total energy of 78 kcal. Egg yolk has a cholesterol content of 200 mg/egg.

FIBER

By definition, fiber is a non-starch polysaccharide that, though non-digestible with negligible food value, helps in digestion of food stuffs. It is a constituent of plant cell and forms bulk of diet.

Fiber-containing Foods

Important fiber-containing foods include:
- Cereals—whole wheat in particular
- Pulses and legumes
- Sprouted seeds
- Nuts—groundnut, walnut, almonds
- Fruits—whole fruits in particular
- Vegetables, including dried beans, green-leafy vegetables (GLV) in particular.

Types

Two types are:
1. *Fibrous:* Cellulose, hemicellulose, lignin
2. *Viscous:* Pectins, gums, mucilages.

Advantages

- It forms the stool bulk which is important for normal functioning of the gut, including proper movements.
- It is important for preventing and even curing chronic constipation.
- It promotes satiety (stomach contentment).
- It prevents hypercholesterolemia.
- It slows down gastric emptying.
- It flattens glucose tolerance curve.
- It decreases blood glucose level in diabetics.
- It enhances water-holding capacity of gut.
- It safeguards against colonic cancer and diverticulitis.

Disadvantage

Very high fiber intake may interfere with bioavailability of minerals resulting in deficiency diseases, e.g. calcium-deficiency rickets.

Daily Requirement

- *Infants and children:* 300–400 mg/kg/day
- *Adolescents:* Around 30–40 g/day.

FATS

- Fats constitute concentrated energy-giving element, thereby enhancing the calories without much increase in bulk. The minimal requirement is not accurately defined.

- Over and above being major source of energy, fats carry fat-soluble vitamins A, D, E and K and are precursors of hormones and prostaglandins.
- Usually up to 30% of total energy should be from fats (3.5% of calories should be supplied by linoleic acid and 0.3% from linolenic acid). Since human body is incapable of synthesizing this acid, it has got to be supplied in diet. Its deficiency in infants causes dryness and thickening of the skin with desquamation and intertrigo.
- Important lipids are:
  - Triglycerides (fats and oils)
  - Phospholipids (lecithin) and
  - Sterols (cholesterol).
- Depending on the length of the carbon, triglycerides may be:
  - Short-chained
  - Medium-chained triglycerides (MCT)
  - Long-chained triglycerides (LCT)
- Depending on the saturation, triglycerides may be:
  - *Saturated:* Obtained from meat and coconut oil. Human body can also produce them from carbohydrates and proteins.
  - *Unsaturated:* Monounsaturated and polyunsaturated, obtained from vegetables, nuts and seeds.
- Whereas monounsaturated fatty acids (MUFA) such as oleic acid may also be produced by the body, polyunsaturated fatty acids (PUFA), also called **essential fatty acids** (EFA), must be provided by the dietary sources. PUFA consists of omega-6 fatty acids (linoleic acid, arachiodonic acid) present in normal balanced diet and omega-3 fatty acids, e.g. linolenic acid, eicosapentaenoic acid (EPA) and docosahexaenoic acid (DHA) which are present in fish and seafood.
- Essential fatty acids deficiency manifests as growth failure, alopecia, diarrhea, and fragile bone from decreased calcium absorption and deposit in bones.
- Lecithin is a major component of cell membrane. It is synthesized by the liver.
- Cholesterol, an important component of cell membrane, may be produced by the human liver. Additionally, its dietary sources include animal fats (egg, meat especially kidney and liver, cheese, desi ghee). It may be transformed to hormones, vitamin D and bile. The daily intake of cholesterol should not exceed 250–300 mg. Just one egg provides near 200–250 mg of cholesterol. Hence consumption of more than one full egg/day is not rationally good.
- Energy value of fats is 9 kcal/g. No more than 7% total fats in diet should be saturated.

GLYCEMIC INDEX

The term, *glycemic index* (GI), is defined as the extent of ability of a carbohydrate item to raise blood glucose level. Hence, higher the glycemic index of a carbohydrate foodstuff, more is the chance of its making a rapid rise in blood glucose level. Likewise, lower the GI of a carbohydrate foodstuff less is the chance of its making a rapid rise in blood glucose level.

High GI foodstuffs include glucose and rice. The low GI foodstuff includes wheat, maize and pulses. These food items are preferred for diabetic patients.

Advantages of Low Glycemic Index Food Items

- Supply and maintenance of blood glucose level for longer time, resulting in prolonged physical endurance.
- Reduction in hunger.
- Facilitation of reduction in weight.
- Reduction in blood glucose level.
- Increased sensitivity to insulin.
- Reduced risk of cardiovascular disease.

VITAMINS

Requirements of vitamins that are essential for maintenance of good health are listed in Table 8.

MINERALS/ MICRONUTRIENTS/TRACE ELEMENTS

Macrominerals are cations like calcium, magnesium, sodium, potassium and anions like phosphorus, sulfur and chloride that are needed in amounts exceeding 100 mg/day.

Elements like iron, zinc, copper, cobalt, iodine, selenium, molybdenum and chromium which are needed in very small amounts (up to 100–200 µg/g

Table 8: Daily requirement for vitamins.

Vitamins	Requirement
A	1,500–5,000 IU
B_1 (Thiamine)	0.5–1.5 mg
B_2 (Riboflavin)	0.5–2.5 mg
B_3 (Niacin, ninacinamide, nicotinamide, nicotinic acid)	0–2 mg
Pantothenic acid	1.7–5 mg
B_6 (Pyrdoxine)	0.4–1.4 mg
B_7 (Biotin)	5–25 µg
B_9 (Folic acid)	1–1.5 µg
B_{12} (Cyanocobalamine)	25–1,000 µg
C (Ascorbic acid)	30–50 mg
D_3 (Cholecalciferol)	400 IU
E	4–5 IU

(IU: international unit)

matrix) are called *microminerals, micronutrients* or *trace elements*. The recommended intake of important minerals is given in Table 9. Table 10 lists salient features of important minerals.

Table 9: Daily requirement for minerals.

Mineral	Requirement
Iron	• Infants: 1mg/kg (6–10 mg) • 1–years: 15 mg • 3–12 years: 10 mg • 12–18 years: 18 mg
Calcium	• Infants: 400–600 mg • 1–10 years: 0.7–1.0 g • Over 10 years: 1.2–1.5 g
Magnesium	• Infants: 40–70 mg • 1–3 years: 100–150 mg • 3–12 years: 200–300 mg • 12–18 years: 300–350 mg
Potassium	1.5 mEq/kg (1–2 g)
Sodium	2.0 mEq/kg
Zinc	0.3 or more mg/kg
Iodine	0.2 mg
Copper	0.05–0.1 mg/kg
Fluorine	0.5–1 mg

Table 10: Salient features of important minerals/trace elements/micronutrients.

Mineral/trace element	Source	Deficiency	Excess
Iron	Green vegetables, meat, yolk, whole grains, nuts, legumes, milk, especially, breastmilk, is a poor source	Microcytic-hypochromic anemia	Hemosiderosis, poisoning
Zinc	Cheese, nut, grains, meat, fish	Dwarfism with iron-deficiency anemia, hyperpigmentation, hepatosplenomegaly, hypogonadism, acrodermatitis enteropathica: poor wound healing, depressed immunocompetence, ITS, LBW	Gastrointestinal upset, copper deficiency, reduced high density lipoprotein
Copper	Legumes, nuts, whole grains, meat, liver, oyster (shell-fish)	Refractory anemia, osteoporosis, neutropenia, depigmentation, ataxia, raised serum cholesterol	ICC

Contd...

Contd...

Mineral/trace element	Source	Deficiency	Excess
Magnesium	Cereals, legumes, nuts, meat, milk	Tetany	None
Calcium	Milk and its products, fish, green leafy vegetables	Tetany, rickets	Renal stones, heart block
Phosphorus	Milk and its products, fish, green leafy vegetables	Rickets	Tetany
Iodine	Seafood, vegetables from iodine-rich soil, iodized salt	Goiter, cretinism	Goiter
Fluoride	Seafood, tea	Dental caries	Fluorosis
Chromium	Drinking water, animal foods, yeast	Impaired glucose tolerance, diabetes mellitus in animals	None

(ITS: infantile tremor syndrome; LBW: low birth weight; ICC: Indian childhood cirrhosis)

Table 11: Foods affecting absorption of iron from the gut.

Absorption enhanced	Absorption reduced
Vitamin C-rich foods	• Tea • Coffee • Maize • Phytates (whole meal bread)
• Guava • Lemon • Orange • Indian gooseberry	
Foods containing heme iron	
• Liver • Meat • Chicken • Fish	
Fermented/germinated foods	

Iron

Two types of iron is available from food: ***heme*** and ***nonheme***. Heme iron is found in nonvegetarian foods, say meat, liver, chicken and fish. Around 15–35% heme iron gets absorbed from the gut. Nonheme iron is present in plants, legumes, eggs, milk and cereals. Its absorption is much less, i.e. hardly 1%. Several factors influence its absorption (Table 11). During adolescence, iron needs enhance. This is especially true in case of menstruating teenagers.

Zinc

Zinc is normally present in our body in sufficient amount. No supplementation is, therefore, required by healthy individuals. In certain situations, say diarrhea (especially persistent diarrhea), malnutrition, infantile tremor syndrome

(ITS), and acrodermatitis enteropathica, zinc deficiency coexists. Therefore, zinc supplementation is strongly recommended to hasten recovery in these conditions. Normal daily requirement of zinc is 4–6 mg/day. Excess of zinc intake may be complicated by copper deficiency.

FREE RADICALS AND ANTIOXIDANTS

Free Radicals Causing Tissue Damage

By definition, *free radicals* are atoms or molecules that contain one or more unpaired electrons that are capable of altering (usually enhancing) their chemical reactivity and cause tissue damage. These are produced in large amounts during all tissue activities (infection, phagocytosis, tissue injury, and ischemia-perfusion). Examples of free radicals are superoxide anions, singlet oxygen, peroxide anion, hydroxyl radical and hydrogen peroxide. Excess of free radicals results either from their higher production or from inadequate antioxidant defense. Disorders in which free radicals appear to play a significant role are listed in Box 4.

Antioxidants

Antioxidants are defined as substances in food that significantly decrease the adverse effects of free radicals. Examples of antioxidants are superoxide dismutase, transferrin, glutathione peroxidase, vitamin C (ascorbic acid), vitamin E (tocopherol), β-carotene, selenium, zinc, iron, manganese, nicotinamide, riboflavin and lycopene.

Recently, a number of synthetic antioxidants N-acetyl cysteine (NAC), glutathione, glutathione peroxidase analogue (ebselen), coenzyme Q derivatives and

Box 4: Free radicals in the pathogenesis of various disorders.

- Retinopathy of prematurity
- Rh hemolytic disease
- Hemolytic anemia of the newborn
- HIE
- IVH
- BPD
- ARDS
- Cystic fibrosis
- NEC
- IBD
- Rheumatoid arthritis
- Severe edematous PEM (kwashiorkor)
- Cholestatic liver disease
- Pancreatitis
- Iron-overload (hemochromatosis)
- Copper-overload (Wilson disease, ICC)
- Storage disorders
- Malignancies.

(HIE: hypoxic-ischemic encephalopathy; IVH: intraventricular hemorrhage; BPD: bronchopulmonary dysplasia; ARDS: acute respiratory distress syndrome; NEC: necrotizing enterocolitis; IBD: inflammatory bowel disease; PEM: protein energy malnutrition; ICC: Indian childhood cirrhosis; Rh: rhesus disease)

superoxide dismutase are available. These are yet to be successfully tried in humans.

Types of antioxidants are:
- *Intracellular antioxidant:* Superoxide dismutase and glutathione peroxidase.
- *Extracellular antioxidant:* Transferrin, haptoglobin, albumin, extra-cellular superoxide dismutase and catalase, bilirubin, mucus, glucose, vitamin C, urate.
- *Lipoprotein antioxidant:* Vitamin E, beta-carotene, retinyl stearate and lycopene.
- *Membrane antioxidant:* Vitamin E, beta-carotene and coenzyme O.
- *Nutritional antioxidants:* Vitamin E (tocopherols and tocotrienols), beta-carotene, vitamin C, phytochemicals like flavonoids, flavones, flavanols, cinnamic acid, cumarin derivatives, phytoalexin derivatives and selenium as a cofactor for glutathione peroxidase, cysteine, taurine.
- Selenium compounds like glutathione peroxidase, food additives like propyl gallate, butylated hydroxyanisole, antioxidant drugs like allopurinol, desferrioxamine and NAC.

Several exogenous substances such as natural dietary components (β-carotenoids, vitamin E, vitamin C, selenium) and pharmaceutical agents (desferrioxamine, allopurinol) can function as antioxidants. However, so far exogenous supplementation of antioxidants is yet to establish its clear-cut role in prevention of disease. Nutritionists, therefore are of the opinion that a mixed well-balanced diet, vegetables, fruits that supply vitamins and other micronutrients is the most feasible and the best way to ensure a sufficient supply of antioxidants.

IMMUNONUTRITION

Immunonutrition (IMN), a relatively new concept, is defined as enteral feeding formulas supplemented with immunonutrients comprising of amino acids, antioxidants, micronutrients and probiotics, etc. aimed at providing beneficial effects of enhanced immune function and, thereby cutting down risk of infectious complications.[9]

Commonly-employed Immunonutrients

The most commonly employed and researched immunonutrients are:
- Amino acids—arginine (a nonessential amino acid), glutamine (precursor for nucleotide)
- Nucleotides
- Fatty acids—omega-3 polyunsaturated fatty acids
- Taurine
- Vitamins—A, C and E
- Micronutrients—iron, zinc, selenium
- Prebiotics and probiotics.

Till date, most experience revolves around ***glutamine supplementation***. Glutamine is a precursor for nucleotide synthesis, a substrate for liver gluconeogenesis and an important fuel source for cell with rapid turnover, say gastrointestinal epithelium, lymphocytes, fibroblasts, reticulocytes, etc.

Arginine, a nonessential amino acid, is a conditionally essential amino acid during catabolic states such as sepsis and trauma (just like glutamine). It has a wide range of biological actions that are beneficial to the body.

Role
- *Nucleotides* play a key role in T-cell function and cell-mediated immunity.
- *Omega-3 fatty acids* (linolenic acid), found in fatty fish oil, has considerable effect on the immune system in the form of immunologic benefit and anti-inflammatory effect.
- *Taurine* is a conditionally semi-essential amino acid in neonates, especially preterms. Currently, it is employed in most infant formulas.
- *Vitamins* A, C, E and micronutrients, iron, zinc, selenium are well known for their immunologic role.
- *Prebiotics and probiotics* exert their beneficial immunologic effect by varied mechanisms, including enhancement of the mucosal immune defense.

Administration
Immunonutrients having favorable effect on the immune system are added to standard nutritional support solutions for deriving immunological benefits. They are usually administered in supranormal doses enterally. At times, they may be added parenterally for modulating response to surgery, trauma or sepsis.

Indications
Undoubtedly, immunonutrition has the potential to cut down morbidity and mortality in critically ill children with:
- Gastrointestinal diseases—inflammatory bowel disease (IBD)
- Immune deficiency disorders
- Polytrauma
- Sepsis.

There is an evidence that immunonutrition may have a promising role in cancer prevention.

Future Prospects
Immunonutrition has bright prospects and potentials for cutting down morbidity and mortality in critically ill children with the above indications. Nevertheless, more work is warranted to establish their efficacy and safety in children.

DIETARY INTAKE BY CHILDREN: INDIAN SCENARIO

Survey conducted by the National Nutrition Monitoring Bureau (NNMB) indicates that diet of the Indian preschoolers is grossly deficient in each and every category of food (Table 12).

Overall, it is the deficiency of calories (energy), whereas protein intake is, by and large, satisfactory. A noteworthy observation is that diet of children belonging to the higher strata of society show intake of protein that is in excess. It is, therefore, important to lay stress on total intake of food rather than just protein as is often done in practice.

Table 13 presents the recommended balanced diets for children. Table 14 gives the nutritive value of some commonly used foods in India as per the

Table 12: National Nutrition Monitoring Bureau (NNMB) survey data on actual vis-a-vis recommended dietary consumption by Indian preschoolers as per Indian Council of Medical Research (ICMR) document.

Dietary item	Actual intake	Recommended intake
Cereals (g)	147	150–200
Pulses (g)	16	40–50
Leafy vegetables (g)	4	50–75
Other vegetables (g)	14	30–50
Fruits (g)	7	40–50
Milk and milk products (g)	80	200
Fats and oils (g)	4	20–25
Flesh foods (g)	4	30
Sugar and jaggery (g)	5	30–40
Calories (kcal)	758	1200–1700
Protein (g)	22–30	22–30
Iron (mg)	6.9	11.5–18.4
Calcium (mg)	193	400
Vitamin A (mg)	220	400
Riboflavin (mg)	–	0.7–1.0

Table 13: Balanced diets for children.

	Preschool children				School children			
	1–3 years		4–6 years		7–9 years		10–12 years	
	Veg. (g)	Nonveg. (g)	Veg. (g)	Nonveg. (g)	Veg. (g)	Nonveg. (g)	Veg. (g)	Nonveg. (g)
Cereals	150	150	200	200	250	250	320	320
Pulses	50	40	60	50	70	60	70	60
Green leafy vegetables	50	50	75	75	75	75	100	100
Other vegetables/roots and tubes	30	30	50	50	50	50	75	75
Fruits	50	50	50	50	50	50	50	50
Milk	300	200	250	200	250	200	250	200
Fats and oils	20	20	25	25	30	30	35	35
Meat fish and eggs	–	30	–	30	–	30	–	30
Sugar and jaggery	30	30	40	40	50	50	50	50

Indian Council of Medical Research (ICMR) with minor modifications. Fruits, vegetables and nuts and seeds are rich in vitamins, micronutrients, minerals, antioxidants and fiber (Figs. 2 to 7).

Table 14: Nutritive value of commonly used food (per 100 g).

Foodstuffs	Calories	Proteins	Foodstuffs	Calories	Proteins
Cereals			**Nuts**		
• Wheat	346	11.8	• Coconuts (dry)	662	6.8
• Rice	346	6.5	• Cashew nut	596	21.2
• Maize	325	4.7	• Groundnut	549	26.7
• Wheat-flour	348	11.0	• Apple	55	0.3
• Soyabean	432	43.2	• Pineapple	46	0.4
• Green gram	348	24.5	• Orange	53	0.3
• Black gram (dal)	347	24.0			
Pulses			**Fruits**		
• Bengal gram (whole)	360	17.1	• Guava	51	0.9
• Bengal gram (dal)	372	20.8	• Tomato (ripe)	20	0.9
• Peas (dry)	315	19.7	• Pomegranate	65	1.6
			• Apricot	51	0.6
			• Mango (ripe)	53	1.0
			• Lemon	57	1.0
			• Litchi	61	1.1
Leafy vegetables			**Flesh foods**		
• Onion tops	61	4.7	• Egg	173	13.5
• Spinach	26	2.0	• Goat meat	118	21.4
• Mustard leaves	34	4.0	• Mutton	194	18.5
• Cabbage	27	1.8	• Chicken	300	25
• Cauliflower leaves	67	5.9	• Fish	80–100	18–20
Roofs and Tubers			**Milk products**		
• Onion	49	1.4	• Cow's milk	66	3.2
• Carrot	48	0.9	• Buffalo's milk	110	4.3
• Potato	97	1.6	• Human milk	66	1.1
• Turnip	29	0.5			
Other vegetables			**Miscellaneous**		
• Amla (Indian gooseberry)	58	0.5	• Bread	245	7.8
• Cauliflower	30	2.6	• Sago	351	0.2
• Pumpkin	25	1.4	• Sugar	398	0.1
• French beans	48	3.8	• Jaggery	383	0.4
			• Oil or ghee	900	Nil

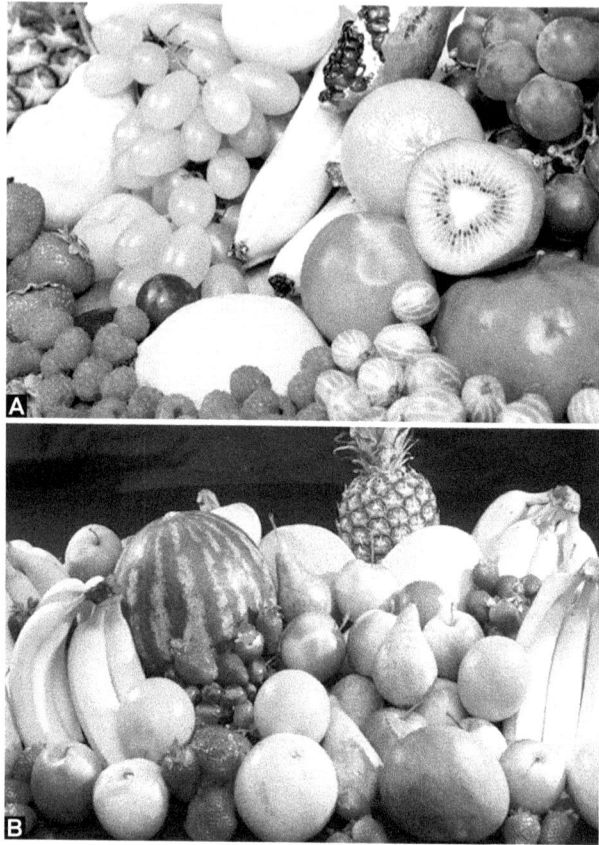

Figs. 2A and B: Fruits are a rich source of vitamins, minerals and antioxidants.

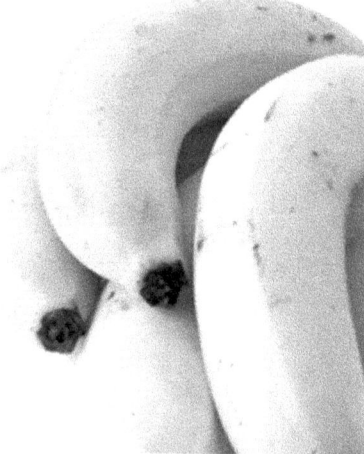

Fig. 3: Bananas are a rich source of carbohydrates (energy), each medium-sized banana providing around 100 kcalories. Also provided are potassium, manganese, vitamin C, vitamin B_6, antioxidants, fiber, and phytonutrients. Fats and cholesterol are virtually negligible.

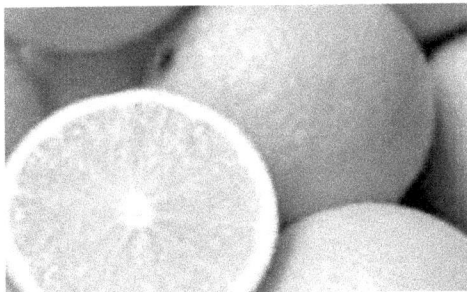

Fig. 4: Orange and other citrus fruits provide plenty of vitamin C.

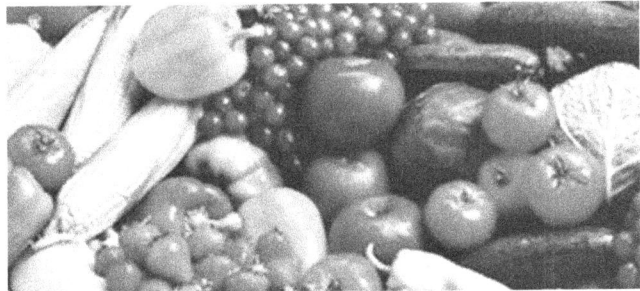

Fig. 5: Vegetables are a rich source of vitamins and minerals.

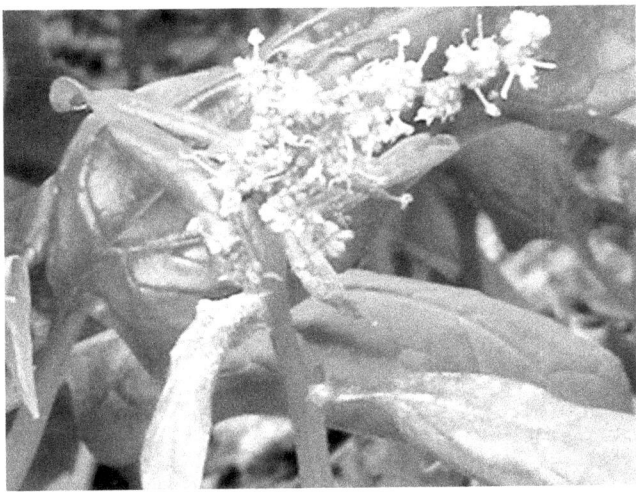

Fig. 6: Dark green leafy vegetables (DGLVs) such as amaranthal, spinach (palak) and fenugreen are a rich source of minerals (iron, zinc, calcium, phosphorous, potassium), vitamins (A, B-complex, C, E, folate, K), fiber and antioxidants. Spinach has been designated as the world's healthiest vegetable.

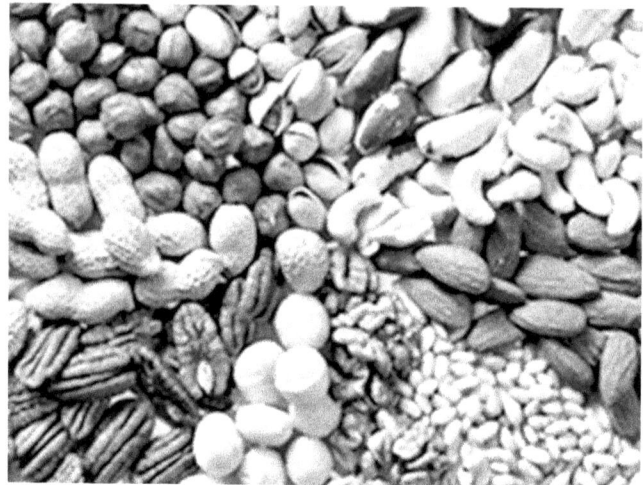

Fig. 7: Mixed nuts and seeds are rich source of unsaturated fat and vitamin E.

CONCLUSION

Nutritional requirements of carbohydrates, proteins and fats as well as minerals in childhood are at peak in the first 3 years of life because of the rapid growth and again during adolescence when the growth spurt occurs. Antioxidants like superoxide dismutase, transferrin, glutathione peroxidase, vitamin C (ascorbic acid), vitamin E (tocopherol), β-carotene, selenium, zinc, iron, manganese, nicotinamide, riboflavin and lycopene too are needed to counter the adverse effects of free radicals. Though immunonutrients have bright prospects and potentials for cutting down morbidity and mortality in critically ill children, more work is needed to establish their efficacy and safety in children.

KEY LEARNING POINTS

- An appreciation of the requirements carbohydrates, fats, proteins, minerals, including macrominerals and microminerals (micronutrients or trace elements) in health and disease is important.
- Nutrition needs are at peak in the first 3 years of life because of the rapid growth and adolescence when the growth spurt occurs.
- Antioxidants (superoxide dismutase, transferrin, glutathione peroxidase, vitamin C (ascorbic acid), vitamin E (tocopherol), β-carotene, selenium, zinc, iron, manganese, nicotinamide, riboflavin and lycopene) are required to decrease the adverse effects of free radicals.
- Immunonutrition carries a promise for cutting down morbidity and mortality in critically ill children though more work is warranted to establish its efficacy and safety in pediatric practice.

REFERENCES

1. Kleinman RE, Greer FR. (For American Academy of Pediatrics Committee on Nutrition). *Pediatrc Nutrition*, 7th edn. Illinois: American Academy of Pediatrics 2013.
2. Bang A, Tiwari SK. Nutritional requirements. In: Gupte S (Ed): *Pediatric Nutrition*, 2nd edn. New Delhi: Peepee 2012:1-9.
3. Vani S, Gupte S. Nutritional requiurements. In: Gupte S (Ed): *The Short Textbook of Pediatrics*, 12th edn. New Delhi: Jaypee 2016:173-182.
4. Indian Council of Medical Research: *Nutrient Requirements and Recommended Dietary Allowances for Indians: Report of Expert Group of the Indian Council of Medical Research*. Hyderabad: National Institute of Nutrition/ICMR 1990.
5. Bhatia J, Griffin I, Anderson D, Kler N, Domellof M. Requirement of iron, copper and zinc in preterm infants. *J Pediatr* 2013:162:48-55.
6. Elizabeth KE. *Nutrition and Child Development* 5th edn. Hyderabad: Paras 2014.
7. Ghosh S. *Nutrition and Child Care*: A *Practical Guide*. New Delhi: Jaypee 2000.
8. Mehta MN, Mehta NJ. *Nutrition and Diet for Children Simplified*. New Delhi: Jaypee, 2014.
9. Bavdekar SB, Suvarna J. Immunonutrition. In: Gupte S (Ed): *Pediatric Nutrition*, 2nd edn. New Delhi: Peepee 2012:274-289.

2

Antioxidants

GS Latha

ABSTRACT

In recent years, there has been a great deal of attention towards the field of free radical chemistry. Free radicals reactive oxygen species and reactive nitrogen species are generated by our body by various endogenous systems, exposure to different physiochemical conditions or pathological states. A balance between free radicals and antioxidants is necessary for proper physiological function. If free radicals overwhelm the body's ability to regulate them, a condition known as oxidative stress ensues.

Free radicals adversely alter lipids, proteins, and DNA and trigger a number of human diseases. Oxidative stress is thought to contribute to the development of a wide range of diseases including heart disease, cancer, the pathologies caused by diabetes, rheumatoid arthritis, and neurodegeneration in motor neuron diseases.

External source of antioxidants can help in coping this oxidative stress. Recent growth in the knowledge of free radicals and reactive oxygen species (ROS) in biology is producing a medical revolution that promises a new age of health and disease management.

The present article on antioxidants provides a brief overview on oxidative stress mediated cellular damages and role of dietary antioxidants as functional foods in the management of human diseases.

Keywords: Antioxidants, Dietary antioxidants, Free radicals, Human disease, Oxidative stress, Reactive oxygen species.

INTRODUCTION

An antioxidant is a molecule stable enough to donate an electron to a rampaging free radical and neutralize it, thus reducing its capacity to damage. These antioxidants delay or inhibit cellular damage mainly through their free radical scavenging property.[1] Oxygen is an element indispensible for life.[2] Oxygen is used by the cells to generate energy. Free radicals are created as a consequence of ATP production by the mitochondria. These products are reactive oxygen species (ROS), results from the cellular redox process and play a dual role as both toxic and beneficial compounds. At low or moderate levels, ROS exert beneficial effects on cellular responses and immune function. Whereas, at higher concentration, generate oxidative stress, a deleterious process that can damage all cellular structures.[3]

Free radicals are substances normally produced by the human as one of the defense mechanisms against harmful substances. When the rate of their production exceeds the antioxidant capacity of the body, oxidative stress occur.[4]

Oxidative stress plays a major role in the development of chronic and degenerative diseases such as cancer, arthritis, hypertension, atherosclerosis, diabetes mellitus, autoimmune disorders, cardiovascular and other neuro-degenerative diseases.[5-9]

The human body has several mechanisms to counteract oxidative stress by producing antioxidants.

ANTIOXIDANTS

Antioxidants are molecules that inhibit the oxidation of other molecules. It is a chemical reaction that can produce free radicals, leading to chain reactions that may damage cells. Antioxidants terminate these chain reactions. The oxidative damage can trigger a low grade silent inflammation throughout the body that lingers for years or decades leading to the production of inflammatory hormones and chemicals, which turn on genes causing fat storage and disease and simultaneously turn off genes reducing inflammation and health risk.[10]

History

Antioxidants are known in the medical literature in the early 19th and 20th centuries. Such as vitamin A and vitamin C were first researched by doctors, Henry Mattill during 1920's–1950's, used to explain why animal fed on whole foods lived longer and healthier.[11]

Antioxidants came to public attention in the 1990s, when scientists began to understand that free radical damage was involved in the early stages of artery-clogging atherosclerosis and may contribute to cancer, vision loss, and a host of other chronic conditions.[12-13]

People with low intakes of antioxidant-rich fruits and vegetables were at greater risk for developing these chronic conditions than were people who ate plenty of these fruits and vegetables.

Antioxidants are either naturally produced in situ or externally supplied through foods and/or supplements. Endogenous and exogenous antioxidants act as free radicals scavengers by preventing and repairing damage caused by ROS, and therefore can enhance the immune system and lower the risk of cancer and degenerative diseases.[4]

Characteristic Features of Free Radicals

Free radicals are less stable and very short lived than non-radical species, although their reactivity is generally stronger. A molecule with one or more unpaired electron in its outer shell is called a free radical.[14]

Free radicals include hydroxyl (OH•), superoxide ($O_2^{•-}$), nitric oxide (NO•), nitrogen dioxide ($NO_2^•$), peroxyl (ROO•) and lipid peroxyl (LOO•). Also, hydrogen peroxide (H_2O_2), ozone (O_3), singlet oxygen ($^1O_2$), hypochlorous acid (HOCl), nitrous acid (HNO_2), peroxynitrite ($ONOO^-$), dinitrogen trioxide (N_2O_3), lipid peroxide (LOOH) are not free radicals and generally called oxidants, but can easily lead to free radical reactions in living organisms.[15]

As free radicals are unstable, they are difficult to measure. But, detrimental effect caused by them can be measured by estimating their byproducts.

Foods

Fruits and Vegetables

Over recent years considerable epidemiological evidence has been gathered to suggest an association between consumption of fruits and vegetables. Antioxidant vitamins are found in vegetables, fruits, eggs, legumes and nuts.

Dietary supplements representing antioxidant from 5 to 7 servings of fruits and vegetables has shown to increase the major antioxidants nutrients in human plasma concentrations similar to those obtained through inclusion of fruit and vegetables in the diet. Lycopene and ascorbic acid concentration were maintained or increased even though the amounts supplied by the supplements were minimal.[16]

Foods Rich in Antioxidants

Antioxidant rich foods like vitamin A, vitamin C, beta-carotene, flavonoids and lycopene, herbs and supplements include green leafy vegetables, artichokes, cocoa, wild berries, green tea, sea vegetables like Kelp, spirulina, quercetin or essential oils like lavender.

- Vitamin A from foods rich in beta-carotene (e.g. carrot, beetroot, sweet potato, spinach).
- Vitamin C from citrus fruits, berries, raw cabbage and broccoli.
- Vitamin E from whole grains, nuts, fish oil, and green leafy veggies.
- Beta-carotene and its related carotenoids (e.g. lycopene, lutein) from fruits and veggies of a red, yellow, and orange color.
- Selenium and manganese minerals from seafood, lean meat, nuts, and whole grains.
- Flavonoids from tea, coffee, and berries.
- Resveratrol from red wine and dark grapes.
- Phytoestrogens from peanuts and soybeans.

Herbs

Clove, cinnamon, oregano, turmeric, cocoa, cumin, ginger, thyme, garlic, cayenne, pepper and green tea.

Fruits

Gojjiberries, wild blue berries, elder berries, cranberries, blackberries, cilantro, dried raisins.

Table 1: Dietary sources of antioxidant vitamins.

Antioxidant vitamins	Foods containing high levels of antioxidant vitamins[17]
Vitamin C (ascorbic acid)	Fresh or frozen fruits and vegetables
Vitamin E (tocopherols, tocotrienols)	Vegetable oils, nuts, and seeds
Carotenoids (carotenes as provitamin A)	Fruit, vegetables and eggs

The processed foodstuffs contain fewer antioxidant vitamins than fresh and uncooked food since preparatory process exposes food to heat and oxygen. Vitamins A, C, and E can be destroyed by long-term storage or prolonged cooking.[18]

In a study, results from the evaluation of the antioxidant activity of various plant parts, the traditional preparations and extracts from various kinds of fruits and leaves demonstrate that among varieties also may be some differences. Extracts of dry fruits of rose water without boiling showed a high antioxidant value, also 'honeys' prepared by extraction of flower from elderberry and dandelion. Whereas, leaves of ramsons-wild garlic showed very low levels of antioxidant activity.[19]

Recommended Allowance

No official recommended daily allowance for antioxidants or antioxidant foods. But, more consumption of foods every day from naturally occurring foods in the diet, the better.

Level of antioxidants in any substance or food is evaluated with an "ORAC Score"(Oxygen radical absorption capacity).

Relation to Diet

It is known that antioxidants, (vitamins) are required in the diet, for good health. There is a considerable debate whether antioxidant rich foods or supplements in having a role in preventing diseases or anti-disease activity. If they are beneficial it is still unknown that which antioxidant is needed in the diet and in what amount is required beyond the dietary intake.[20-22,39-41]

Polyphenols which often have antioxidant properties in vitro are not necessarily antioxidants in vivo due to extensive metabolism.

Drugs

Tirilazad is an antioxidant steroid derivative that inhibits the lipid peroxidation that is believed to play a key role in stroke and head injury.[23] This activity was demonstrated in animal models of stroke, but trials on human showed no beneficial effect on mortality or other outcomes in subarachnoid hemorrhage[24] and worsened results in ischemic stroke.[25,26]

A 2016 systematic review examined antioxidant medications such as allopurinol and acetyl cysteine, as add on treatment for schizophrenia.[27] Evidence was insufficient to determine benefits. Even there was no benefit seen with vitamin E supplementation[28] for physical performance. Six weeks of vitamin E supplementation had no effect on muscle damage in ultra marathon runners.[29]

ROLE OF ANTIOXIDANTS IN MALNUTRITION

Investigations over the last 20 years suggest that increased activity of free radicals and a low concentration of antioxidant and oxidative stress play a role in the pathogenesis of kwashiorkor. This results in the overproduction of reactive oxygen species. These ROS will lead to membrane oxidation and thus an increase in lipid peroxidation such as malondialdehyde (MDA) and protein oxidation by product protein mainly polycarboxyl (PC).[30]

Some results show that lower glutathione concentration (GSH) also vitamin E, or precursor of amino acids of GSH, like cysteine, carotene, selenium and polyunsaturated fatty acids with a decreased NADPH/NADP+ ratio are reduced and elevated glutathione-S transferase activity in kwashiorkor.[31-35]

Another study measures low levels of enzymatic antioxidants like superoxide-dismutase and glutathione peroxidase.[36] All data from these studies shows that protective antioxidative system is impaired in children with kwashiorkor.

Also it has been noted that leukotriene metabolism is known to be redox regulated, studies conducted shows that impaired synthesis of leukotriene, likely to contribute to the pathophysiologic characteristics of kwashiorkar, particularly generalized edema and the susceptibility to infections.[31-35] If so much beneficial, can antioxidants can be used as a therapy in the treatment and prevention of malnutrition. Antioxidant supplementation at the dose provided did not prevent the onset of kwashiorkor.[37] This finding does not support the hypothesis that depletion of vitamin E, selenium, cysteine or riboflavin has a role in the development of kwashiorkor. The study suggests that antioxidant depletion may be a consequence rather than a cause of kwashiorkor.[38]

There has been growing evidence over the past three decades showing malnutrition (dietary deficiency of proteins, selenium, zinc) or excess of certain nutrients (e.g. iron and vitamin C) gives rise to the oxidation of biomolecules and cell injury.[39]

Further research is needed before antioxidants can be included in the WHO treatment protocol for malnutrition (2012).

Role of Dietary Supplements

Supplementation of antioxidant should improve the health and help in preventing certain diseases. But dietary supplements do not improve health nor they are effective in preventing diseases as shown by randomized clinical trials including supplements of beta-carotene, vitamin A and vitamin E, singly or in different combinations having no effect on mortality rate nor cancer risk.[40] Supplementation of selenium or vitamin does not reduce cardiovascular disease.[41] Oxidative stress is thought to contribute to the development of a wide range of diseases. Dietary antioxidants have been investigated for potential effects on neurodegenerative diseases such as Alzheimer's disease, Parkinson's disease and amyotrophic lateral sclerosis, rheumatoid arthritis, diabetes. In many of these cases, it is unclear if oxidants trigger the disease, or if they are produced as a secondary consequence of the disease and from general tissue damage.[42-45]

Potential Hazards of Antioxidants

Antioxidants can interfere with health. The first linking came in a large trial of beta-carotene conducted among men in Finland who were heavy smokers found that there was significant increase in lung cancers among those taking supplements compared to those taking placebo.[46]

In another trial among heavy smokers and people exposed to asbestos beta-carotene was combined with vitamin A increase in the lung cancer was seen in in the supplement group.[47]

ROLE OF ANTIOXIDANTS IN VARIOUS OTHER CONDITIONS

Many decades of research have produced a significant amount of data showing an increased oxidative stress in asthma and chronic obstructive pulmonary disease (COPD) and indicating a potential role of oxidants/antioxidants imbalance in the pathogenesis of these diseases. In COPD patients, oxidative stress may amplify the inflammatory process and also reduce responsiveness to glucocorticoids, so that the development of more effective antioxidant compounds in the management of asthma and COPD and that such potentiality deserves to be deeply explored.[48]

Acute respiratory distress syndrome (ARDS) are deficient in, antioxidant status and N-acetyl cysteine (NAC) treatment can successfully improve intracellular GSH and enhance overall antioxidant power and outcome of patients. Present human study finding supports the previous animal study on the effectiveness of NAC on oleic acid-induced lung injury model.[49]

Study was conducted to know the response of the dietary antioxidants vitamin E and vitamin C to oxidative stress in pre-eclampsia. Administration of vitamin E therapy is of no benefit after the onset of pre-eclampsia, (Stratta et al. 1994) use of vitamin C under similar circumstances has not been studied.[50]

CONCLUSION

Oxidative stress and low grade silent inflammation caused due to free radicals in the body as a result of the unavailability of antioxidants is the underlying cause of chronic diseases.

Small-molecule antioxidants containing sulfur and selenium can ameliorate oxidative damage, and are known for their antioxidants activities are quite distinct. Findings of several recent clinical, epidemiological and in vivo studies highlight the need for future studies that specifically focus on the chemical mechanisms of sulfur and selenium antioxidant behavior.[51]

The intake of foods from the carotenoid-rich vegetables, oils, fats and oilseeds food groups increased the levels of plasma thiols and the intake of foods from the group of cereals decreased the plasma concentration of phenols. Studies should be conducted to investigate the association between the intake of antioxidant-rich foods and the plasma antioxidant profile, as a way to protect against the aging process.[52]

Antioxidant dietary supplements do not improve health nor are they effective in preventing diseases as shown by randomized clinical trials including supplements of beta-carotene, vitamin A, and vitamin E singly or in different combinations having no effect on mortality rate[53,54] or cancer risk.[55,56] Supplementation with selenium or vitamin E does not reduce the risk of cardiovascular disease.[41]

Antioxidant supplementation at the dose provided did not prevent the onset of kwashiorkor.[38]

Possible Reasons for Failure of Antioxidant Treatment

It is possible, however, that the lack of benefit in clinical studies can be explained by differences in the effects of the tested antioxidants when they are consumed as purified chemicals as opposed to when they are consumed in foods, which contain complex mixtures of antioxidants, vitamins, and minerals.[57] Until more is known about the effects of antioxidant supplements in cancer patients, these supplements should be used with caution. Randomized, placebo-controlled trials which, when performed well, provide the strongest evidence offer, only little support that taking vitamin C, vitamin E, beta-carotene, or other single antioxidants provides substantial protection against heart disease, cancer, or other chronic conditions. The results of the largest such trials have been mostly negative. The studies so far are inconclusive, but generally do not provide strong evidence that antioxidant supplements have a substantial impact on disease. The most of the trials conducted up to now have had fundamental limitations due to their relatively short duration and having been conducted in persons with existing disease. Also, using multiple oxidants and different reactivity and selectivity contribute to etiology.[58] Healthy subjects have limited potential beneficial effect of antioxidant supplements. Choice, dose, duration of antioxidant supplement is also important. At the same time evidence suggests that eating whole fruits, vegetables, and whole grains—all rich in networks of antioxidants and their helper molecules—provides protection against many of these secours of aging.

Oxidative stress can be considered as either a cause or consequence of some diseases, an area of research stimulating drug development for antioxidant compounds for use as potential therapies.

In the future, a therapeutic strategy to increase the antioxidant capacity of cells may be used to fortify the long-term effective treatment. Meantime, it is reminded that avoiding oxidant sources (cigarette, alcohol, bad food, stress, etc.) must be considered as important as taking diet rich in antioxidants. Indeed, our health also depends on our lifestyle choice.[59]

> **KEY LEARNING POINTS**
>
> - Radical scavenging antioxidants play an essential role in maintenance of health and protect against free radicals that can cause damage.
> - Oxygen is one of the most essential components for living. Under certain situations has deleterious effects on the human body. Oxygen utilization by the cells produce free radicals which can cause damage.
> - A balance between free radicals and antioxidants is necessary for proper physiological function.
> - Oxidative stress, arises as a result of an imbalance between free radical production and antioxidant defenses, which is associated with damage to a wide range of molecular species including lipids, proteins, and nucleic acid.
> - Health problems such as heart disease, macular degeneration, diabetes, cancer are all contributed by oxidative damage.
> - Oxidative stress is thought to contribute to the development of a wide range of diseases including Alzheimer's disease, Parkinson's disease, the pathologies caused by diabetes, rheumatoid arthritis and neurodegeneration in motor neuron disease.
> - The implication of oxidative stress in the etiology of several chronic and degenerative diseases suggests that antioxidant therapy represents a promising avenue for treatment.
> - Diets high in fruits and vegetables are rich sources of antioxidants and are good for health.
> - Antioxidant dietary supplements do not improve health nor are they effective in preventing diseases as shown by randomized clinical trials.
> - Antioxidants should be beneficial when given to the right subject at right time.
> - Like conventional medicines, dietary supplements may cause side effects, or interaction. If possible, it is best to get the antioxidants from a diet rich in fruits and vegetables rather than from supplements.

REFERENCES

1. Halliwell B. How to characterize an antioxidant. An update. *Biochem Soc Symp* 1995;61:73-101. [PubMed]
2. Mohammed AA, Ibrahim AA. Pathological roles of reactive oxygen species and their defence mechanism. *Saudi Pharm J* 2004;12:1-18.
3. Halliwell B, Gutteridge JMC. Free radicals in biology and medicine. 4th edn. Oxford, UK: Clarendon Press; 2007.
4. Lien Ai Pham Huy, Hua He, Chuong Pham-Huy. Free Radicals, Antioxidant in Disease and Health. *Int J Biomed Science* 2008;4(2):89-6. [PubMed Abstract]
5. Valko M, Rhodes CJ, Moncol J, Izakovic M, et al. Free radicals, metals and antioxidants in oxidative stress-induced cancer. Mini-review. *Chem Biol Interact* 2006;160:1-40. [PubMed]
6. Valko M, Morris H, Cronin MTD. Metals, toxicity and oxidative stress. *Curr Med Chem* 2005;12:1161-208. [PubMed]

7. Parthasarathy S, Santanam N, Ramachandran S, Meilhac O. Oxidants and antioxidants in atherogenesis: an appraisal. *J. Lipid Res* 1999;40:2143-57. [PubMed]
8. Frei B. Reactive oxygen species and antioxidant vitamins. Linus Pauling Institute. Oregon State University. 1997 http://lpi.oregonstate.edu/f-w97/reactive.html.
9. Chatterjee M, Saluja R, Kanneganti S, et al. Biochemical and molecular evaluation of neutrophil NOS in spontaneously hypertensive rats. *Cell Mol Biol* 2007;53: 84-93. [PubMed]
10. Gunjalli G, Kumar KN, Jain SK, et al. Total salivary anti-oxidant levels. Dental development and oral health status in childhood obesity. *Journal of International Oral Health* 2014;6(4):63-67.
11. Valko M, Leibfritz D, Moncola J, Cronin MD, et al. Free radicals and antioxidants in normal physiological functions and human disease. Review. *Int J Biochem. Cell Biol* 2007;39:44-84. [PubMed]
12. Van Gaal LF, Mertens IL, De Block CE. Mechanisms linking obesity with cardio-vascular disease. *Nature*. 2006;444(7121):875-80. Bibcode:2006Natur.444..875V. PMID 17167476. doi:10.1038/nature05487.
13. Aviram M. Review of human studies on oxidative damage and antioxidant protection related to cardiovascular diseases. *Free Radical Research* 2000;33: S85-97. PMID 11191279.
14. Bahorun T, Soobrarree MA, Luximon-Ramma V, Aruoma OI. Free radicals and antioxidants in cardiovascular health and disease. *Internet J Med Update* 2006;1: 1-17.
15. Genestra M. Oxyl radicals, redox-sensitive signalling cascades and antioxidants. Review. *Cell Signal* 2007;19:1807-1819. [PubMed]
16. Record IR, Dreosti IE, McInerney JK. Changes in plasma oxidant status following consumption of diets high or low in fruit and vegetables or following dietary supplementation with an antioxidant mixture. *British Journal of Nutrition* 2001;85:459-464.
17. Beecher GR. Overview of dietary flavonoids: nomenclature, occurrence and intake. *The Journal of Nutrition* 2003;133(10):3248S-54S. PMID 14519822.
18. Rodriguez-Amaya DB. Food carotenoids: analysis, composition and alterations during storage and processing of foods. *Forum of Nutrition* 2003;56:35-37. PMID 15806788.
19. Ing J.Brindza, Ing.E.Ivanisova. Antioxidants from plants in human nutrition and improving of health. *Acupuncture and Natural Medicine* 2/2015:40-51.
20. Stanner SA, Hughes J, Kelly CN, Buttriss J. A review of the epidemiological evidence for the 'antioxidant hypothesis. *Public Health Nutrition* 2004;7(3):407-422. PMID 15153272. doi:10.1079/PHN2003543.
21. Shenkin A. The key role of micronutrients. *Clinical Nutrition* 2006;25(1):1-13. PMID 16376462. doi:10.1016/j.clnu.2005.11.006.
22. Woodside JV, McCall D, McGartland C, Young IS. Micronutrients: dietary intake v. supplement use. *The Proceedings of the Nutrition Society* 2005;64(4):543-553. PMID 16313697. doi:10.1079/PNS2005464.
23. Bath PM, Iddenden R, Bath FJ, Orgogozo JM. Tirilazad for acute ischaemic stroke. *The Cochrane Database of Systematic Reviews* 2001;(4): CD002087.PMID 11687138. doi:10.1002/14651858.CD002087.
24. Sena E, Wheble P, Sandercock P, Macleod M. Systematic review and meta-analysis of the efficacy of tirilazad in experimental stroke. *Stroke; A Journal of Cerebral Circulation* 2007;38(2):388-394. PMID

25. Zhang S, Wang L, Liu M, Wu B. Tirilazad for aneurysmal subarachnoid haemorrhage. *The Cochrane Database of Systematic Reviews* 2010;(2): CD006778. PMID 20166088. doi:10.1002/14651858.CD006778.pub2.
26. Magalhães P, Dean O, Andreazza A. Antioxidant treatments for schizophrenia. *Cochrane Database. Syst Rev* 2016;(1): CD008919.pub2. doi:10.1002/14651858. CD008919.pub2.CD002087. PMID 11687138. doi:10.1002/14651858.CD002087.
27. Robinson AE. Tilirazid in ischemic stroke. *Eur Bull Stroke.* 2017;4:97–102.
28. Takanami Y, Iwane H, Kawai Y, Shimomitsu T. Vitamin E supplementation and endurance exercise: are there benefits? *Sports Medicine* 2000;29(2):73-83. PMID 10701711. doi:10.2165/00007256-200029020-00001.
29. Mastaloudis A, Traber MG, Carstensen K, Widrick JJ. Antioxidants did not prevent muscle damage in response to an ultramarathon run. *Medicine and Science in Sports and Exercise* 2006;38(1):72-80. PMID 16394956. doi:10.1249/01. mss.0000188579.36272.f6
30. https://www.researchgate.net/publication/262021590_Free_Radicals_and_ Antioxidant_Status_in_Protein_Energy_Malnutrition [accessed Aug 23, 2017].
31. Golden MH. Oede thesematous malnutrition. *Br Med Bull* 1998;54:433-444.
32. Golden MH, Ramdath D. Free radicals in the pathogenesis of kwashiorkor. *Proc Nutr Soc.* 1987;46:53-68.
33. Becker K, Bötticher D, Leichsenring M. Antioxidant vitamins in malnourished Nigerian children. *Int J Vitam Nutr Res* 1994;64:306-310.
34. Becker K, Leichsenring M, Gana L, Bremer HJ, Schirmer RH. Glutathione and associated antioxidant systems in protein energy malnutrition: results of a study inNigeria. *Free Radic Biol Med* 1995;18:257-263.
35. Leichsenring M, Sütterlin N, Less S, Bäumann K, Anninos A, Becker K. Polyunsaturated fatty acids in erythrocyte and plasma lipids of children with severe protein-energy malnutrition. *Acta Paediatr* 1995;84:516-520.
36. Shaaban SY, Nassar MF, Ibrahim SA, Mahmoud SE. Impact of nutritional rehabilitation on enzymatic antioxidant level in protein energy malnutrition. *Eastern Mediterranean Health Journal* 2002;8(2-3):290-297.
37. Ciliberto H, Ciliberto M, Briend A, Ashorn P, Bier D, Manary M. Antioxidant supplementation for the prevention of kwashiorkor in Malawian children: randomised, double blind, placebo controlled trial. *British Medical Journal* 2005; 330(7500):1109-1113.
38. Daniel Jahn063597, *Seminar Human Nutrition* (330060);Spring semester 2012.
39. Food, Nutrition, Physical Activity, and the Prevention of Cancer: a Global Perspective. *World Cancer Research Fund* (2007). ISBN 978-0-9722522-2-5.
40. Hail N, Cortes M, Drake EN, Spallholz JE. Cancer chemoprevention: a radical perspective. *Free Radical Biology & Medicine* 2008;45(2):97-110. PMID 18454943. doi:
41. Rees K, Hartley L, Day C, Flowers N, Clarke A, Stranges S. Selenium supplementation for the primary prevention of cardiovascular disease. *The Cochrane Database of Systematic Reviews* 2013;1 (1): CD009671. PMID 23440843. doi:10.1002/14651858. CD009671.pub2
42. Nunomura A, Castellani RJ, Zhu X, Moreira PI, Perry G, Smith MA. Involvement of oxidative stress in Alzheimer disease. *Journal of Neuropathology and Experimental Neurology.* 2006;65(7):631-641. PMID 16825950. doi:10.1097/01. jnen.0000228136.58062.bf

43. Wood-Kaczmar A, Gandhi S, Wood NW. Understanding the molecular causes of Parkinson›s disease. *Trends in Molecular Medicine* 2006;12(11):521-8. PMID 17027339. doi:10.1016/j.molmed.2006.09.00740.
44. Davì G, Falco A, Patrono C. Lipid peroxidation in diabetes mellitus. *Antioxidants & Redox Signaling* 2005;7(1-2):256-268. PMID 15650413. doi:10.1089/ars.2005.7.256
45. Giugliano D, Ceriello A, Paolisso G. Oxidative stress and diabetic vascular complications. *Diabetes Care* 1996;19(3):257-267. PMID 8742574.
46. Albanes D, Heinonen OP, Taylor PR, et al. Alpha-tocopherol and beta-carotene supplements and lung cancer incidence in the alpha-tocopherol, beta-carotene cancer prevention study: effects of base-line characteristics and study compliance. *J Natl Cancer Inst* 1996;88:1560-1570.
47. Omenn GS, Goodman GE, Thornquist MD, et al. Effects of a combination of beta-carotene and vitamin A on lung cancer and cardiovascular disease. *N Engl J Med* 1996;334:1150-1155.
48. Psarras S, Caramori G, Contoli M, Papadopoulos N, Papi A. Oxidants in asthma and in chronic obstructive pulmonay disease (COPD). *Current Pharmaceutical Design* 2005;11:2053-2062.
49. Mohammad Sadegh Soltan-Sharifi, Mojtahedzadeh M, Natafi A, Khajavi MR, et al. Improvement by N-acetylcysteine of acute respiratory distress syndrome through increasing intracellular glutathione, and extracellular thiol moleculets and ante-oxidant power: evidence for underlying toxicological mechanisms. *Human and Experimental Toxicological* 2007;26;697-703.
50. Bowen RS, Mars M, Chuturgoon AA. The response of the dietary anti-oxidants vitamin E and vitamin C to oxidative stress in pre-eclampsia. *Journal of Obstetrics and Gynecology* 1998;18(1):9-13.
51. Battia EE, Brumaghim LL. Antioxidant activity of sulfur and selenium: A review of reactive oxygen species scavenging, glutathione peroxidase, and metal-binding antioxidants mechanisms. *Cell Biochem Biophys* 2009;55:1-23.
52. Boventura BCB, DIPietro PF, DEAssis MAA. Antioxidant biomarkers and food intake in elderly women. *The Journal of Nutrition Health and Aging* 2012;16(1):2012.
53. Bjelakovic G, Nikolova D, Gluud C. Meta-regression analyses, meta-analyses, and trial sequential analyses of the effects of supplementation with beta-carotene, vitamin A, and vitamin E singly or in different combinations on all-cause mortality: do we have evidence for lack of harm? *PLoS ONE* 2013;8(9):e74558. Bibcode: 2013PLoSO...874558B. PMC 3765487. PMID 24040282. doi:10.1371/journal.pone.0074558.
54. Abner EL, Schmitt FA, Mendiondo MS, Marcum JL, Kryscio RJ. Vitamin E and all-cause mortality: a meta-analysis. *Current Aging Science*. 2011;4(2):158-170. PMC 4030744. PMID 21235492. doi:10.2174/1874609811104020158.
55. Cortés-Jofré M, Rueda JR, Corsini-Muñoz G, Fonseca-Cortés C, Caraballoso M, Bonfill Cosp X. Drugs for preventing lung cancer in healthy people. The *Cochrane Database of Systematic Reviews* 2012;10: CD002141. PMID 23076895. doi:10.1002/14651858. CD002141.pub2.
56. Jiang L, Yang KH, Tian JH, Guan QL, Yao N, Cao N, et al. Efficacy of antioxidant vitamins and selenium supplement in prostate cancer prevention: a meta-analysis of randomized controlled trials. *Nutrition and Cancer* 2010;62(6):719-27. PMID 20661819. doi:10.1080/01635581.2010.494335.

57. Bouayed J, Bohn T. Exogenous antioxidants—double-edged swords in cellular redoc state: health beneficial effects at physiologic doses versus deleterious effects at high doses. *Oxidative Medicine and Cellular Longevity* 2010;3(4):228-237. [PubMed Abstract]
58. Lawenda BD, Kelly KM, Ladas EJ, et al. Should supplemental antioxidant administration be avoided during chemotherapy and radiation therapy? *Journal of the National Cancer Institute* 2008;100(11):773-783.
59. Lien Ai Pham Huy, Hua He, Chuong Pham-Huy. Free Radicals, Antioxidant in Disease and Health. *Int J. Biomed Science* 2008;4(2):89-96.

3 Assessment of Nutritional Status

Suraj Gupte, Utpal Kant Singh

ABSTRACT
Assessment of nutritional status is an important component of pediatric practice. In identifying cases of borderline nutritional disturbances such as mild moderate malnutrition, its role assumes special significance. Besides individual levels as in a health facility, it may be needed in large groups and segments of child population, e.g. times of natural calamities/disasters (earthquake, floods and starvation outbreaks). Its major components include dietary history, clinical signs, anthropometry, investigations, associated disorders and vital statistics. *Weight for age* is the most common and simple criteria employed in practice. *Weight for height* is useful when actual age is in doubt. *Height for age* is of no use for detecting early PEM. Its value lies in detecting chronic malnutrition and stunting. If age of he child is unknown, the age-independent indices of nutritional status are recommended.

Keywords: Anthropometry, Body mass index, Ecological factors, Height for age, Mid upper arm circumference, QUAC stick, Shaker's tape, Skinfold thickness, Stunting, Vital statistics, Weight for age, Weight for height.

INTRODUCTION

Though frank cases of kwashiorkor and marasmus cause little difficulty in their identification, assessment of nutritional status may be rather difficult, especially in borderline nutritional disturbances such as mild moderate malnutrition.[1-4] Furthermore, assessment of nutritional status concerns:
- Individual levels as in hospital/health facility
- Large groups and segments of child population, e.g. times of natural calamities/disasters (earthquake, floods and starvation outbreaks).[1,2]

The overall criteria employed for assessment of nutritional status are listed in Box 1.

Box 1: Major criteria for assessment of nutritional status in children.

- Dietary history
- Clinical signs
- Anthropometry
- Investigations
- Associated disorders
- Vital statistics
- Ecological factors

DIETARY HISTORY

The assessment must begin with the dietary history. Details about intake of cereals, vegetables, pulses, fruits, eggs and meat, etc. and thereby average daily consumption of proteins and calories should be obtained. A rough idea about the adequacy of vitamins and minerals in the diet should also be formed.

CLINICAL SIGNS

Deficiency signs such as hair changes, anemia, varying grades of edema (Box 2), xerosis, cheilosis, angular stomatitis, rachitic rosary, bleeding spongy gums and dental caries, etc. should be actively looked for.

The observations on the deficiency signs should, however be interpreted very cautiously. As for instance, phrynoderma (toad skin), though traditionally thought to be due to vitamin A deficiency, may also be a feature of scurvy and deficiency of linoleic acid.

ANTHROPOMETRY

Anthropometry is a very valuable index for evaluation of nutritional status and have stood the test of time in various studies.[4-7]

Age-dependent Indices

- *Weight for age* is by far the simplest, the most widely used and the most reliable index, provided that it is recorded correctly and is related to the correct age of the individual. Also, what is more important is the serial record of child's weight periodically on a growth chart.
- *Weight for height* is useful when actual age is in doubt.
- *Height for age* is of no use for detecting early protein-energy malnutrition (PEM). Its value lies in detecting chronic malnutrition and stunting.

Age-independent Indices

Since, it is often difficult to find true age of the child in the underprivileged and ignorant sections of society, the certain truly or relatively age-independent indices of nutritional status are recommended (Box 3).

Box 2: Grading of edema according to severity.

- **Grade 1 (Mild):** Both feet and ankles
- **Grade 2 (Moderate):** Both feet and ankles + legs, forearms and hands
- **Grade 3 (Severe):** Generalized including face

Box 3: Age-independent indices for assessment of nutritional status.

- Weight for height
- Mid-upper arm circumference
- Mid-upper arm muscle circumference
- Triceps skinfold thickness
- Chest/head circumference ratio
- Quaker upper arm circumference (QUAC) stick method
- Mid-upper arm/height ratio
- Shakir's tape
- Bangle method
- Dugdale index
- Rao's weight/height ratio
- Kanawati index
- Body mass index
- Poneral index
- Quetlet index

- ***Weight for height***, which is only partially age-independent, is calculated as follows:

$$\text{Percentage weight for height} = \frac{\text{Actual weight} \times 100}{\text{Expected weight for actual height}}$$

- ***Nabarrow's thinners chart***, based on weight for height, is recommended by **save the children fund**. The child is made to stand against the chart which bears the expected weight for height. The child's head touches the upper red zone in the presence of severe PEM.
- ***Mid-upper arm circumference (MUAC)*** is measured midway between the point of the shoulder (tip of acromion process) and olecranon process of ulna. For all practical purposes, the maximum circumference of the upper arm measured when the left arm is hanging by the side of the body would do. Between 1 and 5 years, it remains constant between 16.25 and 16.75 cm. This is because of replacements of the baby fat with muscle tissue. Any child in this age group with a circumference less than 11.5 cm of the reference international standard is to be considered suffering from severe malnutrition, between 11.5 cm and 12.5 cm from moderate malnutrition, and between 12.5 and 13.5 cm from mild malnutrition.
- ***Mid-upper arm muscle circumference (MUAMC)*** is calculated by the following formula:

$$\text{MUAMC} = \text{MAC} - \pi \times \text{triceps skin fold thickness}$$

- *Triceps skin fold thickness* is measured by a standard caliper (Lange, Herpenden). Tanner chart gives the normal values at different ages. On an average it exceeds 10 mm in 1–6 years age group. A measurement between 6 and 10 mm points to mild and moderate malnutrition and under 6 mm to severe malnutrition.
- *Chest/head circumference ratio less than* one after first year of life indicates malnutrition.
- *Mid-upper arm/height ratio* of less than 0.29 indicates gross malnutrition, the normal being 0.32–0.33.
- *Quaker upper arm circumference (QUAC) stick method* is a simple, easy, inexpensive and yet reliable method of detecting early malnutrition of acute onset in a large number of children in a brief span of time in the community settings, especially during natural calamities such as floods and earthquakes. The instrument is a stick graduated with figures for MUAC in relation to height (Box 4 and Fig. 1).
- *Shakir tape method* is a simple and age-independent tool for assessing malnutrition. This special tape has colored zones—red, yellow and green, corresponding to less than 12.5 cm (wasted), 12.5–13.5 cm (borderline) and over 13.5 cm (normal) MUAC. Now, new tapes showing less than 11.5 cm as severe malnutrition are replacing the old ones in keeping with the World Health Organization (WHO) recommendations.
- *Bangle method*, another method not needing age and useful in preschool children, consists of slipping a bangle with a diameter of 4 cm up the forearm. An attempt is made to move it over to the upper arm. In case it can slip over the elbow, malnutrition is present. The method, though simple and easy, is not quite reliable.
- *Dugdale index* too is based on relationship between weight and height. It is expressed as:

$$\text{Dugdale index} = \frac{\text{Weight (kg)} \times 1.6}{\text{Height (cm)}}$$

Normal value varies between 0.88 and 0.97. An index of less than 0.79 suggests malnutrition.

Box 4: Quaker upper arm circumference (QUAC) stick method.

- **QUAC stick** is an abbreviation for Quacker upper arm circumference measuring stick. The instrument consists of a stick graduated with figures for mid-upper arm circumference in relation to height. For this test, maximum left-upper arm circumference (the arm hanging by the side of the body) is recorded. Then, the child is made to stand in front of the QUAC stick. From the graduations in the stick, his nutritional status in terms of 50, 60, 70 or 80% of the standard can be easily read (Fig. 1).
- **Modified QUAC stick** utilizes a rod or stick that is colored green (normal nutrition), yellow (borderline nutrition) and red (severe malnutrition).

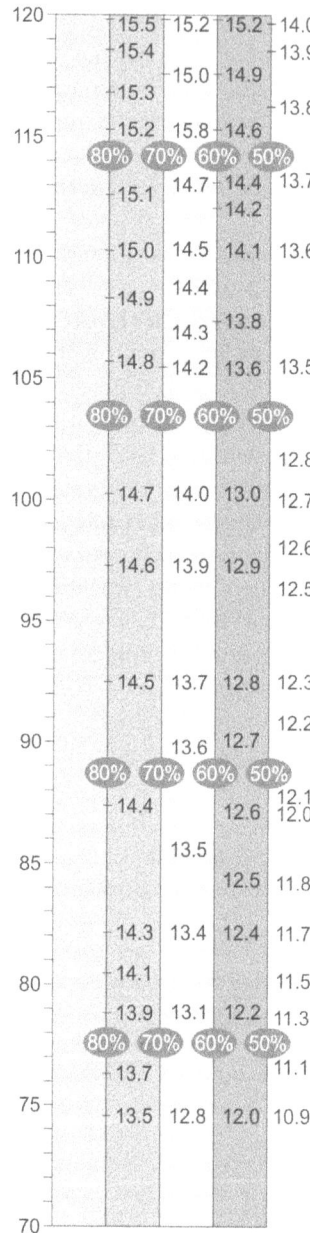

Fig. 1: Quaker upper arm circumference (QUAC) stick method: Quaker upper arm circumference.

- ***Rao's weight/height ratio*** is expressed as:

$$\text{Rap's ratio} = \frac{\text{Weight (g)}}{\text{Height (cm)}^2} \times 100$$

Normal value is above 0.0015. A value of 0.0013-0.0015 indicates moderate malnutrition and less than 0.0013 indicates severe malnutrition.
- **Kanawati index**, based on MUAC and head circumference ratio, varies between 0.32-0.33. A ratio of less than 0.25 points to severe malnutrition.
- **Body mass index (BMI):**

$$BMI = \frac{Weight\ (kg)}{Height\ (m)^2} = kg/m^2$$

  - *Normal:* 18.5-22
  - *Overweight:* 22-25
  - *Obesity:* 25-30
  - *Morbid obesity:* More than 30
  - *Borderline malnutrition:* 15-18.5
  - *Moderate malnutrition:* 13-15
  - *Severe malnutrition:* Less than 13.
- **Ponderal index** is expressed as:

$$Ponderal\ index = \frac{Weight\ (g)}{Length/height\ (cm)^3}$$

An index less than 2 points to asymmetrical intrauterine growth retardation (IUGR), more than 2 symmetrical IUGR, 2-2.5 borderline malnutrition, and less than 2 severe malnutrition, and more than 2.5 appropriate for gestational age (AGA).
- **Quetlet's index** is expressed as:

$$Quetlet's\ index = \frac{Weight\ (g)}{Length/height\ (cm)}$$

Normal value varies between 0.14 and 0.16. In gross malnutrition, it is less than 0.14. It is quite reliable. It is similar to BMI, except that here we take height in centimeters rather than meters.

INVESTIGATIONS

- **Laboratory investigations** include complete blood picture especially, hemoglobin, erythrocyte sedimentation rate (ESR), serum proteins and blood levels of nutrients like vitamins, iron, etc.
- **Tuberculin (Mantoux) test** to exclude tuberculosis.
- **Chest X-ray (CXR)** for superadded lower respiratory infection (say pneumonia) and tuberculosis, etc.
- **Special biochemical tests** may detect subclinical malnutrition that could not be revealed by anthropometry.

- *Amino acid level* in blood and urine may be helpful in borderline cases. Hydroxyproline is the most commonly used among the amino acids. Hydroxyproline levels are an indicator of collagen content. Conditions that increase collagen turnover can elevate serum and urine hydroxyproline levels. Urine and serum hydroxyproline levels can be used as a marker for bone resorption.
- *Hydroxyproline assay kit* is suitable for hydroxyproline detection in cell and tissue culture supernatants, urine, plasma, serum, and other biological samples. Salivary protein, salivary ferritin and free α-amino nitrogen in leukocyte are reduced in malnutrition.
- *Skeletal radiographs* may reveal some retardation of bone age, osteoporosis or classical signs of nutritional rickets or scurvy. Some workers have described transverse lines of arrested growth at the growing ends of long bones months prior to onset of frank PEM.

ASSESSMENT FOR ASSOCIATED DISORDERS

While assessing the nutritional status, one must ascertain for evidence of intestinal parasitic infestations, malabsorption and tuberculosis, etc.

VITAL HEALTH STATISTICS

For evaluation of the nutritional status of a community, the above measures should be supported by vital statistics such as under five mortality, infant mortality, neonatal mortality, perinatal mortality, stillbirth rate and life-expectancy as also the ecological background.

ECOLOGIC FACTORS

Malnutrition is the result of a multitude of ecologic factors. Understandably, it is important to obtain ecologic information on factors such as:
- Food consumption by the community.
- Socioeconomic factors such as knowledge, attitudes, practices (KAPs), beliefs about feeding, education and income.
- Health and education services, e.g. feeding programs, immunization facilities, etc.
- Conditioning influences, e.g. infections that are known causes of precipitating malnutrition.

CONCLUSION

Assessment of nutritional status, an integral part of pediatric practice, is important in identifying cases of borderline nutritional disturbances and severe malnutrition. Besides individual levels as in a health facility, it may be needed in large groups of child population in such emergencies as earthquake, floods and starvation outbreaks. Dietary history, clinical signs, anthropometry, investigations, associated disorders and vital statistics are the chief components. *Weight for age* is the most common and simple criteria employed in practice. *Weight for height* is useful when actual age is in doubt. *Height for age* is of no use for detecting early PEM. Its value lies in detecting chronic malnutrition and stunting. Age-independent indices of nutritional status are recommended when child's age is not clear.

> **KEY LEARNING POINTS**
>
> ¤ In identifying cases of borderline nutritional disturbances such as mild-moderate malnutrition, assessment of nutritional status is unique.
> ¤ It is required in individual cases as well as large groups and segments of child population at times of natural calamities/disasters.
> ¤ Its major components include dietary history, clinical signs, anthropometry, investigations, associated disorders and vital statistics.
> ¤ *Weight for age* is the most common and simple criteria employed in practice. *Weight for height* is useful when actual age is in doubt.
> ¤ *Height for age* is useful in detecting chronic malnutrition and stunting.
> ¤ If age of he child is unknown, the age-independent indices of nutritional status are recommended.
> ¤ Age-independent indices are helpful when child's age is not known.

REFERENCES

1. Gupte S, Gomez EM, UK Singh. Normal growth. In: Gupte S (Ed): *The Short Textbook of Pediatrics*, 18th edn. New Delhi: Jaypee 2018:38-65.
2. Gupte S, Gomez EM. Malnutrition. In: Gupte S (Ed): *The Short Textbook of Pediatrics*, 18th edn. New Delhi: Jaypee 2018:197-225.
3. Elizabeth KE. *Nutrition and Child Development*, 5th edn. Hyderabad: Paras 2014.
4. Mehta MN, Mehta NJ. *Nutrition and Diet for Children Simplified*. New Delhi: Jaypee 2014.
5. Ramachandran P, Gopalan SH. Assessment of nutritional status in Indian preschool children using WHO 2006 Growth Standards. *Indian J Med Res* 2011;134:47-53.
6. Tiwari S. Nutritional status of preschool children. *South Asian J. Multidisciplinary Studies* 2015;1(3). Availble at: http:// www.gjms.co.in/index.php/SAJMS/article/view/930. Accessed on 12 January 2018.
7. Sharda K, Babel G. Assessment of nutritional status of pre-school children (2- 5 years) in Girwah tehsil of Udaipur city. *Asian J Home Sci* 2017;12:124-126.

PART 2: VITAMINS

4 Vitamins: Essentials and Therapeutics in a Nutshell

Novy Gupte, Suraj Gupte, Utpal Kant Singh

ABSTRACT

Vitamins, organic compounds that are needed in limited quantities, are essential for maintenance of normal health. These must be provided from external (usually dietary) sources. Besides controlling protein synthesize, vitamins function as hormones, antioxidants and regulators of a tissue growth and differentiation.

The 13 vitamins that are universally recognized comprise 9 water-soluble (vitamins B complex and C) and fat-soluble (vitamins A, D, E and K).

Water-soluble vitamins are not stored in the body in any appreciable quantity. Their excessive consumption causes no particular toxicity, the surplus being excreted. On the contrary, fat-soluble vitamins are stored in liver. Their excessive consumption may, therefore, cause toxicity.

Vitamin deficiencies may occur individually, in combination with other members of the group, or in combination with other nutritional problems such as protein-energy malnutrition (PEM), micronutrient deficiency (say, iron-deficiency anemia), etc.

Keywords: Ascorbic acid, Biotin, Cyanocobalamine, Folic acid, Nicotinic acid, Pantothinic acid, Pyrdoxine, Riboflavine, Thiamne, Vitamin A, Vitamin B_1, Vitamin B_2, B_3, B_6, Vitamin B_6, Vitamin B_{12}, Vitamin C, Vitamin D, Vitamin E, Vitamin K.

INTRODUCTION

Vitamins are the organic compounds that are essentially needed in only small amounts for maintenance of normal health.[1-3] These must be provided from external (usually dietary) sources.

Functions of vitamins include:[1-4]
- *As hormones:* Vitamin D
- *As antioxidants:* Vitamin E
- *As regulators of tissue growth and differentiation:* Vitamin A
- *As coenzymes*: B complex vitamins, e.g. pyridoxine for nicotinic acid
- *For control of protein synthesis*: Vitamin A, D, E and K.

Currently, 13 vitamins stand universally recognized. The two major categories are:
1. *Water-soluble:* Vitamins B complex and C (9 in toto)
2. *Fat-soluble:* Vitamins A, D, E and K (4 in toto)

Water-soluble vitamins are not stored in the body in any appreciable quantity. Their excessive consumption causes no particular toxicity, the surplus being excreted. On the contrary, fat-soluble vitamins are stored in liver. Their excessive consumption may, therefore, cause toxicity.

Vitamin deficiencies may occur:
- Individually,
- In combination with each other members of the group, or
- In combination with other nutritional problems such as protein-energy malnutrition (PEM), micronutrient deficiency such as iron deficiency anemia.

WATER-SOLUBLE VITAMINS

Water-soluble vitamins are[5-9]
- B-complex Group
  - Thiamin (Vitamin B_1)
  - Riboflavine (Vitamin B_2)
  - Nicotinic acid (Vitamin B_3)
  - Pantothenic acid (Vitamin B_5)
  - Pyridoxine (Vitamin B_6)
  - Biotin (Vitamin B_7)
  - Folic acid (Vitamin B_9)
- Vitamin C

Thiamine (Vitamin B_1)

- *Functions:* It has a role in nerve conduction, as a coenzyme in transketolation and decarboxylation of alpha-ketoacids, in carbohydrate and protein metabolism.
- *Dietary source:* Milk, whole grain cereals, pulses, dried yeast, oilseeds (Fig. 1), fruits and eggs. Green vegetables and meat are relatively poor in thiamine.
- *Daily requirement:* 0.4 mg/1000 kcal.

Deficiency

- *Etiology:* Thiamine deficiency occurs either because of poor intake in the diet, malabsorption states, or prolonged illness.
- *Clinical features:* Thiamine deficiency leads to the disease, **beriberi**. It occurs usually in infants *(wet beriberi)* though older infants and children may also suffer from its chronic form *(dry beriberi)*. Meningitis form is also known.

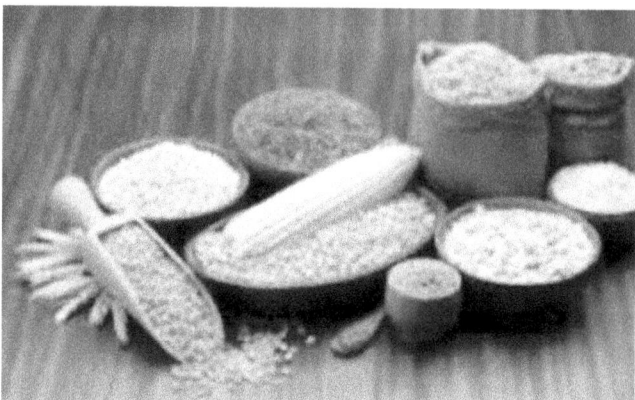

Fig. 1: Sources of thiamine (vitamin B_1).

The earliest symptoms occurring in early infancy (especially if the mother is providing thiamine-deficient breast milk), include restlessness, bouts of excessive crying (as if the infant is having an abdominal colic), vomiting, abdominal distention, flatulence, constipation and insomnia.

- In the *acute cardiac form* (wet beriberi), the infant may develop congestive cardiac failure in the form of tachycardia, gallop rhythm, dyspnea, cyanosis, hepatomegaly, cardiomegaly, edema and pulmonary edema. The possibility of thiamine deficiency should always be considered in endemic areas in subjects presenting with intractable congestive cardiac failure.
- In the *chronic neurologic form* (dry beriberi), the manifestations may include anorexia, weight loss, weakness, diarrhea, constipation and edema. The child is usually drowsy and apathetic. Ataxia is common. There may be peripheral neuritis and various palsies, including hoarseness due to vocal cord paralysis, and nystagmus. Deep tendon reflexes are usually absent.
- In the *meningitic form*, the clinical picture is dominated by bulging anterior fontanel, dilated pupils, head retraction and coma. Convulsions may occur, leading to a mistaken diagnosis of encephalitis or meningitis. Cerebrospinal fluid (CSF) reveals no abnormality.

In addition to all this, thiamine dependency has been incriminated in the etiology of:
  - Anomalies of branched chain ketoacid decarboxylase system, e.g. maple syrup urine disease.
  - Syndrome of optic atrophy, intermittent ataxia, lactic acidosis and hyperalaninemia due to pyruvate decarboxylase deficiency.

Differential Diagnosis

Differentiation needs to be made from pyloric stenosis and other high obstruction in the presence of troublesome vomiting. Endomyocardial fibroelastosis, congenital heart disease and glycogen storage disease involving the heart (Pompe disease) may be considered in the presence of congestive cardiac failure (CCF). Chronic neurologic form would require differentiation from lead poisoning. Meningitic form may be confused with meningitis or encephalitis; a normal CSF may prove most helpful in such a situation.

Diagnosis

It is more or less clinical. However, if facilities are available, the following investigations may be done:
- **Blood thiamine level:** Less than 4 µg/dL (normal is 10 ± 5 µg/dL) is suggestive.
- **Milk thiamine level:** Less than 7 µg/dL.
- **Red cell transketolase level:** The level is low. A dramatic response, within a few hours, to an intramuscular injection of 25 mg of thiamine is a good therapeutic test.

Treatment

As soon as the diagnosis is convincingly made, the child must receive 10 mg of thiamine intravenously. In the subsequent three days, he should be given 10 mg of the vitamin intramuscularly twice daily. Over the next six weeks, 10 mg daily should be administered orally. The breastfeeding mother should receive thiamine therapy simultaneously.

Prognosis

It is excellent, provided reasonable intake of thiamine is ensured.

Prevention

Ensuring that at least 0.4 mg of thiamine is provided in the daily diet (thrice the quantity in case of pregnant and lactating women) prevents beriberi.

Riboflavin (Vitamin B$_2$)

- **Function:** As a constituent of flavoprotein coenzymes [flavin adenine dinucleotide (FAD) and flavin mononucleotide (FMN)], it plays an important role in the intermediary metabolism of carbohydrates.
- **Dietary sources:** Both animal and vegetable foods such as liver, fish, egg, kidney, meat, beans, yeast, green leafy vegetables (GLV), cereals, legumes, groundnut (Fig. 2) and milk (5 times more in cow milk than in human milk).
- **Daily requirement:** 0.6 mg/1,000 kcal.

Deficiency

Deficiencies of thiamine and riboflavin may be coexisting.
- **Etiology:** Since both breast milk and cow milk provide sufficient riboflavin for infant's needs, its deficiency usually occurs in children on restricted protein intakes or with dominant protein malabsorption states.

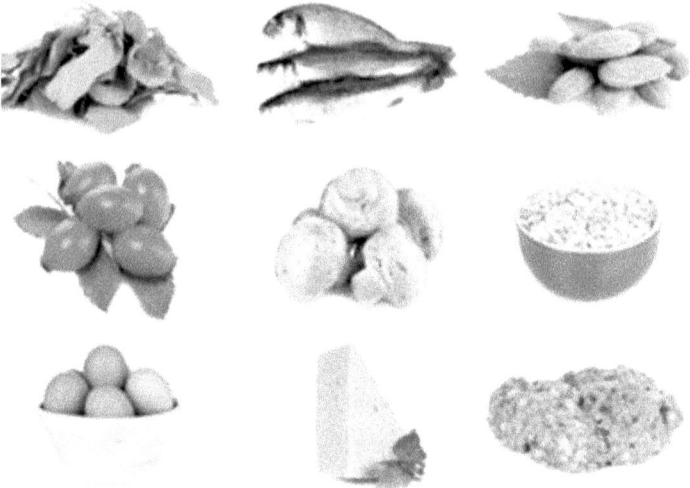

Fig. 2: Sources of riboflavin (vitamin B$_2$).

Most subjects are vegetarian. Its deficiency may also occur in neonates under phototherapy because of its being subject to photodegradation.
- **Clinical features:** Manifestations include angular stomatitis (Fig. 3), cheilosis (fissuring of lips), nasolabial seborrhea and occasionally purplish-red (magenta) stomatitis with smooth tongue (Fig. 4). There may occur corneal injection (vascularization) at the limbus, leading to excessive lacrimation, photophobia, eye pain and later interstitial keratitis.

Diagnosis

It is essentially clinical. Laboratory investigations include:
- Urinary excretion of riboflavin less than 30 µg/24 hours.
- Excretion of less than 125 µg of riboflavin/g of creatinine in a random urine sample.
- Increased erythrocyte glutathione reductase activity after the addition of FAD.

Treatment

Therapy consists of administering riboflavin, 3–10 mg orally or 2 mg intramuscularly daily for a few days. This should be followed by 10 mg orally daily for about three weeks. With this regimen, response is good. Complete recovery occurs provided that adequate intake of vitamin B$_2$ is ensured in the weeks and months ahead.

Prevention

In order to prevent riboflavin deficiency, it should be ensured that the daily diet provides at least 0.6 mg riboflavin per 1,000 kcal. It is advisable

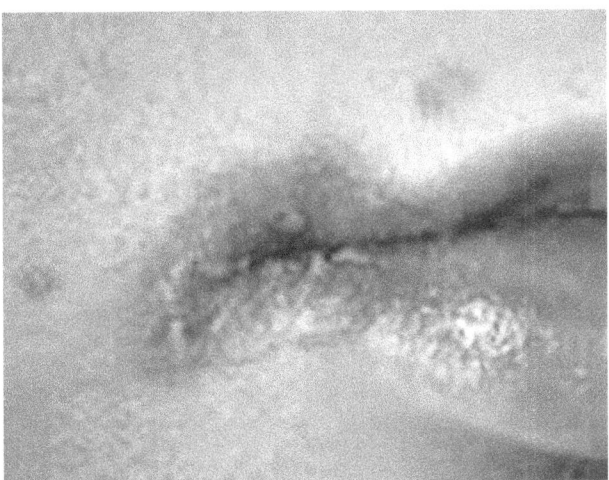

Fig. 3: Angular stomatitis and cheilosis from riboflavin (vitamin B$_2$ deficiency). Note the lesions at the corners of the mouth (angular stomatitis) along with fissuring of the adjoining lips (cheilosis). Most common in pure vegetarians.

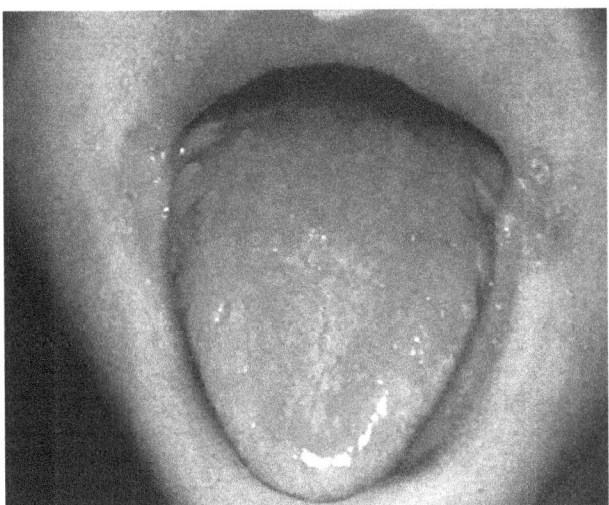

Fig. 4: Glossitis with stomatitis from riboflavin deficiency. Note the typical smooth and magenta tongue. There is also an evidence of angular stomatitis.

to administer supplements of riboflavin (the whole B-complex may be still better) to the infants and children belonging to vulnerable categories.

Nicotinic Acid (Niacin, Nicotinamide, Vitamin B$_3$)

- *Functions:* Nicotinic acid (niacin) or vitamin B$_3$ is also involved in the carbohydrate metabolism and plays a vital role in the functioning of the skin, gastrointestinal tract, central nervous system and hematopoietic system.

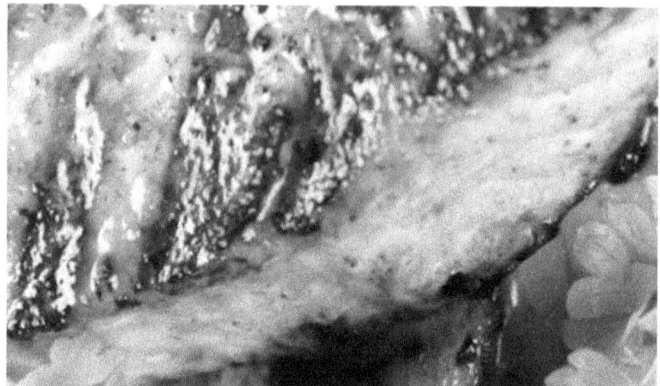

Fig. 5: Meat, fish and pouttry are by and large, the best source of nicotinic acid.

- **Dietary sources:** This vitamin may be obtained either from the natural food sources or from the tryptophan endogenously. The natural food sources include milk, liver, pork, fish, cheese, egg, yeast, cereals and vegetables, etc. (Fig. 5).
- **Daily requirement:** 6.6 mg/1,000 kcal.

Deficiency

- **Etiology:** Nicotinic acid deficiency is usually encountered in children receiving a maize diet as staple, in chronic diarrhea, in malabsorption states, and in anorexic states. Pyridoxine deficiency may also contribute to nicotinic acid deficiency and pellagra-like lesions.
- **Clinical features:** Pellagra usually occurs in children of school-going age. The manifestations are briefed as **4Ds** (Dermatosis, Diarrhea, Dementia and Death).
    - The characteristic lesions are seen over the exposed areas of the skin, such as limbs, neck (Casal necklace) and cheeks (Fig. 6). The lesions are symmetrical of desquamating pigmentary dermatitis type and are aggravated by sunlight.
    - Gastrointestinal symptoms in the form of red and sore tongue, dysphagia, nausea, vomiting and diarrhea.
    - Dementia is encountered much less in childhood than in adults. Most children with pellagra are simply apathetic.
    - Anemia as also other signs of malnutrition is usually present.

Diagnosis

It is purely clinical.

Differential Diagnosis

At times, severe PEM in the form of kwashiorkor may warrant differentiation. Remember that in kwashiorkor the skin lesion tend to be around pressure

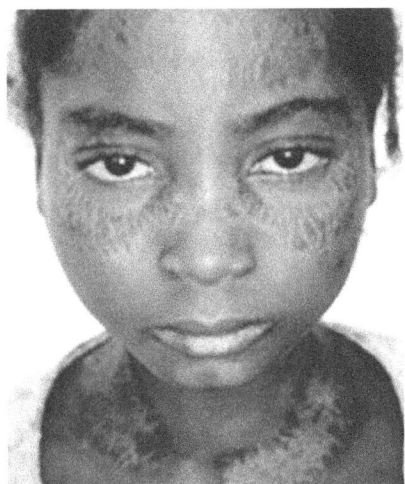

Fig. 6: Pellagra. Note the characteristic skin lesion, especially necklace-like involvement of the neck.

sites and flexure surfaces in the trunk, groin and knee rather than over the exposed parts as is typical of pellagra.

Treatment
Nicotinamide, 50–300 mg daily in divided doses orally, given for two weeks followed by adequate supply of B complex vitamins in diet brings about complete recovery.

Prevention
The disease may be prevented by providing a balanced diet containing 5–10 mg daily supply of nicotinamide.

Pantothenic Acid (Vitamin B_5)
It is synthesized by microbes from pantoic acid and β-alanine in addition to food sources.
- *Function:* It plays an important role in the synthesis of fatty acids, cholesterol and steroids, metabolism of pyruvate and alpha-ketoglutarate.
- *Dietary sources:* Almost all naturally occurring foods, especially germinated wheat; liver, dried yeast, egg yolk and fish.
- Daily requirement:
  - *Infants:* 1.5–2.5 mg and 2–5 mg
  - *Children:* 5–8 mg
  - *Adolescents:* 10 mg.
- *Clinical uses:* Burning feet syndrome, hair loss, seborrhea, premature graying of hair, obesity and multiple sclerosis.

Deficiency
- ***Etiology:*** Usually in combination with other B complex deficiencies.
- ***Clinical features:*** Burning-feet syndrome, gastrointestinal tract (GIT) upset, sleep disturbances (especially insomnia), headache and muscle cramps.

Treatment
Calcium D-pantothenate 10–50 mg/day is suggested.

Pyridoxine (Vitamin B_6)
- ***Functions:*** Vitamin B_6 plays a vital role in the metabolism of proteins and fatty acids. It is claimed to have a role in blood formation, in proper functioning of the nervous system and in conversion of tryptophan to nicotinic acid.
- ***Dietary sources:*** Its natural sources include liver, egg yolk, meat, wheat germ, soyabeans, yeast, peas, pulses and cereals. It is found in only small quantity in most vegetables and milk (Fig. 7).
- ***Daily requirement:*** 1–1.5 mg.

Deficiency
- ***Etiology:*** Pyridoxine deficiency of nutritional origin is rare in childhood—in fact, in humans as such. Deficiency may, however, complicate:
    - Prolonged isoniazid or cycloserine therapy in tuberculosis
    - Penicillamine therapy in Wilson disease
    - Use of contraceptives.

  Pyridoxine-responsive convulsions and anemia have been described. Pyridoxine-dependent inborn errors of metabolism, e.g. homocystinuria, cystathioninuria, xanthurenic aciduria, kynureninase deficiency and hyperoxaluria, are also reported.

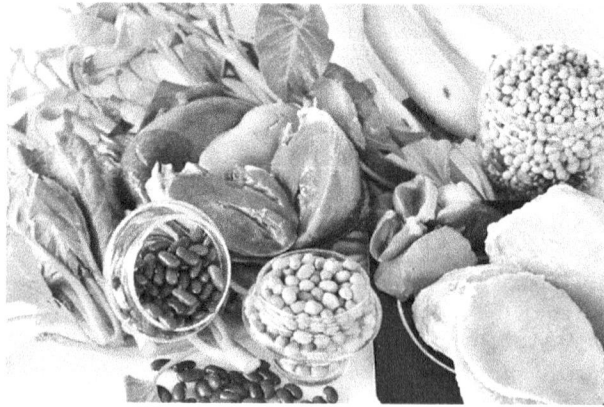

Fig. 7: Sources of pyridoxine (B_6).

- **Clinical features:** Manifestations include:
  - Convulsions refractory to usual therapy
  - Microcytic-hypochromic anemia refractory to iron therapy
  - Growth retardation
  - Gastrointestinal symptoms like diarrhea
  - Seborrheic dermatitis around nose and eyes
  - Sensory neuropathy (uncommon in children)
  - Cheilosis and glossitis (infrequent in childhood).

Diagnosis

High index of suspicion of vitamin B_6 deficiency in infants with persistent convulsions, provided that hypoglycemia, hypocalcemia and birth injury have been excluded would help to diagnose this condition.

Such an infant should receive 50–100 mg of pyridoxine intravenously. If the response is gratifying, diagnosis is quite probable. The confirmation of diagnosis may be done by the tryptophan loading test. The same applies to anemia refractory to iron deficiency.

Treatment

Administration of 5 mg of pyridoxine intramuscularly followed by 0.5 mg daily orally for two weeks causes complete recovery.

Excess/Toxicity

Ataxia, stiffness in the feet followed by the cumbrous hands and night-time restlessness.

Biotin (Vitamin B_7)

A relatively less-understood vitamin, it is mainly produced by the gastrointestinal flora.
- **Functions:** Biotin acts as a coenzyme in carboxylation reactions (Box 1).
- **Dietary sources:** Meat (especially liver), egg (yolk), milk and yeast extract.
- **Daily requirement:** 0.15 mg.

Deficiency

- **Etiology:** Most common cause is consumption of large number of raw eggs. The white (yolk) of egg is supposed to be rich in a glycoprotein, **avidin**. Avidin binds to biotin (avidin-biotin complex) so that its absorption is hindered. Prolonged parenteral nutrition (PN), without supplements of

---

Box 1: Carboxylation reactions needing biotin as a coenzyme.

- Acetyl-CoA carboxylase → malonnyl-CoA in fatty acid synthesis
- Pyruvate carboxylase → oxaloacetate in Krebs cycle
- Propionyl-CoA carboxylase → in methylmalonyl-CoA in Krebs cycle
- Methylcrotonyl-CoA carboxylase in catabolism of leucine

biotin may cause biotin deficiency. Infants of biotin-deficient mothers may develop biotin deficiency.
- **Clinical features:** These include anorexia, vomiting, premature hair-fall, hyperkeratotic skin, glossitis, muscle pains, hyperesthesia, anemia, hyperlipidemia (hypercholesterolemia). Maternal deficiency may cause deficiency signs in infants and children and may even contribute to dysmorphism.

Treatment
- **Mild deficiency:** 2–5 mg/day (orally) for 2–3 weeks.
- **Severe deficiency:** 200 µg/day parenterally for 2–5 days.

Prevention
Parenteral nutrition given over a prolonged time should have biotin incorporated.

CYANOCOBALAMIN (Vitamin B_{12}, Extrinsic Factor of Castle)
Cyanocobalamin is primarily produced by intestinal microbial flora.
- **Functions:** It is a coenzyme for conversion of homocysteine into methionine and L-methylmalonyl-CoA to succinyl-CoA for important metabolic reactions and synthesis of deoxyribonucleic acid (DNA) in bone marrow.
- **Dietary sources:** Animal origin foods such as meat (richest source is liver), fish, eggs; fresh milk and cheese milk powders (Fig. 8).
- **Daily requirement:**
    - *Infants:* 0.3 µg
    - *Children:* 1 µg
    - *Adolescents:* 1.5–2 µg.

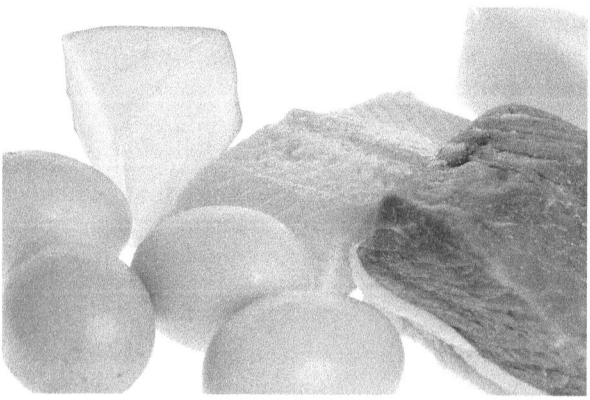

Fig. 8: Sources of vitamin B_{12}.

Deficiency

- ***Etiology:*** Strict vegetarianism; malabsorption syndrome (especially endemic tropical sprue, blind loop syndrome, inflammatory bowel disease), infantile tremor syndrome; drugs like neomycin, colchicine, para-amino salicylic acid (PAS) deficiency of intrinsic factor (pernicious anemia).
- ***Clinical features:*** Megaloblastic anemia (Fig. 9) manifesting with pallor, skin pigmentation (Fig. 10), smooth, red and painful tongue, neurologic manifestations (ataxia, paresthesias, hyporeflexia, tremors, peripheral neuropathy, subacute combined degeneration) and depression, etc.

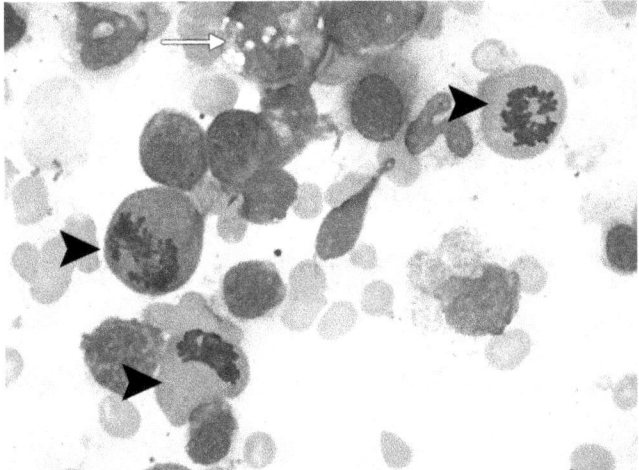

Fig. 9: Vitamin B_{12} deficiency. Note the megaloblastosis in the bone marrow of a child suffering from vitamin B_{12} deficiency as a part of endemic tropical sprue. Besides manifestations of malabsorption, he had skin pigmentation.

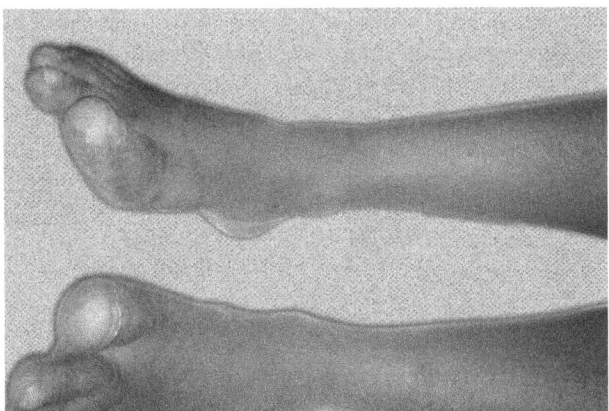

Fig. 10: Vitamin B_{12} deficiency: Note the pigmentation of skin, including soles.

Diagnosis

- Macrocytic/megaloblastic erythropoiesis
- Serum B_{12} level less than 100 µg/mL with increased level of serum lactic acid dehydrogenase (LDH)
- Methyl malonic aciduria is a sensitive and reliable index
- Schilling test.

Treatment

- For megaloblastic anemia, vitamin B_{12} 1 mg (1,000 µg) intramuscular (IM) leads to prompt hematological response (reticulocytosis) in 2–4 days.
- For neurologic involvement, same IM dose should be repeated daily for two weeks followed by a monthly maintenance dose (same dose and again IM) throughout life.

Folic Acid (Folacin, Folate, Vitamin B_9)

- *Functions:* Essential for maturation of red blood cells (RBCs). Moreover, it assists in protecting DNA and ensuring its replication when under attack by free radicals.
- *Dietary sources:* Meat (liver, kidney), egg, yeast, green leafy vegetables (GLVs)(spinach, cabbage, turnip greens), asparagus, mushrooms, beans, peas, sunflower seeds, whole grains (Fig. 11).
- *Daily requirements:*
  - *Infancy:* 40 µg
  - *Children:* 100 µg
  - *Adolescents:* 200 µg
  - *Pregnancy and lactation:* 400 µg.

Deficiency

- *Etiology:* Inadequate dietary intake or a disease process, e.g. malabsorption. It may occur in isolated form or in combination with other deficiencies such as vitamin B_{12}, iron, protein and PEM. Deficiency causes impairment of DNA synthesis resulting in defective cell division. Rapidly dividing cells such as in bone marrow and intestinal mucosa are adversely affected.

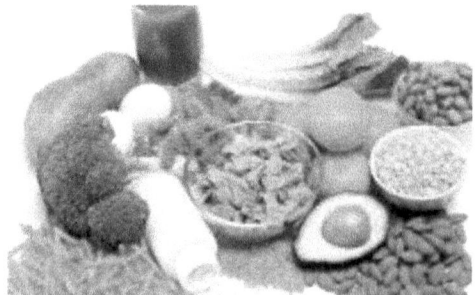

Fig. 11: Sources of folic acid.

- **Clinical features:** Megaloblastic anemia, neural tube defects (NTDs) (Fig. 12), cleft lip/palate. In adults, it is implicated in Alzheimer disease, dementia, depression, and hearing loss.

Diagnosis
By and large clinical.

Treatment
0.5–1 mg of folic acid daily.

Prevention
For prevention of NTDs, periconceptional folic acid therapy one month before and 2–3 months after conception.

Since folic acid is available as only 5 mg tablets, its one tablet daily is prescribed for periconceptional therapy. No adverse effects are known even with this high dose.

Vitamin C (Ascorbic Acid)
This structurally glucose-related vitamin is not synthesized by the body. It is known for its unique property of reversible oxidation-reduction.
- **Functions:** Ascorbic acid which structurally resembles a monosaccharide sugar is known to play important role in oxidation of tyrosine and phenylalanine, information of hydroxyproline, in preventing depolymerization of collagen, maintaining integrity of ground substance, and in hemopoiesis.
- **Dietary sources:** Citrus fruits–Indian gooseberry (amla), guava, lemon, orange, grapes, GLVs, soaked cereals (Fig. 13).

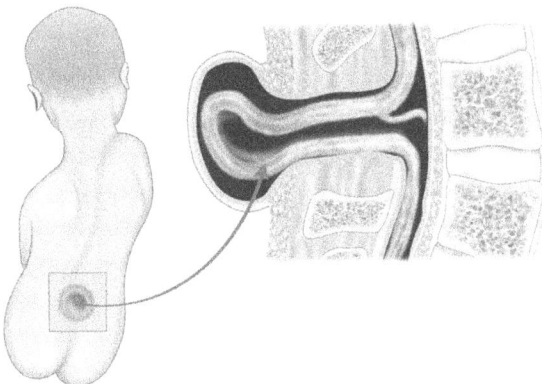

Fig. 12: Maternal folic acid deficiency. Note the neural tube defect (meningocele) in the infant born to such a mother. Periconceptional folic acid therapy has now become a universal recommendation.

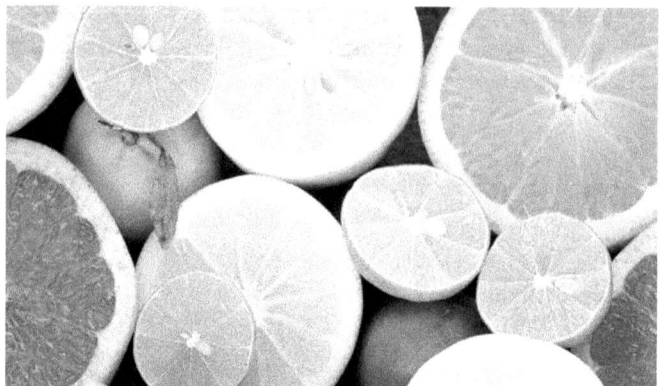

Fig. 13: Sources of vitamin C.

- **Daily requirement:**
  - **Infants and children:** 30–40 mg
  - **Pregnancy and lactation:** 60 mg.

Deficiency

Deficiency of vitamin C, though quite common in its subclinical form, has virtually disappeared in its overt form from the affluent countries. However, frank cases still continue to be seen from time to time in some parts of the developing regions.

FAT-SOLUBLE VITAMINS

Vitamin A (Retinol)[10-13]

Vitamin A, a fat-soluble alcohol, is derived primarily from a plant pigment, β-carotene, which plays a vital role in the photochemical basis of vision. Conversion of carotene to vitamin A occurs in the intestinal wall and its absorption into the lymphatic system is facilitated by bile. It is concerned with the maintenance of epithelial tissue in the body, especially that of eye, skin and mucous membrane.

- **Dietary sources:** Shark and cod-liver oil, dark green leafy vegetables (DGLV), e.g. fenugreek, carrot, oranges, tomatoes; fortified infant formulas and foodstuffs (Fig. 14).
- **Daily requirement:**
  - **Infants:** 300–400 µg
  - **Children:** 400–600 µg
  - **Adolescents:** 750 µg.
  It may be noted that 1 µg = 3.3 IU
- **Functions:** Maintenance of vision, epithelium and differentiation of various tissues in utero.

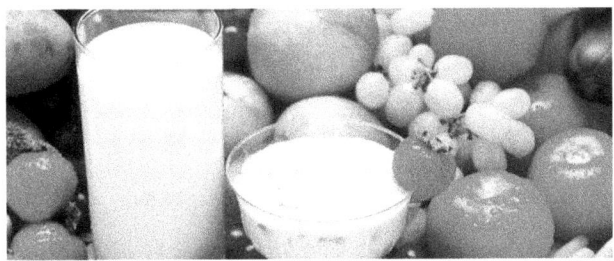

Fig. 14: Sources of vitamin A.

Box 2: World Health Organization (WHO) classification of xerophthalmia.

- *XN:* Night blindness
- *X1A:* Conjunctival xerosis
- *X1B:* Bitot spot
- *X2:* Corneal xerosis
- *X3A:* Corneal ulceration/keratomalacia <1/3rd corneal surface
- *X3B:* Corneal ulceration/keratomalacia >1/3rd corneal surface
- *XS:* Corneal scar
- *XF:* Xerophthalmic fundi (white retinal lesions)

Box 3: Extraoccular manifestations of vitamin A deficiency.

- Dry, scaly skin, especially over the outer aspect of the limbs (follicular hyperkeratosis, toad skin or phrynoderma)
- Hypertrophy or even atrophy of tongue
- Increased susceptibility to infections due to squamous metaplasia of respiratory, gastrointestinal, urinary and vaginal tract epithelium as a result of impaired immune response (both specific and nonspecific)
- Increased susceptibility to renal and vesical calculi
- Growth failure
- Pseudotumor cerebri
- Infertility
- Fetal defects

Deficiency

Deficiency signs of vitamin A deficiency (VAD) may be ocular or extraocular (details vide infra) and also clinical or suclinical depending on the magnitude of deficiency.

Ocular Manifestations

The ocular manifestations are listed in Box 2.

Extraocular Manifestations

The extraocular manifestations of VAD are listed in Box 3.

Treatment

Box 4 presents the WHO/UNICEF-recommended treatment schedule for xerophthalmia.

Box 4: WHO/UNICEF treatment schedule of xerophthalmia.

Children 1 to 6 years and above	
• Immediately on diagnosis	200,000 IU vitamin A(O)
• The following day	200,000 IU vitamin A(O)
• Four weeks later	200,000 IU vitamin A(O)
Children under 1 year and under 8 kg weight at any age	
• Half the doses as indicated for	10,000 IU vitamin A(O) for
• Children 1–6 years and above	2 weeks
• For night blindness of bitot spot, with a daily dose of	

Note: If there is a persistent vomiting or profuse diarrhea, an intramuscular injection of 100,000 IU of water-miscible vitamin A (but not an oil-based preparation) may be substituted for the first dose.

Excess/Toxicity (Hypervitaminosis A)

Abuse of vitamin A (more than 20,000 IU daily over several months) may cause toxicity (hypervitaminosis A).

- **Manifestations** include hyperirritability, anorexia, lassitude, headache, alopecia and/or coarsening of scalp hair, desquamation of skin (note in VAD it is hyperkeratosis), fever, benign raised intracranial pressure (ICP) (pseudotumor cerebri), hepatosplenomegaly and tender swellings of the bones.
- **X-ray** shows cortical hyperostosis of long bones (ulna, tibia, etc.), most marked in the middle of the shaft with sparing of the metaphysis.

Even teratogenicity in the form of malformations (often resulting in abortions) may be encountered in infants of mothers who are on retinoic acid for acne or cancer during first trimester of pregnancy. **Gulf syndrome** refers to hypervitaminosis A plus D secondary to excessive consumption of fish oil pearls marketed by Gulf countries.

Vitamin D[14-18] (Sunshine Vitamin)

Functions

Vitamin D, a secondary steroid, plays an important role in calcium and phosphorus homeostasis. It is a precursor of 1, 25-dihydroxyvitamin D_3, a hormone synthesized and secreted by kidneys under the control of parathormone and tissue phosphate levels.

The ultraviolet rays of the sunlight are responsible for converting the 7-dehydrocholesterol that is normally present under the skin, into vitamin D_3 or cholecalciferol. The latter is further converted to 25-hydroxycholecalciferol and 25-hydroxyergocalciferol in the liver. The last two forms are essential for maintenance of adequate calcium and phosphorus concentration in the extracellular fluid and for the formation of bone matrix. It is now established that 25-hydroxycholecalciferol is then converted to 1, 25-dihydroxycholecalciferol. The latter is specifically helpful in promoting synthesis of **calcium transport protein** in the intestinal wall.

Maintenance of blood level of 25-hydroxyvitamin D more than 20 ng/mL is important for maximum health benefits. In short, vitamin D has both skeletal (calcitropic) as well as extraskeletal (pleotrophic) role. Extraskeletal benefits are reportedly as anti-infective, in respiratory disease, immunological disease and malignancies, etc.

Sources
Sources of vitamin D include sunshine (90%) and diet (10%), fish, fish oils, egg (yolk), milk, infant formulas and supplements such as cereals and margarine (butter-like product made of vegetable oils) (Fig. 15).

Daily Requirement
Current recommendation is 400 IU of vitamin D per day for all infants, children and adolescents. This is essential to maintain a vitamin D blood level of 20 ng/mL. With the earlier recommendation of just 200 IU, this level is not maintained.

Deficiency
- ***Etiology:*** Vitamin D deficiency may result from several conditions (Box 5).
- ***Clinical features:*** Vitamin D deficiency may produce and/or be associated with:
  - ***Bone-related:*** Rickets and osteoporosis

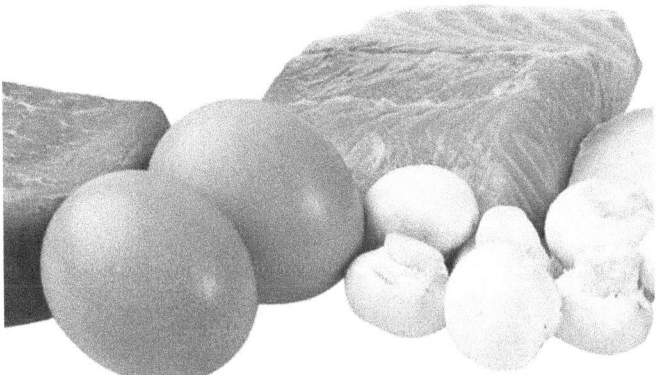

Fig. 15: Sources of vitamin D.

Box 5: Causes of vitamin D deficiency.

- Decreased synthesis by skin
- Decreased nutritional intake
- Prematurity and VLBW
- Decreased maternal stores
- Formula-fed infants
- Malabsorption
- Chronic liver disease—decreased synthesis
- Chronic renal disease
- Drug-induced—antiepileptics, rifampicin, INH
- Tumors

(VLBW: very low birth weight; INH: isonicotinyl hydrazide)

- ***Extraskeletal:*** Susceptibility to infections, muscle pains and weakness, seizures, asthma, malignancies, type II diabetes, hypertension and obesity.

Excess/Toxicity (Hypervitaminosis D)

It produces clinical manifestation via hypercalcemia due to excessive bone resorption when vitamin D is taken more than 1,000 IU/day by infants and 2,000 IU/day by adolescents over several months.

Manifestations include anorexia, excessive irritability, abdominal pain, vomiting, constipation, polyuria, dehydration and hypernatremia, Caffey's disease-like painful cortical thickening of certain bones (mandible, clavicle, ulna, and radius) and ectopic calcification.

Serious adverse effects relate to cardiovascular system (CVS) (hypertension, decreased QT interval, arrhythmias), central nervous system (CNS) (hypotonia, depression, hallucinations, psychosis, coma) and kidneys (chronic renal failure from renal calculi), even pancreatitis may occur.

Gulf syndrome refers to hypervitaminosis D along with A as a result of excessive consumption of fish oil pearls marketed by Gulf countries. Response to withdrawal of vitamin D and calcium and therapy with normal saline, loop diuretics, aluminium hydroxide suffices in most cases.

Prednisolone, calcitonin, chelating agent (sodium versenate), biphosphonates and hemodialysis may be considered in severe hypercalcemia.

Vitamin E

Alpha-tocopherol is the most biologically active among the eight related fat-soluble compounds formed by the tocopherols and their unsaturated derivatives, the tocotrienols.

- ***Dietary sources:*** The compound, i.e. vitamin E, occurs naturally in foods eaten by humans, such as vegetable oils including soyabean, wheat, germ, sunflower oil, egg yolk and leafy vegetables (Fig. 16).
- ***Daily requirement:*** Its requirement should, therefore, be according to the intake of polyunsaturated fats. It is claimed to be 0.5 mg for every gram of linoleic acid. Generally speaking, 5–15 mg daily should suffice.
- ***Functions:*** This vitamin is believed to be important in maintaining the stability of biological membranes. Many of its properties are yet unclear, earning it the designation ***shady lady of nutrition.***

Deficiency

In man, vitamin E deficiency is fortunately uncommon. When it occurs, the causes include prematurity and malabsorption and cholestatic states.

Clinical features: In the ***premature infant,*** vitamin E deficiency produces hemolytic anemia 4–6 weeks after birth. Additional problems include edema,

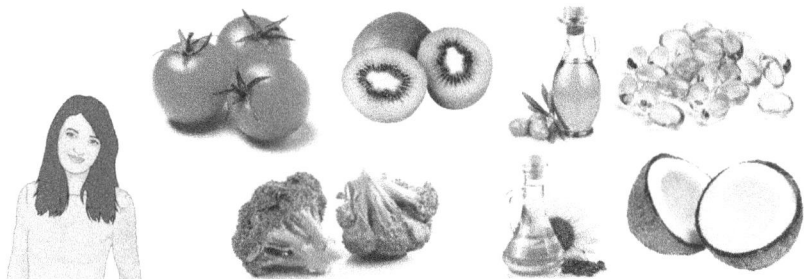

Fig.16: Sources of vitamin E.

skin changes, retinopathy of prematurity (ROP), bronchopulmonary dysplasia and intraventricular hemorrhage. It is worth noting that the deficiency occurs most often in babies who are being fed the milk that is quite rich in linoleic acid. Another factor that may precipitate vitamin E deficiency and hemolytic anemia in the premature infant is the administration of supplementary iron without added vitamin E.

In *children and adolescents*, manifestations include muscular dystrophy (fatty type), growth retardation, impaired reproductive ability, etc.

Treatment

Premature infants fed on formulas rich in linoleic acid and fortified with iron must receive 0.7 IU of vitamin E/100 kcal or 1 IU/g of linoleic acid to avoid occurrence of hemolytic anemia. Generally, it is given 15–25 mg IU/day.

Some authorities recommended administration of vitamin E (IM) once daily for several days after birth in infants who receive excessive concentration of oxygen.

Excess/Toxicity

Neonatal necrotizing enterocolitis.

Vitamin K

- *Function:* Vitamin K is concerned with synthesis of coagulation factors II, VII, IX and X in the liver.
- *Dietary sources:* GLV, soyabeans and fish are its natural sources (Figs. 17A and B). Enough of this vitamin is produced by the intestinal flora.
- *Daily requirement:*
  - *Birth:* 5 µg
  - *Two years:* 10–12 µg
  - *Later:* 12–30 µg
  - Mother's milk provides only 1.5 µg/100 mL of it.

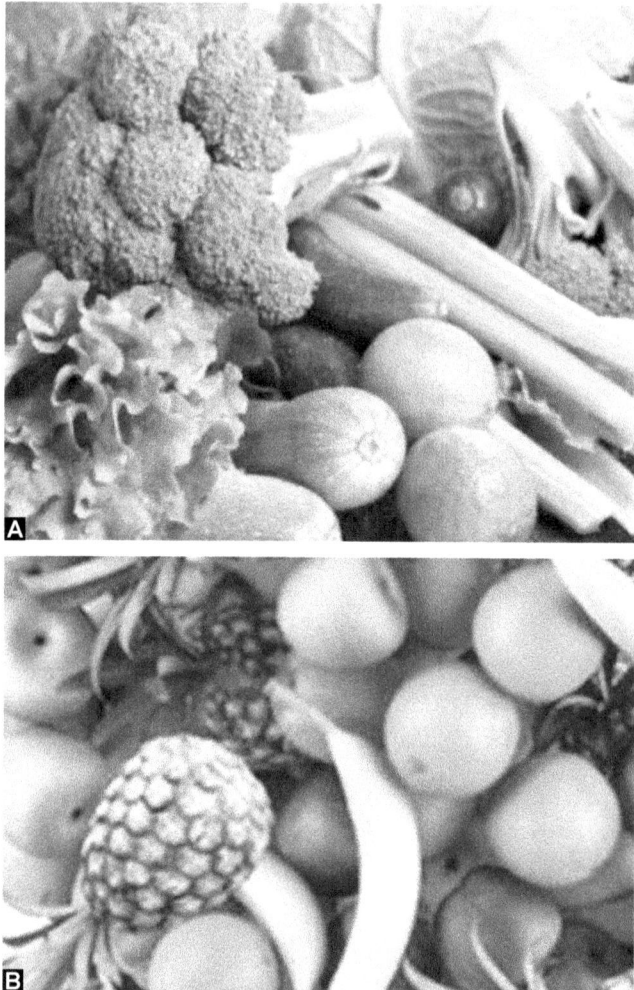

Figs. 17A and B: Dietary sources of vitamin K.

Deficiency

Etiology

Deficiency of vitamin K may occur in the following situations:
- Newborns before adequate colonization of the intestines by bacterial flora have indeed occurred.
- Newborns fed on unsupplemented breast milk. Though both cow and human milk have low content of vitamin K, the former supplies four times more vitamin K than the latter.
- Infants fed on unsupplemented milk formulas based on soyabean isolates.
- Chronic intestinal parasitosis.
- Malabsorption states.
- Biliary obstruction.
- Oral antibiotics.

Clinical Features

These include:
- **Hemorrhagic disease of the newborn (HDN):** This is the most common manifestation of vitamin K deficiency. Generally, bleeding from the GIT, intracerebral hemorrhage or bleeding from the umbilical stump occurs in the first week, usually round about the third day after birth. Therapy consists of blood transfusion and parenteral administration of vitamin K, 2-5 mg.
- **Very-late vitamin K deficiency-related hemorrhagic disease:** This may occur in older neonates, paraneonates and infants. Whereas factors such as persistent/chronic diarrhea, malabsorption, ascariasis, biliary tract obstruction, poor vitamin K intake and broad-spectrum antibiotics could well be the cause or precipitating factor(s) in many cases, there remain some cases without any well-defined etiologic factor.

Prophylaxis

One mg of vitamin K should be given to all newborns intramuscularly soon after birth for prevention of early-onset vitamin K deficiency bleeding (VKDB). This practice has considerably brought down incidence of early-onset VKDB. Hence, VKDB is now mostly seen after 2 weeks of age (late-onset VKDB).

Treatment

2-5 mg parenterally.

Excess/Toxicity

Excessive administration of vitamin K especially in preterm and G-6-PD deficient infants, may cause:
- Hemolytic anemia
- Hyperbilirubinemia
- Kernicterus.

SOME SPECIAL FEATURES OF VITAMINS AT A GLANCE

- A vegetable and fruit-based diet generally has a higher content of vitamins A, C and E and folic acid but is generally poor in vitamins B_{12} and D.
- Vitamins mandatory for energy releasing processes are B_1, B_2, B_3, B_5, B_6, and biotin.
- Vitamins necessary for red blood cell synthesis are B_9, B_6.

Earlier names for riboflavin (vitamin B_2) were lactoflavin, ovoflavin, hepatoflavin and verdoflavin, indicating the sources (milk, eggs, liver and plants) from which the vitamin was first isolated.

Prenatal multivitamin/mineral supplements are associated with a reduced risk of low birth weight infants and with improved birth weight when compared with iron-folic acid supplements.

In observational studies (case-control or cohort design), people with high intake of antioxidant vitamins by regular diet typically have a lower risk of heart attack and stroke than people who do not consume enough.

CONCLUSION

Vitamins are essential for maintenance of normal health and usually need to be provided from external dietary sources. They are important in controlling protein synthesis and acting as hormones, antioxidants and regulators of a tissue growth and differentiation. Deficiencies of vitamins may be as such or secondary to overall malnutrition or disease states. Water-soluble vitamins (B-complex, vitamin C) are not stored in the body in any appreciable quantity and are by and large safe despite excessive intake. Excessive intake of fat-soluble vitamins (A, D, E, K), that are stored in liver, may cause toxicity.

KEY LEARNING POINTS

- Vitamins, organic compounds, needed in limited quantities and are essential for maintenance of normal health, usually need to be provided from usually dietary sources.
- Besides controlling protein synthesizes, vitamins function as hormones, antioxidants and regulators of tissue growth and differentiation. The 13 vitamins that are universally recognized comprise 9 water-soluble (vitamins B complex and C) and fat-soluble (vitamins A, D, E and K).
- Water-soluble vitamins are not stored in the body in any appreciable quantity. Their excessive consumption causes no particular toxicity, the surplus being excreted. On the contrary, fat-soluble vitamins are stored in liver. Their excessive consumption may, therefore, cause toxicity.
- Vitamin deficiencies may occur individually, in combination with other members of the group, or in combination with other nutritional problems such as protein-energy malnutrition (PEM), micronutrient deficiency (say, iron deficiency anemia), etc.

REFERENCES

1. Gupte S. *Pediatric Nutrition.* New Delhi: Peepee 2012.
2. Mehta MN, Mehta NJ. *Nutrition and Diet for Children Simplified.* New Delhi: Jaypee 2014.
3. Elizabeth K. *Nutrition and Child Development,* 5th edn. Hyderabad: Paras 2015.
4. Gupte S. Vitamins. In: Gupte S (Ed): *The Short Textbook of Pediatrics,* 12th edn. New Delhi:Jaypee 2016:225-244.
5. WebMed. Folic acid. Available at: https://www.webmd.com/vitamins-supplements/ingredientmono-1017-FOLIC+ACID.aspx?activeIngredientId=1017&activeIngredientName=FOLIC+ACID Accessed on: 23 January 2018.
6. Burn S. Biotin. Avaiolable at: http://www.massagetherapy.com/articles/index.php/article_id/1091/Biotin-Basics Accessed on: Accessed on: 23 January 2018.
7. WebMed. Pyridoxine HCl. Available at: https://www.webmd.com/drugs/2/drug-5427/pyridoxine-vitamin-b6-oral/details Accessed on: 23 January 2018.

8. Nordavist C. Everything you need to know about vitamin B12. Available at: https://www.medicalnewstoday.com/articles/219822.php Accessed on 23 January 2018.
9. University of Maryland Medical Center. Vitamin C (ascorbic acid). Availableat: https://www.umm.edu/health/medical/altmed/supplement/vitamin-c-ascorbic-acid Accessed on 24 January 2018.
10. Akhtar S, Ahmed A, Randhawa MA, Atukorala S, Arlappa N, Ismail T, et al. Prevalence of vitamin A deficiency in South Asia: Causes, outcomes, and possible remedies. *J Health Popul Nutr* 2013;31:413-423.
11. Kapil U, Sachdev HP. Massive dose vitamin A programme in India--need for a targeted approach. *Indian J Med Res* 2013;138:411-417. Available at: https://www.ncbi.nlm.nih.gov/pubmed/24135191 Accessed on: 24 January 2018.
12. Agrawal A, Shrivastava J. Vitamin A deficiency in children: Is it still prevalent in India? *Indian J Child Health* 2015;2:45-46.
13. Raman JK, Chaudhery DN. Need to revisit vitamin A supplementation programme in India. *Indian J Med Res* 2014; 139: 323-324.
14. Bener A, Hoffmann G. Nutritional rickets among children in a sun rich country. *Int J Pediatr Endocrinol* 2010, 410502 Available at: https://www.ncbi.nlm.nih.gov/pmc/articles/PMC2965426/ Accessed on: 20 January 2018.
15. Prentice, A. Nutritional rickets around the world. *J Steroid Biochem. Mol Biol* 2013; 136:201-206.
16. Thacher TD. Increasing incidence of nutritional rickets: a population-based study in Olmsted County. Minnesota. *Mayo Clin. Proc* 2013;88:176-183.
17. Uush T. Prevalence of classic signs and symptoms of rickets and vitamin D deficiency in Mongolian children and women. *J Steroid Biochem Mol Biol* 2013;136: 207-210.
18. Munns CF. Global consensus recommendations on prevention and management of nutritional rickets. *J Clin Endocrinol Metab* 2016;101:394-415.

5
Vitamin A Deficiency

Suraj Gupte, Kareena Naidu, Isobel Tanapong

ABSTRACT

Vitamin A, a fat soluble vitamin, is mandatory for healthy vision and epithelial tissues. Its precursor is dietary beta-carotene and 3 other carotenoids. As high as 80–90% of vitamin A is stored in liver. Also called retinol, its natural and synthetic compounds are known as retinoids. Normal range of vitamin A/retinol is 28–86 µg/dL.

Vitamin A deficiency is defined as serum retinol levels of below 28 µg/dL. Primary vitamin A deficiency results from prolonged dietary deprivation. Secondary vitamin A deficiency is caused by reduced absorption, storage or transport of vitamin A as a consequence of a disease. Deficiency causes conjunctival and corneal damage ending up as keratomalacia and blindness, hyperkeratotic skin, growth retardation, etc.

VAD is common in underprivileged children. Mercifully, following nationwide prophylactic program, its prevalence in India has considerably come down.

Keywords: Bitot's spots, Corneal scarring, Dark adaptation, Keratomalacia, Blindness, Malabsorption, Night blindness, Phthisis bulbi, Vitamin A deficiency, Xerophthalmia.

INTRODUCTION

Deficiency of vitamin A, *xerophthalmia*, a leading cause of blindness among the underprivileged continues to be a problem of public health magnitude in the resource-poor communities.[1-6] Of the 10 million children suffering every year from xerophthalmia, 5 million belong to Asia. One-fourth of them are eventually blinded. Half a million go blind in India alone every year. Mercifully, vitamin A massive dose prophylaxis has come in handy in controlling the problem.[7-12]

ETIOLOGY

Vitamin A deficiency usually occurs:
A. As a primary deficiency because of decreased intake, or
B. In association with malnutrition and chronic intestinal disorders, such as malabsorption states (celiac disease, tropical sprue, cystic fibrosis),

chronic diarrheal disease, pancreatic disease, chronic giardiasis, and hepatic insufficiency. In these situations, vitamin A absorption or metabolism is disturbed.

Diarrhea is a risk factor for VAD; vice versa also is true. Severe measles too is a risk factor for vitamin A deficiency.[13]

PREVALENCE

The precise incidence of xerophthalmia in the pediatric population defies evaluation. In general, 3-10% of the infants and children in the resource-limited countries suffer from it.

According to the WHO, vitamin A deficiency is a public health problem in more than half of all countries, especially in Africa and South-East Asia, hitting hardest young children and pregnant women in low-income countries.

Following proactive measures on a large scale, prevalence in India has considerably fallen.

CLINICAL FEATURES[1,2]

Ocular Manifestations

The earliest manifestation, **night blindness** or **poor dark adaptation** (**XN**), is due to insufficient formation of the visual purple (rhodopsin), the rose-red pigment in the rods. Often, the mother of the infant observes that he takes considerable time to adjust to dim light or darkness.

Conjunctival xerosis (X1A) is usually the first sign that can be seen on examination. The conjunctiva becomes dry, lusterless, wrinkled and dirty-brown in color. These changes are most obvious in the interpalpebral bulbar conjunctiva (Fig.1). In advanced cases, significantly evident involvement of conjunctiva over the lower lid and lower fornix may be present (Box 1).

Conjunctival xerosis may lead to formation of the so-called **Bitot spot*** (X1B) which consists of an almost triangular area, usually about the lateral aspect of the limbus, covered by fine, white, foamy or greasy substance (Figs. 2 and 3). It is basically a heaped-up dry mass of conjunctival epithelium. The appearance is like grains on chalky, pasty foam. Bitot spots are generally seen in both the eyes and are present far more frequently to the lateral than the medial of the limbus.

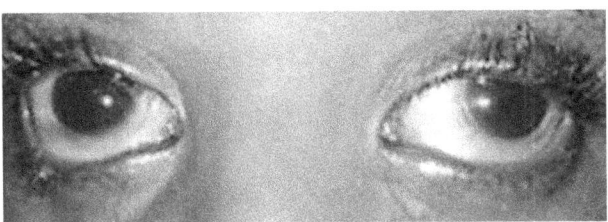

Fig. 1: Xerophthalmia. Note the dry, dull, muddy and wrinkled bulbar conjunctiva (X1A).

---

* After the French physician, Bitot, who described it in 1980s.

Box 1: WHO classification of xerophthalmia.

- **XN:** Night blindness
- **X1A:** Conjunctival xerosis
- **X1B:** Bitot spot
- **X2:** Corneal xerosis
- **X3A:** Corneal ulceration/keratomalacia <1/3rd corneal surface
- **X3B:** Corneal ulceration/keratomalacia >1/3rd corneal surface
- **XS:** Corneal scar
- **XF:** Xerophthalmic fundi (white retinal lesions).

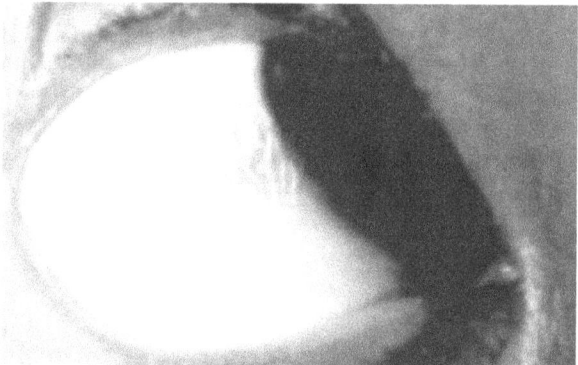

Fig. 2: Xerophthalmia. Note the position of the lesion and its shape in **Bitot's spot (X1B)**. The foamy deposit lies on top of a patch of pigmented conjunctiva.

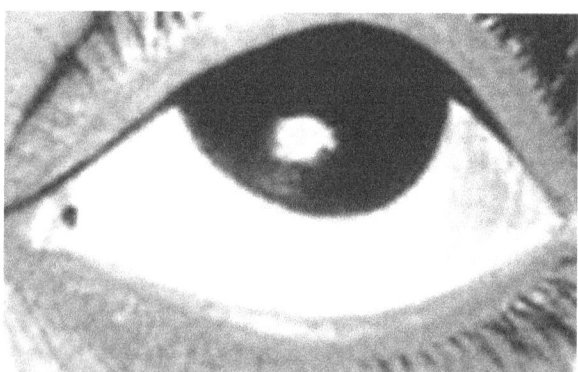

Fig. 3: Xerophthalmia. Bitot's spot with localized xerosis and pigmentation in a 4-year-old boy (X1B).

Corneal xerosis (X2) is the dryness and dullness of the cornea (Fig. 4).

Keratomalacia (X3) is the advanced stage of xerophthalmia. It consists of softening, necrosis and ulceration of the cornea (Figs. 4 and 5). Unlike the preceding stage of corneal xerosis, keratomalacia is irreversible, except for the possible replacement of the grossly damaged cornea by a transplant. Once cornea gets involved, photophobia accompanies the clinical profile.

With the onset of keratomalacia, cornea melts into a dead-white to dirty-yellow structure. Invasion by an infection (which is quite usual) further

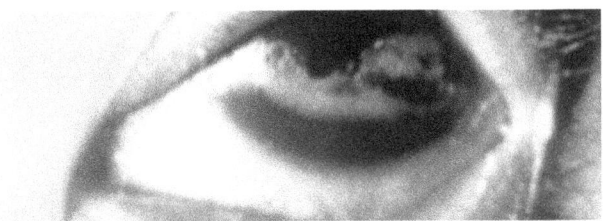

Fig. 4: Xerophthalmia. Note the corneal xerosis with dry and dull cornea (X2).

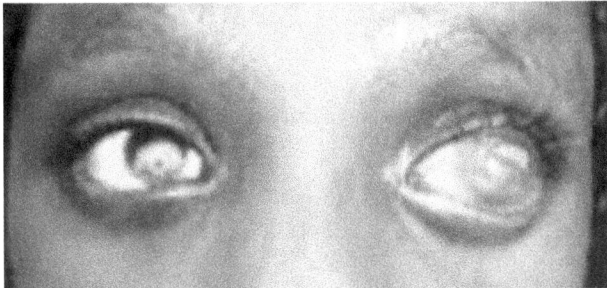

Fig. 5: Xerophthalmia. Note the involvement of a part of cornea of right eye (X3A); opacification of nearly whole of cornea in left eye (X3B).

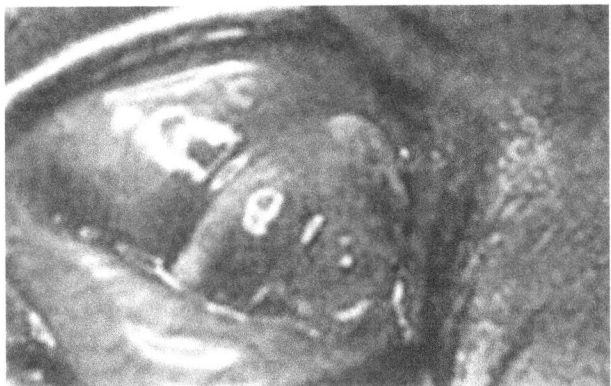

Fig. 6: Xerophthalmia. Bulging staphyloma.

aggravates the situation. If corneal perforation occurs (which again is quite frequent), herniation of the lens and vitreous may result (Fig. 6).

Corneal scarring (XS) as seen in Figure 7 causes complete blindness.

Eventually, **panophthalmitis** leads to almost total destruction of not just the cornea, but that of the whole eyeball. Irreversible blindness (which was entirely preventable) is the final outcome, the eye ending up as a shrunken globe, the so-called **phthisis bulbi** (Fig. 8).

During the course of destruction of the globe, retina does not lag behind in suffering. On fundoscopy, it reveals small white spots and granules, the so-called *fundus ophthalmicus*.

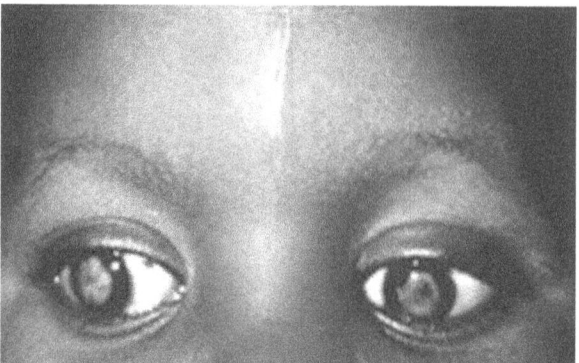

Fig. 7: Xerophthalmia. Bilateral corneal scarring (XS).

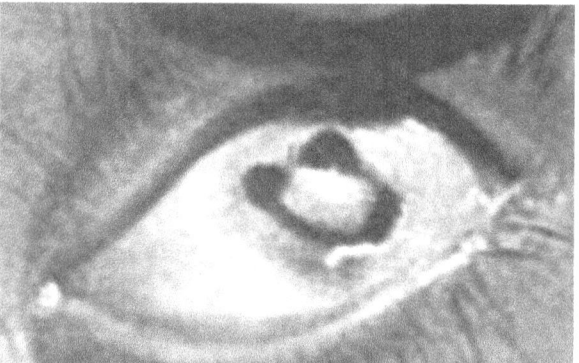

Fig. 8: Xerophthalmia. Phthisis bulbi as a result of vitamin A deficiency.

Extraocular Manifestations

The extraocular manifestations of VAD are listed in Box 2.

Box 2: Extraoccular manifestations of vitamin A deficiency.

- Dry, scaly skin, especially over the outer aspect of the limbs (follicular hyperkeratosis, toad skin or phrynoderma)
- Hypertrophy or even atrophy of tongue
- Increased susceptibility to infections due to squamous metaplasia of respiratory, gastrointestinal, urinary and vaginal tract epithelium as a result of impaired immune response (both specific and nonspecific)
- Increased susceptibility to renal and vesical calculi
- Growth failure
- Pseudotumor cerebri
- Infertility
- Fetal defects

DIAGNOSIS

- High index of suspicion from the clinical picture is the most important diagnostic measure. Support may be obtained from the dark adaptation test.

- Objective tests based on vital staining of xerotic conjunctiva (Rose Bengal, lissamine, kajal or other mascara) or conjunctival impression cytology (CIC) may supplement clinical diagnosis of xerophthalmia.
- Determination of plasma or liver retinol (vitamin A) level is helpful. The normal values are 50–100 IU in infants and 100–300 IU in grown up children.
- Vitamin A absorption test may be carried out by giving 0.2 mL/kg of cod liver oil by mouth. Blood samples are obtained before its administration and thereafter at 3, 5, 7, 9 and 12 hours. Afterwards, a curve is plotted from the vitamin A values obtained on these samples. A flat curve indicates defective absorption.

TREATMENT

The currently recommended World Health Organization (WHO)/United Nation Children Funds (UNICEF) schedule for treatment of xerophthalmia is summarized in Box 3. An oily preparation for oral and a water-miscible preparation for injection is the current recommendation. Steroids may be of help if used early enough in these cases. Almost all cases recover fully without when treatment is given fairly early. Recurrence, though rare, may occur.[14]

PREVENTION[15-17]

- An intake of at least 1500 IU/day in infants and children less than 4 years and 5000 IU/day in grown up children should be ensured. Just milk meets this requirement in infants. Older children need leafy vegetables and red palm oil in addition to milk.
- According to the National Vitamin A prophylaxis program, all children in the age group 9 months to 3 years in the target areas should receive 100,000 IU for less than 1 year and 200,000 IU for more than 1 year of vitamin A (in an oily base) orally every six months a total of five doses. The agent is supplied as syrup of 100,000 units of vitamin A/mL.
- For preventive purposes, use of β-carotene-rich foods, DGLV, say mustard (sarson), spinach (palak), fenugreek (methi), amaranth (chaulai), drumstick

Box 3: WHO/UNICEF treatment schedule of xerophthalmia

Children 1–6 years and above	
• Immediately on diagnosis	200,000 IU vitamin A(O)
• The following day	200,000 IU vitamin A(O)
• Four weeks later	200,000 IU vitamin A(O)
Children under 1 year and under 8 kg weight at any age	
• Half the doses as indicated for:	10,000 IU vitamin A(O) for 2 weeks
– Children 1–6 years and above	
– For night blindness of Bitot spot with a daily dose of	

Note: If there is a presistent vomiting or profuse diarrhea, an intramuscular injection of 100,000 IU of water-miscible vitamin A (but not an oil-based preparation) may be substituted for the first dose.

(sahjan), yellow vegetables (carrot), yellow fruits (mango, orange, papaya) and vitamin A-rich foods, say fish, liver, fresh liver oil, dairy products and edible oils, should be encouraged. **Vision by vegetables** is a good slogan.
- Dark green leafy vegetables are an inexpensive and superb source of β-carotene (precursor of vitamin A). Just 40 g of GLV cooked with 2-3 g of oil provide 1200 μg of β-carotene which is the recommended daily allowance (RDA) as per WHO. Even in malnourished children, absorption of β-carotene is about 70%. Children are able to eat enough GLV from a single traditional meal to meet their vitamin A requirement.
- Fortification of commonly-eaten foods with vitamin A can be an effective prophylactic measure in a population.
- Adequate and timely treatment of PEM, intestinal parasitosis and diarrheal disease, especially with supplementation of the intake with DGLV and edible oil, goes a long way in preventing xerophthalmia.
- The pregnant and lactating mothers should get enough of retinol or carotene in their diets.

CONCLUSION

Primary vitamin A deficiency results from prolonged dietary deprivation. Secondary vitamin A deficiency is caused by reduced absorption, storage or transport of vitamin A in association with malnutrition, liver disease, chronic diarrhea, pancreatic disease, malabsorptive disorders like celiac disease, tropical sprue, cystic fibrosis, etc. Deficiency causes ocular (conjunctival and corneal damage ending up as keratomalacia and blindness) as well as extraocular manifestations (hyperkeratotic skin and growth retardation, pseudotumor cerebri, etc.). VAD is common in underprivileged children. Mercifully, following nationwide prophylactic program, its prevalence in India has considerably fallen.

KEY LEARNING POINTS

- Vitamin A is a fat-soluble vitamin required for healthy vision and epithelial tissues, the precursor being dietary beta-carotene and 3 other carotenoids.
- Also called retinol, its natural and synthetic compounds are known as retinoids. Normal range of vitamin A/retinol is 28–86 μg/dL.
- As high as 80–90% of vitamin A is stored in liver.
- Primary vitamin A deficiency results from prolonged dietary deprivation. Secondary vitamin A deficiency is caused by reduced absorption, storage or transport of vitamin A as a consequence of a disease.
- Deficiency causes conjunctival and corneal damage ending up as keratomalacia and blindness, hyperkeratotic skin, growth retardation, pseudotumor cerebri, etc.
- Diagnosis is usually clinical though biochemical tests are available.
- Prophylactic as well as therapeutic approach is as per recommendations of the WHO/UNICEF.
- Though common in underprivileged children, following nationwide prophylactic program, its prevalence in India has considerably come down.

REFERENCES

1. World Health Organization. Micronutrient deficiencies. Available at: http://www.who.int/nutrition/topics/vad/en/ Accessed on: 23 January 2018.
2. Gupte S. Vitamins. In: Gupte S (Ed). *The Short Textbook of Pediatrics*, 12th edn. New Delhi: Jaypee 2016:224-244.
3. World Health Organization. *Global prevalence of vitamin A deficiency in populations at risk 1995–2005. WHO global database on vitamin A deficiency*. Geneva: WHO 2009.
4. National Nutrition Monitoring Bureau (NNMB). *Prevalence of vitamin A deficiency among rural pre-school children*. Hyderabad: National Institute of Nutrition: 2006. Available at: http://www.nnmbindia.org/vad-report-final-21feb07.pdf Accessed on: 25 January 2018
5. Agrawal A, Shrivastava J. Vitamin A deficiency in children: Is it still prevalent in India? *Indian J Child Health* 2015;2:45-46. Available at: https://www.atharvapub.net/index.php/IJCH/article/view/584 Accessed on: 27 January 2018.
6. Akhtar S, Ahmed A, Randhawa MA, Atukorala S, Arlappa N, Ismail T, et al. Prevalence of vitamin A deficiency in South Asia: Causes, outcomes, and possible remedies. *J Health Popul Nutr* 2013;31:413-423.
7. Kapil U, Sachdev HP. Massive dose vitamin A programme in India—need for a targeted approach. *Indian J Med Res* 2013;138:411-417. Available at: https://www.ncbi.nlm.nih.gov/pubmed/24135191 Accessed on: 24 January 2018.
8. Raman JK, Chaudhery DN. Need to revisit vitamin A supplementation programme in India. *Indian J Med Res* 2014; 139: 323-324.
9. McLaughlin S, Welch J, MacDonald E, Mantry S, Ramaesh K. Xerophthalmia--a potential epidemic on our doorstep? *Eye (Lond)* 2014;28:621-663.
10. Agrawal VK, Agrawal P, Dharmendra Prevalence and determinants of xerophthalmia in rural children of Uttar Pradesh, India. *Nepal J Ophthalmol* 2013;5:226-229. [PubMed]
11. McLaren DS, Kraemer K. Xerophthalmia. *World Rev Nutr Diet* 2012;103:65-75. [PubMed]
12. Dole K, Gilbert C, Deshpande M, Khandekar R. Prevalence and determinants of xerophthalmia in preschool children in urban slums, Pune, India—a preliminary assessment. *Ophthalmic Epidemiol* 2009;16:8-14.[PubMed]
13. Pal R, Sagar V. Antecedent risk factors of xerophthalmia among Indian rural preschool children. *Eye Contact Lens* 2008;34:106-108. [PubMed]
14. Kapil U, Bhadoria AS, Sareen N. Reappearance of Bitot's spots after complete resolution in children between 1 and 5 years of age. *J Trop Pediatr* 2015;61(2):131-134.
15. Girard AW, Self JL, McAuliffe C, Olude O. The effects of household food production strategies on the health and nutrition outcomes of women and young children: A systematic review. *Paediatr Perinat Epidemiol* 2012;26 Suppl 1:205-222.
16. Vijayaraghavan K, Nayak M, Bamji M, Ramana G, Reddy V. Home gardening for combating vitamin A deficiency in rural India. *Food Nutr Bull* 1997;18:337-343.
17. Feroze KB, Kaufman EJ. Xerophthalmia. Treasure Island (FL): StatPearls Publishing 2017 Available at: https://www.ncbi.nlm.nih.gov/books/NBK431094/ Accessed on: 27 January 2018.

6 Vitamin D Deficiency

Harmesh S Bains

ABSTRACT

Vitamin D deficiency, a global public health problem, is caused by decreased dietary intake, decreased synthesis in the skin, lower levels of vitamin D in mothers, exclusive breastfeeding, malabsorption, and liver and kidney diseases. Its diagnosis is established by, in addition to clinical criteria, estimating main circulating vitamin D 25(OH)D in serum. Treatment is required in all cases of vitamin D deficiency, regardless whether the child is asymptomatic or symptomatic.

Keywords: Global public health problem, Malabsorption, Osteomalacia, Rickets, Serum vitamin D 25(OH)D, Vitamin D deficiency.

INTRODUCTION

Today vitamin D deficiency is reported to be a global public health problem,[1,2] including India where there is enough availability of sunshine. Vitamin D not only controls the calcium and bone metabolism but also has a role in various other diseases, including immune diseases, malignancies, cardiovascular and infectious diseases.[2-4] Several factors are involved in causation of vitamin D deficiency, e.g. decreased dietary intake, decreased synthesis in the skin, lower levels of vitamin D in mothers, exclusive breastfeeding, malabsorption, and liver and kidney diseases.[4-7] Treatment is required in both asymptomatic as well as symptomatic cases of vitamin D deficiency.

METABOLISM OF VITAMIN D

Ultraviolet rays (290–320 nm) of sunlight cause conversion of epidermal stores 7-dehydrocholesterol (provitamin D_3) to previtamin D_3.

Previtamin D_3 is converted into vitamin D_3 by a non-enzymatic process.

In liver vitamin D is metabolized to 25 hydroxy vitamin D 25(OH)D by a hepatic mitochondrial and or microsomal enzyme(s). 25(OH)D is not physiologically active in vivo.

Flowchart 1: Metabolism of vitamin D at a glance.

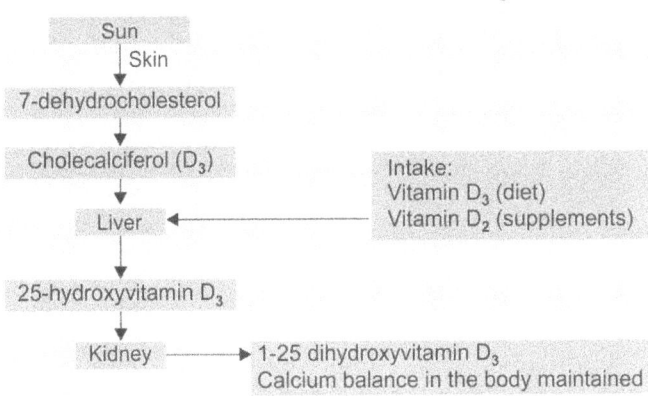

In kidneys 25-OH D is converted into 1 alpha 25 (OH) 2D. Hypocalcemia leads to release of parathormone (PTH) and enhanced activity of renal mitochondrial D 25(OH)D 1alpha hydroxylase which is responsible for this conversion.1 alpha 25 (OH) 2D is bound to vitamin D binding protein and delivered to intestine where it is taken up by specific cytoplasmic receptor protein to stimulate calcium and phosphorus transport from the intestine lumen into the circulation. It acts synergistically with parathyroid hormone (PTH) on bone resorption in physiological conditions. In higher doses it acts directly to increase bone mineral mobilization.

Vitamin D deficiency leads to decreased intestinal absorption of calcium and decreased mobilization of calcium from bones, resulting in hypocalcemia which stimulates increased secretion of PTH which tends to raise plasma calcium levels and increased renal phosphate clearance Flowchart 1.

Risk factors for vitamin D deficiency:
- Dark skin
- Excessive coverage of body by clothes
- Inadequate intake of vitamin D
- Vitamin D deficient mother and exclusively breast fed babies
- Underlying diseases like malabsorption, chronic liver or renal disorders.
- Major impact of vitamin D deficiency is on bones. Figure 1 shows classical radiological changes at the wrist.

Indications for Estimation of Vitamin D Levels

Clinical features of rickets, abnormal investigations, chronic diseases and drugs:
- Bowing of legs
- Knock knees
- Widening of wrist joint and rachitic rosary
- Wide persistent anterior fontanel
- Parietal prominences
- Pot belly
- Cat back

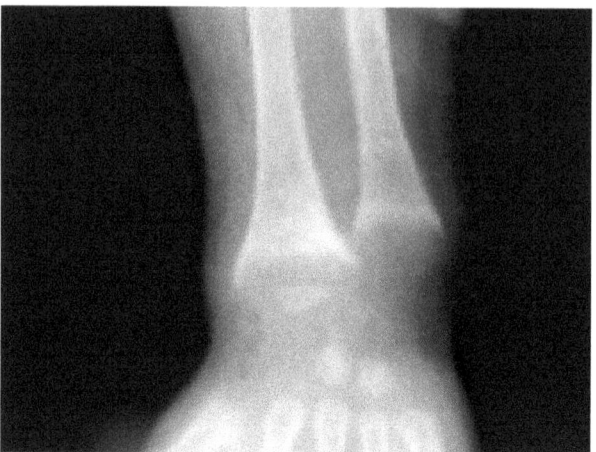

Fig. 1: Cupping, flaring and fraying at wrist in rickets.

- Low levels of plasma calcium or phosphate
- High alkaline phosphatase
- Radiological changes of rickets
- Chronic renal failure
- Chronic liver disease
- Celiac disease
- Phenobarbitone, phenytoin, carbamazepine.

DEFINITION OF VITAMIN D DEFICIENCY

Serum estimation of the main circulating vitamin D (25-OHD) is used for defining vitamin D deficiency. There is no consensus on normal plasma values of vitamin D and its deficiency. The vitamin D status in relation to 25(OH)D levels is shown in Table 1.

BIOCHEMICAL MARKERS IN VITAMIN D DEFICIENCY

The severity of vitamin D deficiency is based on the level of biochemical markers (Table 2).

TREATMENT

Indications for Treatment

- Clinical features of hypocalcemia
- Clinical features of rickets
- Low vitamin D levels even if asymptomatic.

Different Regimens

Table 3 presents the different treatment regimens.

Table 1: Vitamin D status in relation to 25(OH)D levels.

Vitamin D status	Levels
US Institute of Medicine classification	
Severe deficiency	<5 ng/mL
Deficiency	<15 ng/mL
Sufficiency	>20 ng/mL
Risk of toxicity	>50 ng/mL
US Endocrine Society classification	
Deficiency	<20 ng/mL (50 nmol/L)
Insufficiency	21–29 ng/mL (52.5–72.5) nmol/liter
Sufficiency	>30 ng/mL
Toxicity	>150 ng/mL

1 µg = 40 IU; 0.025 µg is 1 IU

Table 2: Biochemical markers in vitamin D deficiency.

Biochemical markers	Severity		
	Mild	Moderate	Severe
Serum calcium	Normal	Normal or decreased	Markedly decreased
Serum phosphorus	Decreased	Decreased	Increased or decreased
ALP	Increased	Increased	Markedly increased
PTH	Increased	Markedly increased	Markedly increased
25 (OH)D	Decreased	Markedly decreased	Markedly decreased
1,25 (OH)D3	Normal	Increased	Normal/increased
Radiography	Osteopenia	Rachitic changes 1+	Rachitic changes 2+

(ALP: alkaline phosphatase; PTH: parathyroid hormone; 25(OH)D: 25-hydroxyvitamin D; 1,25 (OH) D3: 1,25-dihydroxy vitamin D3)

Table 3: Treatment regimens for vitamin D deficiency.

Group	Daily regimen (8–12 weeks)	Weekly regimen (8–12 weeks)	Stoss therapy (oral or IM)	Maintenance
< 1 months old	1,000 IU	50,000 IU	-	400–1,000 IU
1–12 months old	1,000–5000 IU	50,000 IU	1 lakh–6 lakh units over 1–5 days (Preferably 3 lakh)	400–1,000 IU
1–18 years old	5,000 IU	50,000 IU	3–6 lakh units over 1–5 days	600–1,000 IU
>18 years old	6,000 IU	50,000 IU	3–6 lakh units over 1–5 days	1,500–2,000 IU
Obese patients, patients with malabsorption syndrome, or on medications affecting vitamin D	6,000–10,000 IU/ day			3,000–6,000 IU

* To convert (IU) to µg of calciferol divide by 40.

Monitoring Therapy

Estimation of serum calcium, phosphorus and serum alkaline phosphatase levels is recommended 1 month after initiation of therapy. Usually calcium and phosphorus levels become normal within 6-10 days whereas PTH, 25(OH)D levels normalize within 1-2 months and serum alkaline phosphatase by 3-6 months. Complete radiological healing takes longer than one month although evidence of healing is seen within 4 weeks.

RECOMMENDED DAILY VITAMIN D INTAKE

The recommended vitamin D intake is 400 IU/day in infants less than 1 year and 600 IU/day in children more than 1 year of age.

CONCLUSION

The problem of vitamin D deficiency, as a result of decreased dietary intake, decreased synthesis in the skin, lower levels of vitamin D in mothers, exclusive breastfeeding, malabsorption, liver and kidney diseases is widespread in India as elsewhere in the world. Vitamin D 25(OH)D in serum estimation is the most objective parameter for its diagnosis. All cases of vitamin D deficiency, regardless whether asymptomatic or symptomatic, warrant treatment.

> **KEY LEARNING POINTS**
>
> - Vitamin D deficiency is reported to be a global public health problem.
> - Vitamin D deficiency is caused by decreased dietary intake, decreased synthesis in the skin, lower levels of vitamin D in mothers, exclusive breastfeeding, malabsorption, liver and kidney diseases.
> - Serum estimation of the main circulating vitamin D 25(OH)D is used for defining vitamin D deficiency.
> - Treatment is required in all cases of vitamin D deficiency in both asymptomatic as well as symptomatic cases.

ACKNOWLEDGMENT

Thanks are due to Dr Ashneet Singh for help in developing the manuscript.

REFERENCES

1. Pearce SHS, Cheetham TD. Diagnosis and management of vitamin D deficiency. *BMJ* 2010;340:142-147.
2. Jackson AA (chair). *Update on vitamin D: Position statement by the scientific advisory committee on nutrition*. Scientific Advisory committee on nutrition. London 2007. Available at: http://www.sacn.gov.uk/reports/position_statements/ update_on_ vitamin_d.html Accessed on: 14 July 2017.
3. Anonymous. Primary vitamin D deficiency in adults. *Drug and Therap Bullet* 2006;44:25-30.

4. Balasubramanian S, Dhanalakshmi K, Amperayani S. Vitamin D deficiency in childhood: A review of current guidelines on diagnosis and management. *Indian Pediatr* 2013;50:669-675.
5. Holick MF, Binkley NC, Bischoff-Ferrari HA, Gordon CM, Hanley DA, Heaney RP, et al. Evaluation, treatment and prevention of vitamin D deficiency: An Endocrine Society Practice guideline. *J Clin Endocrinol Metab* 2011;96:1911-1930.
6. Lips P. Which circulating level of 25-hydroxyvitamin D is appropriate? *J Steroid Biochem Mol Biol* 2004;89-90:611-614.
7. Ross AC, Manson JE, Abrams SA, et al. The 2011 report on dietary reference intakes for calcium and vitamin D from the Institute of Medicine: What clinicians need to know? *J Clin Endocrinol Metab* 2011;96:53-58.

7 Vitamin D Deficiency Rickets and Other Rickets

Suraj Gupte, Waheeda Shaik, EW Kawasaki

ABSTRACT

Though vitamin D deficiency is the most common and the most important cause of rickets, it is not the only cause of rickets. A number of other conditions may contribute to or be responsible for similar clinical picture. Besides vitamin D deficiency secondary to such disorders as malabsorption syndrome, it may be caused by calcium and phosphate deficiencies. Further, vitamin D dependent and resistant rickets occur though infrequently. Treatment varies with the etiologic diagnosis. Standard treatment for vitamin D deficiency does not work for other rickets where attention to the fundamental defect becomes important, e.g. malabsorption, chronic liver disease, kidney disease, rickets secondary to some tumors, etc. In general, vitamin D resistant rickets needs very high doses of vitamin D. In familial hypophosphatemic rickets, therapy with phosphates in the form of disodium hydrogen phosphate 13.6 g and phosphoric acid 5.9 g/day is required. In place of vitamin D, 1,25(OH)2 vitamin D in a dose of 1 µg/day may be employed for better outcome. In case of vitamin D dependent rickets, the recommended dose of vitamin D is 10,000–50,000 units/day. Alternatively, 1,25 dihydroxyvitamin D_3, 0.5–2.0 µg/day may be employed for vitamin D-dependent rickets (type 1). Rickets accompanying chronic anticonvulsant therapy may be prevented by ensuring adequate dietary intake of calcium and an extra 500–1,000 IU of vitamin D_3 each day.

Keywords: Calcium, Familial rickets, Hypophosphatemic rickets, Rickets, Vitamin D deficiency rickets, Vitamin D-dependent rickets, Vitamin D-resistant rickets.

INTRODUCTION

Vitamin D, a secondary steroid, plays an important role in calcium and phosphorus homeostasis. It is a precursor of 1, 25-dihydroxyvitamin D_3, a hormone synthesized and secreted by kidneys under the control of parathormone and tissue phosphate levels.

The ultraviolet rays of the sunlight are responsible for converting the 7-dehydrocholesterol that is normally present under the skin, into vitamin D_3 or cholecalciferol. The latter is further converted to 25-hydroxycholecalciferol and 25-hydroxyergocalciferol in the liver. The last two forms are essential for maintenance of adequate calcium and phosphorus concentration in the extracellular fluid and for the formation of bone matrix. It is now established that 25-hydroxycholecalciferol is then converted to 1, 25-dihydroxycholecalciferol. The latter is specifically helpful in promoting synthesis of **calcium transport protein** in the intestinal wall.

Maintenance of blood level of 25-hydroxyvitamin D more than 20 ng/mL is important for maximum health benefits. In short, vitamin D has both skeletal (calcitropic) as well as extraskeletal (pleiotropic) role. Extraskeletal benefits are reportedly as anti-infective, in respiratory disease, immunological disease and malignancies, etc.

Sources of vitamin D include sunshine (90%) and diet (10%), fish, fish oils, egg (yolk), milk, infant formulas and supplements such as cereals and margarine (butter-like product made of vegetable oils).

Current recommendation is 400 IU of vitamin D per day for all infants, children and adolescents. This is essential to maintain a vitamin D blood level of 20 ng/mL. With the earlier recommendation of just 200 IU, this level is not maintained.

Vitamin D deficiency may produce and/or be associated with rickets and osteoporosis. *Extraskeletal manifestations include* susceptibility to infections, muscle pains and weakness, seizures, asthma, malignancies, type II diabetes, hypertension and obesity.

Vitamin D deficiency rickets continues to be rampant in resource-limited countries, including those with enough of sunshine with its re-emergence even in the western countries. [1-7]

VITAMIN D DEFICIENCY RICKETS (NUTRITIONAL RICKETS)

Classically, vitamin D deficiency predominantly causes defect of bones, i.e. rickets in growing infants and children before closure of epiphysis. Osteomalacia is characterized by spongy trabecular bones also resulting from demineralization as a consequence of vitamin D deficiency, but after the closure of epiphysis, i.e. in adults.[8]

Etiologic Considerations

Vitamin D deficiency may result from several conditions (Box 1).

Box 1: Causes of vitamin D deficiency.

- Decreased synthesis by skin (especially dark complexion)
- Decreased nutritional intake
- Prematurity and VLBW
- Decreased maternal stores
- Formula-fed infants
- Malabsorption
- Chronic liver disease—decreased synthesis
- Chronic renal disease
- Drug-induced—antiepileptics, rifampicin, INH
- Tumors

(VLBW: very low birth weight; INH: isonicotinyl hydrazide)

Despite such a lot of sunshine, its incidence continues to be high in India and other resource-limited countries. This appears to be due to poor dietary intake of vitamin D and also due to poor exposure to sunlight. The latter seems to be related to the widely-prevalent practice of covering the infants with loads of clothes and from living in slums and crowded places. Poor exposure to sunlight may also be related to the inactivity of the malnourished children.

Disturbed metabolism and poor synthesis of vitamin D from the skin, malabsorption state, diarrheal disease and excessive phytate with low calcium and low phosphate content of the diet may well be other causes of rickets in malnourished children.

Our repeated observations of development of rickets in later age-group too, suboptimal intake of calcium and more gratifying response to a combination of vitamin D and calcium than to vitamin D alone in India strongly indicate that both vitamin D and calcium (and perhaps phosphate too) deficiency contribute to the continuing high incidence of nutritional rickets in India and other developing countries.

Obviously, the problem of calcium deficiency (perhaps, in association with phosphate deficiency), in addition to vitamin D deficiency, in etiology of rickets in developing countries needs greater consideration. The preventive as well as therapeutic implications of this observation are vital.

Predisposing factors for early onset of rickets include:
- Prematurity and low birth weight (LBW)
- Maternal vitamin D deficiency, especially osteomalacia.

Prevalence

Conservatively speaking, vitamin D deficiency rickets should be the problem of temperate climate. It had more or less disappeared from the wester, except in migrant dark-skinned population, in bed-ridden institutionalized children and in areas where milk supply is not fortified with vitamin D. This was ascribed to health education, enrichment of milk with vitamin D, wide use of vitamin D concentrates, and better standard of living and better health and medical care. However, in recent decades it has resurfaced in the Western countries.

The problem of rickets in India is much greater than its extent suggested by the descriptions in various texts. Congenital rickets is a rare entity occurring in neonates of mothers suffering from osteomalacia. However, rickets of premature and very low birth weight (VLBW) infants is frequent.

Clinical Features

Classically, rickets is a disease of rapidly growing period. The peak incidence is encountered in the age group 6 months to 2 years. It is uncommon in infants under 3 months of age, except in premature and/or VLBW infants (rickets of prematurity) and infants of mothers suffering from osteomalacia during pregnancy (congenital rickets). To less extent, rickets may be encountered in toddlers and adolescents as well.

The **earliest manifestations** are quite vague and nonspecific. These include profuse sweating over the forehead (more so during sleep) even in wintery months, irritability and restlessness. The earliest sign is craniotabes.

Head

Bossing [frontal (Fig. 1) and parietal], macrocephaly with flattening of vertex (box head, caput quadratum or hot-cross-bun*), increased size and delayed closure of fontanels (including posterior fontanel), craniotabes [a peculiar softening of occipital and posterior parietal bones which give in like a ping-pong (table-tennis) ball under pressure from thumb]; wide open cranial sutures.

Teeth

Delayed dentition.

Thorax

Rachitic rosary (smooth rounded, nontender costochondral beading as seen in Figure 2), **pigeon-chest deformity** *(pectus carinatum)*, funnel chest deformity (Fig. 3), **Harrison sulcus** or groove which is a depression along the insertion of diaphragm into the ribs, flaring of lower ribs. **Violin-shaped** deformed chest is characteristic.

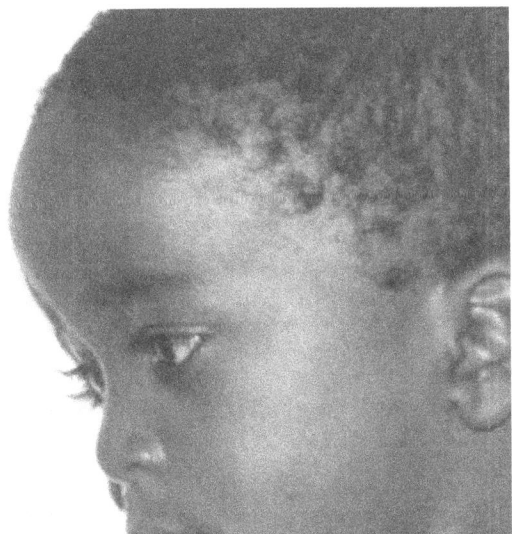

Fig. 1: Bossing of forehead.

---

* Hot-cross-bun may also be seen in chronic hemolytic anemia's, chronic iron-deficiency anemia, congenital (cyanotic) heart disease and skeletal dysplasia. At times, no cause may be forthcoming.

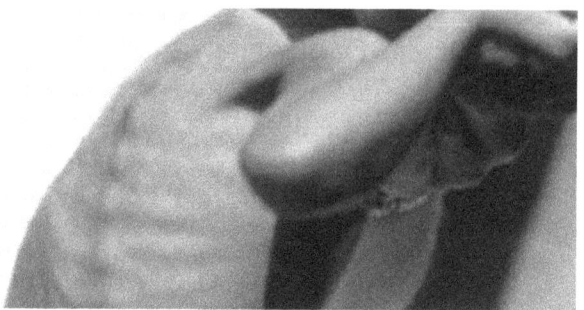

Fig. 2: Rachitic rosary.

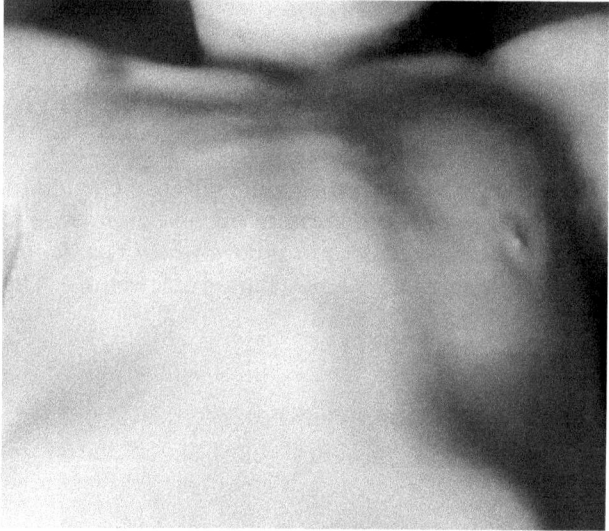

Fig. 3: Pigeon chest deformity (Pectus carinatum). Note the forward protrusion of the sternum.

Infrequently, sternum is unusually depressed, the so-called **pectus excavatum** (Fig. 4). A concavity at inferior angle of scapula may be detected.

Spine

Scoliosis, kyphosis; infrequently lordosis. Severe deformity of the spine may end up with disproportionate short stature of short trunk type.

Extremities

Widening of wrists, ankles (with **double malleoli***) and other epiphyses due to expansion and cupping of growing ends of bones; **genu valgum**

---

* Above the normal medial mallolus, there is appearance of another prominence from widened epiphysis. This may be seen, but is more often felt on palpation. It is termed **Marfan sign**.

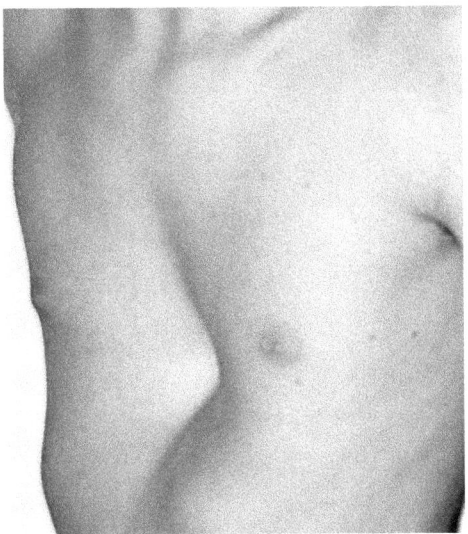

Fig. 4: Funnel-chest deformity (pectus excavatum) in a child with advanced rickets. This deformity is most often familial than because of rickets. In rickets, chest deformity is usually pigeon chest (pectus carinatum) rather than pectus excavatum.

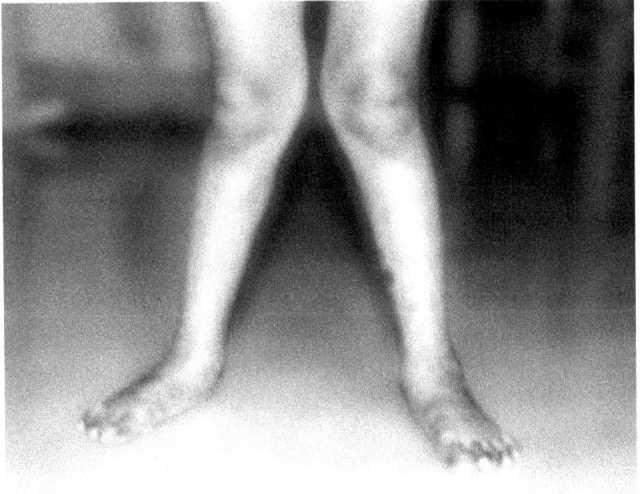

Fig. 5: Genu valgum.

*(knock-knees)*** in older children (Fig. 5) or **_genu varum (bow leg_**s usually anterolateral with the level of bend at junction of middle and lower one-third) in toddlers (Fig. 6); enhanced tendency for green-stick fractures and bending with deformities.

** Intermalleoli distance more than 0 cm.

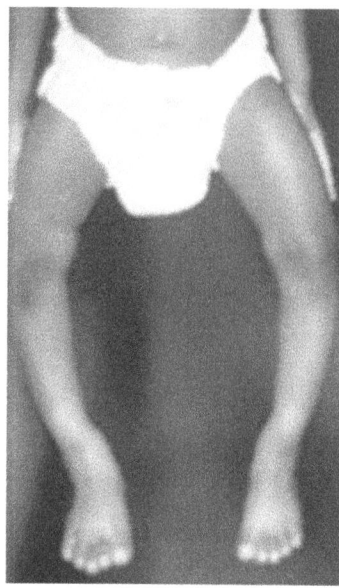

Fig. 6: Genu varus.

Miscellaneous

- As a result of poor muscle tone (more so in the proximal ones) and relaxation of ligaments, the child may have growth failure, delayed milestones, flat feet, and pot-belly.
- Some degree of **visceroptosis** pushes the liver and spleen downward so that these become palpable without having been enlarged. In such a case scenario, though liver may be considerably palpable below right costal margin, its span remains normal. The upper border comes to lay a space or two below the normal level. At times, laxity of ligaments may be of such a magnitude that the limbs can be bent into any position. **Acrobatic rickets** is the name given to this condition.
- **Constipation** is often present and is supposed to be secondary to poor muscle tone.
- Rarely, **tetany** may accompany rickets due to reduced level of ionized calcium in plasma. Even seizures may occur in early infancy. Tetany and seizure suggest a defective vitamin D metabolism defect.
- Inadequate mineralization of the collagen renders long bones vulnerable to *fractures* (green stick in infants and toddlers) and **deformities**.
- Dental caries may be seen in some cases of rickets. **Bony tenderness** may be present in some children. If rickets is not adequately treated in time, bone deformities may be left as scar the so-called **old rickets**.
- **Short stature** may also follow. Short stature secondary to rickets is usually disproportionate. Both **short limb** and **short trunk** can occur

depending on the predominance of deformities occurring in legs or spine.

Differential Diagnosis
- *Physiological bowing of the legs* seen in some healthy toddlers due to normal deposition of adipose tissue over the lateral aspects is not accompanied by other signs of rickets and disappears in due course of time without any treatment.
- *Physiological knock-knee* as a result of slight valgus position of the feet may also need differentiation from rickets which is likely to have other rickets related signs.
- *Scurvy* manifesting with costochondral beading may cause confusion with similar-looking beading in rickets. Classically, beading in rickets is smooth, rounded and nontender. On the contrary, beading in scurvy is sharp, angular and tender since the problem pertains to collagen rather than mineralization. Some evidence of bleeding is invariably present in scurvy.
- *Child abuse and neglect (CAN)* with fractures may sometime be confused with fractures caused in rickets. A detailed history, physical examination and investigations assist in differentiating the two.
- *Fluorosis* is endemic in some parts of India. In children, it may present with clinical features that resemble rickets. Differentiating features which are characteristic of fluorosis such as dental mottling, osteosclerosis and calcification of ligaments and known background of high fluoride water levels in water of the area assist in arriving at correct diagnosis.
- *Metaphyseal dysplasia* may present with bow legs, waddling gait, short stature and even rickets-like radiological findings.
  Remaining differentials include:
  - Renal rickets
  - Hepatic rickets
  - Malabsorptive rickets
  - Drug-induced rickets
  - Oncogenous rickets
  - Vitamin D-dependent rickets
  - Familial hypophosphatemic rickets.

  Salient features of these disorders are described later in this very chapter.

Diagnosis
Biochemical
Biochemical findings include raised alkaline phosphatase (except in malnourished children in whom this may well be normal), usually normal or somewhat low serum calcium and reduced phosphorus.[9]

Today, reduction in the serum 25-hydroxyvitamin D level (<10 µg/mL) is considered a sensitive and reliable index of rickets even in malnourished children. This is the only way to diagnose subclinical vitamin D deficiency.

Radiological

X-ray findings are best seen at the wrist, i.e. lower ends of radius and ulna (Figs. 7 and 8). These include:[10]

- *Cupping (saucer-like concave depression):* The osteoid (matrix minus mineralization), being radiotranslucent is not seen. In fact the space normally occupied by mineralized matrix is empty.
- *Flaring/splaying (widening):* Everted (out-turned) edges.

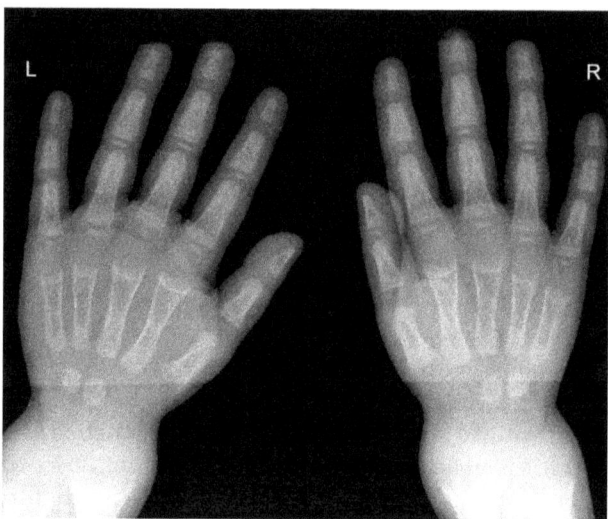

Fig. 7: X-ray changes at wrist in rickets. Note the flaring, fraying and cupping at the metaphysis of ulna and radius.

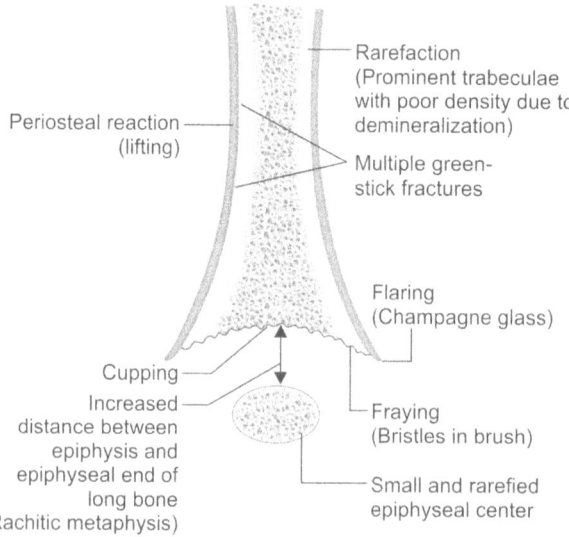

Fig. 8: Rickets. Diagrammatic representation of radiologic picture of radius in vitamin D deficiency rickets.

- *Fraying (rarefaction):* Irregular tooth brush-like margin (bottom of the cup).
- Additionally:
  - There is an increase in the distance between the epiphyseal center and metaphysis of long bones due to radiotranslucency of the osteoid
  - Epiphyseal centers have unclear margins
  - Periosteal reaction in the form of double shadow of outer contour
  - Prominence of trabeculae though the shaft shows rarefaction
  - Green-stick fractures
  - Bending and deformities.

  Overall, long bones have the ***champagne glass*** appearance.

Treatment

Specific Treatment

Stoss therapy consists of administering a single massive dose of vitamin D_3 (3,00,000 units up to 1 year of age; 6,00,000 units for later ages) orally or intramuscularly together with supplementary calcium and phosphorus.

Though serum alkaline phosphatase and phosphorus tend to return to normal within just 5 days, initiation of radiological evidence in the form of appearance of a linear shadow of provisional zone of calcification in 10–14 days with further healing (this zone fusing with the metaphysic as osteoid gets calcified) by 3–4 weeks. Thus, radiologic evidence of healing (say at wrist) is in the form of:

- Appearance of provisional zone of calcification
- Mineralization of *fraying* at the epiphyseal end
- Recalcification of osteoid
- Disappearance of the cupping, fraying and flaring/splaying with adequate mineralization.

In order to achieve real consolidation of cure, it may be desirable to give an additional massive dose of vitamin D after 3–4 weeks. All along, supplements of calcium (100 mg/kg) and phosphorus need to be given. Alternatively, the child may be treated with:

- 60,000 units of vitamin D_3 daily orally for 10 days
- 20,000 units of vitamin D_3 daily orally for 30 days.

Surgical Intervention

Gross orthopedic deformities, especially in adolescents, may occasionally need surgical correction (say osteotomy).

Prognosis

As a rule, response to pharmacotherapy is gratifying. However, in an occasional child, a poor response to adequate doses of vitamin D_3 may be encountered. In such a case scenario, probability of refractory or resistant rickets should be considered and the child investigated for the following conditions:

- Malabsorption state, e.g. celiac disease, endemic tropical sprue, cystic fibrosis
- Renal rickets—chronic renal disease and renal tubular acidosis (Fanconi syndrome, and Lowe syndrome)
- Prolonged anticonvulsant therapy
- Chronic liver disease, etc.
- Magnesium deficiency
- Hereditary vitamin D dependent rickets
- Familial hypophosphatemic rickets
- Oncogenous rickets.

Prevention

Availability of at least 400 IU (not 200 as was believed earlier) of vitamin D through sunshine, diet or supplements must be ensured. Now it is a standard practice to supplement all infants in the first year of life with 400 IU of vitamin D. Health education to parents against overclothing the infants and young children and proper housing is important.

Long-Term Complications (Sequelae)

Most infants and children with vitamin D deficiency rickets recover fully following timely and adequate therapy. Delayed treatment may fail to prevent sequelae which are:
- Skeletal deformities
- Fractures
- Slipped femoral epiphysis
- Short stature (disproportionate; short trunk or short limb).

OTHER TYPES OF RICKETS

(Rickets other than Vitamin D Deficiency Rickets)

Rickets of Prematurity
(Metabolic Bone Disease of Premature Infants)

Significant mineralization of fetal bones occurs in the last trimester of pregnancy. The premature infant, therefore, considerably loses that opportunity. He stands high chances of developing osteopenia and rickets. Use of frusemide and steroids enhances vulnerability to these problems.

Manifestations include poor growth, frontal bossing, craniotabes, costochondral beading, and epiphyseal widening (most prominent at wrist). Response to vitamin D plus calcium and phosphorus is gratifying with appearance of healing line in the X-ray of wrist in 3–4 weeks.

Malabsorptive Rickets (Celiac Rickets)

All major malabsorptive states such as celiac disease, tropical sprue and cystic fibrosis may have rickets associated with them because of poor absorption of vitamin D and minerals.

Drug-induced Rickets

Prolonged therapy with antiepileptic drugs (AEDs)/anticonvulsant drugs like phenobarbital, phenytoin, carbamazepine, valproate and lamotrigine increase vitamin D metabolism and enhance vulnerability to development of rickets. The mechanism involved is induction of hepatic cytochrome P-450 enzyme which converts $25(OH)D_3$ to inactive (polar) vitamin D_3. Anticancer drug, imatinib, and drugs such as outdated tetracyclines may also contribute to development of rickets.

Hepatic Rickets

Children with chronic liver disease such as neonatal cholestasis (say congenital biliary atresia, neonatal hepatitis, chronic hepatitis, cirrhosis) are vulnerable to development of rickets in due course due to decreased intestinal absorption of vitamin D and decreased hydroxylation by liver.

Hereditary Vitamin D-dependent Rickets (Pseudodeficiency Rickets)[12-14]

It is an autosomal recessive disorder involving deficiency of $\alpha\text{-}25(OH)_2D_3$. It is characterized by severe rickets which develop in early infancy (at 3-6 months of age) in spite of adequate vitamin D supplements. It fails to respond to vitamin D therapy up to 4,000 units/day. However, response to long-term massive doses of vitamin D_3 or, still better, to oral therapy with α-hydroxyvitamin D_3 is gratifying.

- *Type I* has enzyme 25-hydroxyvitamin D_1 α-hydroxylase deficiency.
    - *Clinical features*, over and above those of vitamin D deficiency rickets, include hypocalcemic tetany or seizures, anemia, and, at times, respiratory difficulty.
    - *Investigations* show similar findings as in vitamin D deficiency rickets plus very low blood levels of $1,25(OH)D_3$ with normal $25(OH)D_3$.
    - *Treatment* is with α-calcidiol or calcitriol, 1-2 μg/day, preferably along with calcium and phosphate supplements. Within 6-8 weeks, radiologic healing occurs.
- *Type II* is characterized by end-organ resistance to $1,25(OH)_2D_3$ which in spite of high level, becomes redundant in action.
    - *Clinical profile* is characterized by early onset of rickets together with alopecia and ectodermal defects such as milia, epidermal cysts and oligodontia.

- *Investigations* show low blood calcium, secondary hyperparathyroidism and high $1,25(DH)_2D_3$.
- *Treatment* is problematic with poor response to vitamin D analog. Long-term therapy with calcium (oral or IV) may prove beneficial.

Refractory Rickets (Resistant Rickets)[15]

The term, *refractory rickets*, refers to rickets that is resistant to the usually recommended therapeutic doses of vitamin D.

Rickets complicating renal disease, familial hypophosphatemic rickets, oncogenous rickets and magnesium-dependent rickets fall under this broad umbrella. However, some authorities consider vitamin D-dependent rickets, malabsorptive rickets, hepatic rickets and drug-induced rickets too belonging to this category.

Renal Rickets

Rickets may complicate renal disease, e.g.:
- **Chronic kidney disease:** Tubulointerstitial disease with glomerular filtration rate (GFR) less than 30–35 mL/min/1.73 m² may eventually land up with florid rickets. Laboratory tests show high blood creatinine, phosphate and parathormone.
  Treatment is in the form of:
    - Restricting intake of phosphate
    - Supplements of calcium and vitamin D analog.
- In **renal osteodystrophy**, kidneys fail to form $1,25\ (OH)_2D_3$. It is characterized by bone mineralization deficiency, that is a direct result of the electrolyte and endocrine derangements that accompany chronic kidney disease. Renal osteodystrophy can be further divided into metabolic states associated with either high or low bone turnover.
- *Renal tubular acidosis (RTA):* An important cause of refractory rickets, RTA is characterized by hyperchloremic metabolic acidosis, often in association with aminoaciduria, reduced blood phosphate level and low molecular weight proteinuria. Blood urea and creatinine levels remain normal.
- *Fanconi syndrome (cystinosis):* In this condition, cysteine crystals are found throughout the reticuloendothelial system. Renal tubular defects include glycosuria, aminoaciduria, tubular acidosis, phosphaturia, potassium loss, and, at times, uricosuria and sodium loss. Rickets associated with this condition needs heavy doses of vitamin D (50,000–300,000 units/day) for healing.
- *Lowe syndrome:* This condition presenting very early in life (first few months) is known for severe rickets. Additional features include motor and cognitive retardation, hypotonia, congenital glaucoma (buphthalmos) and other ocular defects and seizures. Death usually occurs in early childhood from progressive kidney injury secondary to glomerulosclerosis.

Familial Hypophosphatemic Rickets[10]

This type of refractory rickets has X-linked dominance with variable penetrance. Rarely, autosomal recessive inheritance may be encountered. Sporadic cases are also seen.

- *Pathophysiology:* The fundamental pathological defect revolves around poor tubular reabsorption of phosphate. Blood phosphate levels are low. Yet, blood levels of $1,25(OH)_2D_3$, rather than being high, are low.
- *Clinical features:* Manifestations include short stature, bow legs/knock-knee, coxa vara, craniosynostosis and dental abnormalities with abscesses. Notably, hypocalcemic tetany is absent. The patient's mother is usually short statured with genu varum and fasting hypophosphatemia.
- *Specific laboratory findings:* These include very low blood levels of $1,25(OH)_2D_3$ and high urinary phosphate excretion with low tubular reabsorption of phosphate.
- *Therapy:* It comprises of oral phosphate, 30–50 mg/kg in 5–6 divided doses. The so-called *Joulie's solution* provides 30.4 mg/mL phosphaste. With this dosage, serum phosphate blood level of 3–3.2 mg/dL is achieved. This level is mandatory for optimal outcome.

Along with oral phosphate, vitamin D supplements should be provided. A recommended regimen is alfacalcidol, 25–50 ng/kg/day.

Oncogenous Rickets (Oncogenic Rickets, Tumor-related Rickets)

Tumor-induced rickets is a syndrome characterized by hypophosphatemia, renal phosphate wasting, and decreased serum $1,25(HO)_2D_3$ levels. The tumors secrete a fibroblast growth factor which is phosphaturic and causes total body phosphate depletion, leading to rickets (osteomalacia in adults).

Usually these tumors are benign and of small size. Their diagnosis and localization is often difficult. Whole body magnetic resonance imaging (MRI) may prove useful for their detection.

Resection of the causative tumor leads to gratifying outcome with reversal of the biochemical, radiological and clinical abnormalities. Neurofibromatosis (von Recklinghausen disease), epidermal nevus syndrome, and linear nevus syndrome are examples of such tumors. Occasionally, mesenchymal malignant tumors, such as osteosarcoma and fibrosarcoma may also cause oncogenous rickets.

Magnesium-dependent Resistant Rickets

Occasionally, rickets associated with hypomagnesemia may occur. In them, response to treatment with massive doses of vitamin D fails. However, they show an excellent response to oral magnesium-chloride supplementation. It has been suggested that serum-magnesium levels should be determined in all cases of rickets in those who are resistant to vitamin D therapy.

Broad etiologic classification of dependent rickets is given in Box 2.

Box 2: Broad etiologic classification of vitamin D dependent rickets.

Type I rickets
• **Vitamin D deficiency:** Poor consumption, malabsorption states, poor exposure to sunlight. • **Disturbed vitamin D metabolism from liver disease:** Poor formation of 25(OH) vitamin D_3, degradation of vitamin D_3 to 25(OH)D-26, 23-lactone (chronic anticonvulsant therapy causing stimulation of microsomal enzyme in liver) • **Disturbed vitamin D metabolism from renal disease:**[12-14] Enzyme, 1-hydroxylase, deficiency in tubules interferes with conversion of 25(OH) vitamin D to 1,25(OH)$_2$ vitamin D_3. This is termed **vitamin D-dependent rickets (type I)**. Failure of target cells to form 1,25(OH)$_2$ vitamin D. This is termed **vitamin D-dependent rickets (type II)**. Failure of kidney to form 1,25(OH)$_3$ vitamin D_3. This is termed **renal dystrophy**
Type II rickets
• Poor intake or absorption of phosphates • **Defective reabsorption of phosphates by the renal tubules:** Fanconi syndrome, familial hypophosphatemic vitamin D refractory rickets, isolated phosphaturia, renal tubular acidosis, rickets, oncogenous tumors (oncogenic rickets) as in von Reckinghausen disease, epidermal nevus syndrome or linear nevus syndrome

Table 1 presents the clinical clues to diagnosis of refractory rickets.

Table 1: Clues to diagnosis of refractory rickets.[8,15,16]

Clue	Diagnosis
Clinical	
Familial	Familial hypophosphatemic vitamin D refracting rickets, 1-hydroxylase deficiency, vitamin D-dependent rickets, renal tubular acidosis (distal)
Manifesting before 6 months of age	Familial conditions like Fanconi syndrome, cystinosis, 1-hydroxylase deficiency
Manifesting after 6 months of age but before 12 months	X-linked dominant vitamin D refractory rickets
Manifesting in early childhood	Renal tubular acidosis
Manifesting in late childhood	Renal osteodystrophy, glycine phosphaturia
Gross muscle weakness	Renal tubular acidosis, glycine phosphaturia
Renal/ureteric colic	Renal stone, renal tubular acidosis
Nausea, vomiting, lethargy	Renal osteodystrophy, renal tubular acidosis, hypophosphatasia
Mental deficieny, buphthalmos	Lowe syndrome
Highly pigmented skin, cystine crystals in cornea on slit lamp examination	Cystinosis
Sutural diastais, short ribs, cutaneous dimples, hypotonia, failure to thrive	Hypophosphatasia
Laboratory investigations	
Low phosphate with amino aciduria	Vitamin D deficiency secondary to malabsorption, liver disease, chronic anticonvulsant therapy
Low phosphate without aminoaciduria, isolated phosphaturia, normal pH	Familial hypophosphatemic vitamin D refractory rickets, oncogenic tumors
Low pH	Renal tubular acidosis
High phosphate	Renal osteodystrophy

CONCLUSION

Vitamin D deficiency continues to contribute to bone-related as well as extra-skeletal illnesses in children. Bone-related problems are concentrated around vitamin D deficiency rickets and osteoporosis. Extraskeletal manifestations include susceptibility to infections, muscle weakness and pains, seizures, asthma, malignancies, type II diabetes, hypertension and obesity. Etiologic factors include decreased synthesis by skin, decreased nutritional intake, prematurity and VLBW, decreased maternal stores, formula-fed infants, malabsorption, chronic liver disease (decreased synthesis), chronic renal disease, medication (antiepileptics, rifampicin, INH), tumors, etc. Apart from vitamin D deficiency, calcium and phosphorus deficiency may too contribute to development of rickets. Of the various therapeutic modalities, Soto's massive dose vitamin D regimen is the most accepted and popular treatment. In rickets secondary to such conditions as malabsorption, antiepileptic drugs, tumors, etc. amelioration of the primary condition in addition to vitamin D is warranted. Vitamin D resistant and dependent rickets need much higher doses of vitamin D plus additional measures.

> **KEY LEARNING POINTS**
>
> - Vitamin D deficiency results from decreased synthesis by skin (as in dark complexion), decreased nutritional intake, prematurity/VLBW, decreased maternal stores, breast feeding, vitamin D-free formula-feeding, malabsorption, chronic liver disease (decreased synthesis), chronic renal disease, medication (antiepileptics, rifampicin, INH), tumors, etc.
> - Rickets is the most important manifestation of vitamin D deficiency in children, the others being susceptibility to infections, muscle weakness, pains and weakness, seizures, asthma, malignancies, type II diabetes, hypertension and obesity.
> - A number of other conditions (calcium/phosphate deficiency, genetic enzyme deficiency) may contribute to or be responsible for similar clinical picture.
> - Whereas Soto's massive dose vitamin D regimen is the most accepted and popular treatment for vitamin D deficiency rickets, additionally amelioration of the causative condition, e.g. malabsorption, chronic liver disease, kidney disease, rickets secondary to some tumors, etc. becomes important.
> - In general, vitamin D resistant rickets needs far higher doses of vitamin D.
> - In familial hypophosphatemic rickets, therapy with phosphates in the form of disodium hydrogen phosphate 13.6 g and phosphoric acid 5.9 g/day is required. In place of vitamin D, $1,25(OH)_2$ vitamin D in a dose of 1 μg/day may be employed for better outcome.
> - In case of vitamin D-dependent rickets, the recommended dose of vitamin D is 10,000–50,000 units/day. Alternatively, 1,25 dihydroxyvitamin D_3, 0.5–2.0 μg/day may be employed in type 1.

REFERENCES

1. Creo AL, Thacher TD, Pettifor J, et al. Nutritional rickets around the world: An update. *Pediatr Int Child Health* 2016; 37: 84-98.

2. Wheeler BJ, Dickson NP, Houghton LA, et al. Incidence and characteristics of vitamin D deficiency rickets in New Zealand children: A New Zealand Pediatric Surveillance Unit study. *Aust N- Z J Public Health* 2015;39:380-383.
3. Bener A, Hoffmann G. Nutritional rickets among children in a sun rich country. *Int. J. Pediatr. Endocrinol* 2010, 410502 Available at: https://www.ncbi.nlm.nih.gov/pmc/articles/PMC2965426/ Accessed on: 20 January 2018.
4. Prentice A. Nutritional rickets around the world. *J. Steroid Biochem. Mol Biol* 2013; 136: 201-206.
5. Thacher TD. Increasing incidence of nutritional rickets: a population-based study in Olmsted County. *Minnesota. Mayo Clin. Proc* 2013;88:176-183.
6. Uush T. Prevalence of classic signs and symptoms of rickets and vitamin D deficiency in Mongolian children and women. *J. Steroid Biochem Mol Biol* 2013;136: 207-210.
7. Munns CF. Global consensus recommendations on prevention and management of nutritional rickets. *J Clin Endocrinol Metab* 2016;101:394-415.
8. Gupte S. Vitamins. In: Gupte S (Ed): *The Short Textbook of Pediatrics*, 12th edn. New Delhi: Jaypee 2016.
9. Mersch J. Rickets (Calcium, Phosphate, or Vitamin D Deficiency). Available at: https://www.medicinenet.com/rickets/article.htm Accessed on: 23 January 2018.
10. Shore RM, Chesney RW. Rickets: Part I. *Pediatr Radiol* 2012;43:140-151.
11. Linglart A, Biosse-Duplan M, Briot K. Therapeutic management of hypophosphatemic rickets from infancy to adulthood. Available at: http://www.endocrineconnections.com/content/3/1/R13.full Accessed on: 18 January 2018.
12. Takeda E, Yamamoto H, Taketani Y, Miyamoto K. Vitamin D-dependent rickets type I and type II. *Acta Paediatr Jpn* 1997;39:508-513.
13. Takeda E1, Yamamoto H, Taketani Y, Miyamoto K. Vitamin D-dependent rickets type I and type II. Available at: https://www.ncbi.nlm.nih.gov/pubmed/9316302 Accessed on: 20 January 2018.
14. Choudhury S, Jebasingh K F, Ranabir S, Singh T. Familial vitamin D resistant rickets: End-organ resistance to 1,25-dihydroxyvitamin D. *Indian J Endocr Metab* [serial online] 2013 Available at: http://www.ijem.in/text.asp?2013/17/7/224/119579 Accessed on 30 March 2018.
15. Litman NN, Ulstrom RB. Westin WW. Vitamin D resistant rickets. *Calif Med* 1957;86: 248-53.
16. Garabedian M. Vitamin D resistant rickets. Available at: https://www.medicinenet.com/rickets/article.htm Accessed on: 20 January 2018.

PART 3: MINERALS

8 Micronutrients and Macrominerals

Novy Gupte, Suraj Gupte, Utpal Kant Singh

ABSTRACT

The term, micronutrients (trace elements, minor minerals), denotes substances which are needed by the body in minute quantities. Micronutrients include vitamins. These are considered the "magic wands" because of their ability to produce enzymes, hormones and other substances essential for proper growth and development. The consequences of their deficiency are critical. Of all micronutrients, deficiency of iron, iodine and vitamin A, most important in global public health terms, represents a major threat to the health and development of child populations in particular in resource-limited countries.

The term, trace elements (microminerals), is by and large synonymous with micronutrients. Minerals are naturally occurring, homogeneous, inorganic substances required by humans in amounts of 100 mg/day or more. Minor minerals are iron, zinc, copper, chromium, cobalt, iodine, fluorine, manganese and selenium, etc. Major or macro minerals include sodium, potassium, calcium, phosphorous and magnesium.

Keywords: Arsenic, Calcium, Iodine, Iron, Macrominerals, Magnesium, Microminerals, Micronutrients, Molybdenum, Potassium, Silicone, Trace elements, Vandium, Zinc.

INTRODUCTION

Micronutrients, also termed trace elements or microminerals, are needed only in minuscule amounts, i.e. μg or mg/day rather than g/day to perform various physiologic functions.[1-5]

Notably, less than 0.01% of human body is formed by them.

These are considered the "magic wands" because of their ability to produce enzymes, hormones and other substances essential for proper growth and development. The consequences of their deficiency are critical.

Of all micronutrients, deficiency of iron, iodine and vitamin A, most important in global public health terms, represents a major threat to the health and development of child populations particularly in resource-limited countries.[6-9]

The term, trace elements (microminerals), is by and large synonymous with micronutrients.

Minerals are naturally occurring, homogeneous, inorganic substances required by humans in amounts of 100 mg/day or more. Minor minerals (same as micronutrients) are iron, zinc, copper, chromium, cobalt, iodine, fluorine, manganese and selenium, etc. Macrominerals include sodium, potassium, calcium, phosphorous and magnesium. Vitamins fall under the umbrella of micronutrients.

The so-called "rainbow revolution"[4] aims at promoting consumption of green, yellow, orange, red (GYOR) vegetables and fruits which are rich sources of micronutrients through intensified campaign.

MICRONUTRIENTS

Iron

Human body contains just 3-4 g iron: 75% in hemoglobin, 20% in stores and 5% in myoglobin. Storage as ferritin and hemosiderin is in bone marrow, liver and spleen.

- *Functions:* Hemoglobin formation, normal growth and maintenance of normal immune function. Iron-protein complex in muscle comes in handy in time of need.
  Cellular iron is involved in respiratory chains of mitochondria for cellular metabolism. It is critical in brain development.
- *Dietary sources:* Green leafy vegetables (amaranth richest around 30 g/100 g)*, pulses, beans, dried fruits, nuts, cereals, molasses; meat, egg yolk and fish. Milk is a poor source of iron, providing just 0.2 mg/dL.
- *Daily requirements (10-20 mg/day):* Preterm and low birth weight (LBW) infants require 1.5-2 mg/kg for the whole first year.

Deficiency

Iron deficiency, a major nutritional problem, exists in two forms:
1. Iron deficiency anemia (IDA) with overt manifestations such as pallor (Fig. 1), poor growth and development, reduced learning capacity, cognitive function and work capacity.
2. Iron-deficient stores which sooner or later end up as IDA.

Preterm and LBW infants are at high risk of developing iron deficiency since iron requirement is enhanced on account of rapid postnatal growth.

Excess

Accidental ingestion in excess may cause severe stomatitis and gastritis. Excess supplementation predisposes to risk of infection and hinder absorption and metabolism of other micronutrients.

---

* Spinach, believed to be very rich in iron, provides only 1.14 mg% iron against amaranth 22.9%, mustard leaves 16.3% and mint 15.6%.

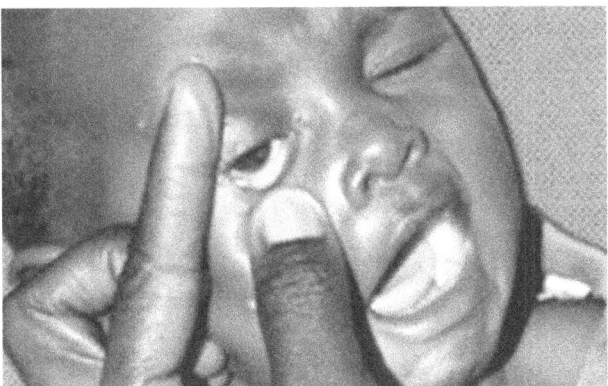

Fig. 1: Iron-deficiency anemia. Note severe pallor of palpebral conjunctiva. Over and above protein-energy malnutrition, the child had multiple vitamin deficiency signs and heart failure.

Chronic overload occurs in thalassemia major with multiple blood transfusions, leading to iron deposits in viscera, especially liver, pancreas, heart, skin and pituitary gland, the so-called *hemosiderosis* and *hemochro-matosis*. Iron-chelating agents (e.g. desferrioxamine) may be used in such situations.

For more details about IDA, *See* Chapter 9 (Iron Deficiency Anemia).

Iodine

Iodine is essential for production of thyroid hormones, i.e. triodothyroxine (T_3) and thyroxine (T_4).

- *Functions:*
  - Synthesis of thyroid hormones which eventually influence the physical and mental growth and development.
  - Regulation of metabolism of nutrients of the body.
  - Regulation of functioning of nerves and muscles.
- *Sources:* Water, iodized salt, seafoods, fresh-water and fish.
- *Daily requirement:* 90–150 mg/day depending on age.
  - Less than 6 year: 90 mg,
  - 6–12 years: 120 mg,
  - 12 years: 150 mg.

Requirement in pregnant and lactating mothers is enhanced, i.e. 200–250 mg daily. Most of the requirement is met from drinking water.

Deficiency

- *Etiology:* Iodine deficient drinking water
- *Clinical features:* It manifests as iodine deficiency disorder (Box 1).

Excess

Goiter, iodism (ptyalism, coryza, frontal headache, emaciation, and skin eruptions).

Box 1: Iodine deficiency disorder (IDD).

Etiology
Enlargement of the thyroid gland (Table1) as a result of iodine deficiency. It is endemic in sub-Himalayan belt extending from Ladakh through Himachal Pradesh, Uttar Pradesh, Bihar, Bengal, Sikkim, Bhutan, Assam, Arunachal Pradesh, Meghalaya and Nagaland to Burma. Isolated pockets are being increasingly identified, e.g. Rajasthan, Gujarat, Maharashtra, Madhya Pradesh, Andhra and Kerala. Since sea-water is a rich source of iodine, goiter is rare in population living along the sea coast.

Clinical features
Subclinical deficiency of iodine may manifest in the form of goiter only at puberty or confining to the periods of stress. The public health importance of goiter lies in the high incidence of deafmutism, mental retardation (often accompanying frank cretinism), ataxia and spasticity in the endemic areas.
- *Intrauterine life:* Abortion, stillbirth, congenital defects, perinatal mortality; congenital hypothyroidism (cretinism).
- *Newborn:* Mental retardation, goiter and neonatal hypothyroidism.
- *Infants, children and adolescents:* Goiter, growth retardation, poor cognition and subclinical hypothyroidism.

Prevention
As per India's National Goiter Control Program (in operation since 1962), availability of iodized salt (common salt fortified with sodium or potassium iodate in a ratio of 1 in 40,000) is the most economic, convenient and effective means of mass prophylaxis in endemic areas.
An alternative to iodized salt is iodized oil capsules at 6–10 months interval, iodized oil given as an intramuscular injection once in three years, Lugol's iodine periodically and iodization of water supply. Double fortified salts iodine plus iron are also available.

Table 1: Clinical grading of thyroid (revised).

Clinical grading	Characteristics
Grade 0a	Thyroid not palpable or if palpable, not larger than normal
Grade 0b	Thyroid distinctly palpable, but usually not visible with the head in a normal or raised position and considered to be definitely larger than normal, i.e. at least as large as the distal phalanx of the subject's thumb
Grade I	Thyroid easily palpable with the head in either a normal or raised position. The presence of a discrete node qualifies a patient for inclusion in this grade
Grade II	Thyroid easily visible at a distance
Grade III	Goiter visible at a distance
Grade IV	Monstrous goiter

Zinc

Next to iron, zinc is the most abundant trace element in the human body. Its concentration in hair is deemed to reflect the zinc status of a subject. It is also present in erythrocytes, prostate, eye, bone and endocrine glands. Total body zinc content of a newborn is about 60 mg and that of an adult about 1,600 mg.
- *Functions:* It is an essential component (cofactor) of at least 20 enzymes, including alkaline phosphatase, carbonic anhydrase and pancreatic carboxypeptidase required for growth and immunity. It plays a vital role in protein synthesis and ribonucleic acid (RNA).

- *Dietary sources:* Meat, liver, fish nuts, grains, dry beans and legumes.
- *Daily requirement (5-15 mg/day):* 1-2 mg/kg in preterm infants.

Deficiency

- *Etiology:* Zinc deficiency may occur in protein-energy malnutrition (PEM), malabsorption states, regional ileitis, rheumatoid arthritis, sickle-cell anemia, achondroplasia, chronic blood loss, excessive sweating and hyperzincuria in catabolic states or viral hepatitis. Prolonged parenteral nutrition, if not supplemented with zinc, may also cause zinc deficiency state. Consumption of fibers and phylates in excess hampers zinc absorption.
- *Clinical features:* Clinical manifestation of zinc deficiency include (Fig. 2):
  - *Growth retardation, hypogonadism, anemia and hepatosplenomegaly:* This peculiar syndrome called *adolescent nutritional dwarfing* has been described particularly from Iran and Egypt, though cases have been seen in India and other developing countries. However, a convincing cause and effect relationship between this syndrome and zinc deficiency remains to be established. Also, it has been said that zinc deficiency in such cases may well be due to poor absorption because of phylates, calcium and other dietary components rather than low dietary intake.
  - *Gastrointestinal manifestations:* Protracted diarrhea, delayed wound healing, anorexia, failure to thrive, pica, impaired taste perception (hypogeusia).

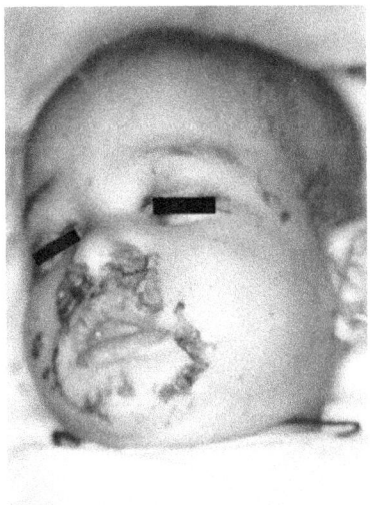

Fig. 2: Acrodermatitis enteropathica. Note skin lesions and alopecia in an infant with protracted diarrhea, similar skin lesion over perianal area, photophobia, atrophic nails, and failure to thrive. Response to therapy with zinc was gratifying.

- *Dermatological manifestations:* Hyperkeratotic skin.
- *Acrodermatitis enteropathica* is an autosomal recessive inborn error of zinc metabolism in which there are skin lesions (dry and scaly, eczematous or vesicobulbous) at the extremities and around the orifices (perioral, perianal), protracted diarrhea, alopecia, atrophy of nails, eye changes (conjunctivitis, blepharitis, photophobia), irritability, stomatitis and failure to thrive. It usually manifests shortly after weaning and shows dramatic and sustained response to therapy with zinc.
- *Infantile tremor syndrome* (ITS) characterized by tremors (in wakeful hours), anemia, regression of milestones, and mental retardation is also believed to be related to zinc deficiency.

Diagnosis

Diagnosis is usually clinical [prolonged low intake, clinical features, malabsorption and total parenteral nutrition (TPN)]. The laboratory confirmation for zinc deficiency may be obtained from a plasma zinc level of below 70 µg/dL or a hair zinc level of below 70 µg/g dry weight.

Treatment

It consists of giving zinc sulfate, 0.2–1 mg of elemental or 1–5 mg of the salt as such per kg body weight per day orally (O). In very severe deficiency states, as high a dose as 20–40 mg/day of elemental zinc may be administered.

Now, 10 mg daily in infants less than six months and 20 mg more than six months in all infants and children with diarrhea is an accepted strategy.

Prophylaxis

Zinc fertilizer strategy is a promising approach to enhance crop volume as well as address zinc deficiency in human.

Excess

Zinc in some excess is fairly safe, except that gastrointestinal upset and copper deficiency may occur. Large accidental ingestion may cause acute kidney injury and copper deficiency syndrome.

Copper

Copper, rightly called the *iron twin*, plays a vital role in the utilization of iron stores and in the activity of many important enzymes, including cytochrome oxidase, monoamine oxidase, dopamine beta-hydroxylase, delta-aminolevulinic acid dehydrogenase, ascorbic acid dehydrase, uricase and tyrosinase.

Total body copper content of a newborn is about 14 mg and that of a young adult about 100 mg. Thus, there is an average growth requirement of 10 µg/day. It is distributed in all tissues of body, including kidney, liver, brain, heart, bone marrow and bones.

Whereas in a newborn as much as 50% of body copper is found in the liver, the corresponding figure in a young adult is only 5%. Thus, just, as is the case with iron, copper stores of an infant are sufficient for the first six months of life. In the liver, copper is incorporated into a protein complex, *ceruloplasmin*.

- *Functions:* Utilization of iron stores and activity of several enzymes.
- *Dietary sources:* Copper is widely distributed in foodstuffs (especially seafood, meat, liver, nuts, seeds) with the exception of milk; breast milk contains 40 µg/dL (levels are high in early milk and gradually decline with lactation) and cow milk 20 µg/dL of it.
- *Daily requirement:* 1-2 mg. In preterm infants 30 µg is enough for maintain normal growth though some authorities recommend a higher intake (120/150 µg).

Deficiency

- *Etiology:* Deficiency may be encountered in the following situations:
  - PEM including nutritional rehabilitation employing predominantly soy milk and zinc supplementation in excess
  - Malabsorption states
  - Chronic diarrheal disease
  - Prolonged parenteral feeding without copper supplements
  - Premature infants being fed low-copper milk preparations. The maximum risk of copper deficiency in breastfed preterm infants is between age five week and eight months when copper levels in milk decline compared to the early milk.
- *Clinical features:* Failure to thrive (FTT), anemia (microcytic-hypochromic that is refractory to iron therapy), neutropenia, vascular abnormalities, hypopigmental hair and skin, seborrhea-like lesions; osteoporosis, metaphyseal fraying and fractures. Deficient immune function may occur.

Excess

Usually genetic in origin, is associated with Wilson disease, Menkes kinky hair disease, and Indian childhood cirrhosis (ICC) now a rare entity.

Cobalt

It is a part of vitamin B_{12} and is required for iodine utilization. It increases iron absorption.
- *Function:* Iodine utilization and iron absorption
- *Deficiency:* Anemia and goiter.

Excess

Dilated cardiomyopathy (which is indistinguishable from primary dilated cardiomyopathy) and goiter.

Selenium

Selenium, an integral part of enzymes, glutathione peroxidase is linked to vitamin E. Being an important antioxidant, it protects cells and membrane against oxidative damage. Selenium and vitamin C both antioxidants are known to spare each other.

Since it is found in the soil, overcultivation leads to depletion of selenium content in the crops.

- *Function*: As an antioxidant, it is cardioprotective as well as liver protective.
- *Dietary sources*: Meat, chicken, fish, egg, seafood; cheese, milk; cashew nuts, Brazil nuts; grains, whole wheat bread; sunflower seeds, garlic and onion. Vegetables and fruits are poor in selenium.
- Daily requirement:
  - *Children:* 20–30 µg
  - *Adolescents:* 50–55 µg
  - *Pregnancy and lactation:* 60–70 µg.

Deficiency

- *Etiology*: Malnutrition, TPN, low soil content.
- *Clinical features:* Growth retardation, myalgia, myopathy, cardiomyopathy and liver necrosis, selenium-related dilated cardiomyopathy [Endemic dilated cardiomyopathy (DCM)/Keshan disease] used to be common in certain geographical parts of China. It was first described in 1979 and may occur in young children and women. It is a preventable cardiomyopathy, but once DCM sets in, total reversal to normality is not possible even with selenium supplementation. Four forms of Keshan's disease are recognized—an acute variety with shock, a subacute variety with both hypotension and congestive heart failure (CHF), a chronic variety with CHF and the fourth one, which presents as asymptomatic cardiomegaly. It is virtually indistinguishable from various presentations of primary DCM.

Excess

Dental caries, alopecia and garlic odor in breath.

Chromium

This micronutrient has an important role in glucose tolerance and in facilitating insulin action.

- *Dietary sources*: Vegetables, fruits, nuts, cereals, pulses, yeast and liver
- *Daily requirement*: 10–70 mg/day.

Deficiency

- *Etiology:* Malnutrition and TPN
- *Clinical features:* Hyperglycemia, glycosuria, peripheral neuritis; poor glucose tolerance complicating malnutrition TPN, and neuropathy. It facilitates insulin action.

Excess
Dermatitis and renal failure.

Manganese
Manganese is an enzyme cofactor in superoxide dismutase, oxidative phosphorylation and bone mineralization.
- *Daily requirement:* 1-5 mg
- *Dietary sources:* Nuts, vegetables, pulses and cereals.

Deficiency
Growth retardation, weight loss, red hair, hypocholesterolemia, increased prothrombin time. Deficiency usually is associated with PEM and TPN.

Excess
Cholestasis, encephalopathy, basal ganglia disorder, goiter and cardiomyopathy.

Fluorine
Fluorine is mainly a component of bone and teeth wherein it is found as calcium salt. Only up to 1 ppm in drinking water is desirable; more than 2 ppm in water may cause fluorosis.
- *Function:*
    - Protection of dental enamel and inhibition of dental caries
    - Calcification of bones
    - Antibacterial against *Streptococcus mutans*, known for causing dental decay.
- *Dietary source:* Drinking water, seafoods (fish), cheese and tea.
- Daily requirement:
    - *Children:* 7-1 mg/day
    - *Adolescents:* 2-3 mg/day.

Deficiency
Dental caries manifesting as loss of luster of enamel, yellow brownish staining and even pitting.

Excess
Fluorosis, both dental (chalky white mottled with brownish staining) and skeletal (fluorine deposits in vertebral column, spine, pelvis, lower limbs; eventually neurologic signs and symptoms, deformities and crippling develop).

Molybdenum
Molybdenum, a component of xanthine oxidase is considered the last trace element.

- *Function:* Important in uric acid metabolism and in preventing dental decay.
- *Dietary sources*: Meat, green leafy vegetables (GLVs), dried beans, dried peas, pulses and whole grain cereals.
- *Daily requirement:* 100–500 µg/day.

Deficiency

- *Etiology:* TPN, poor content
- *Clinical features:* Tachycardia, irritability, central scotoma and upper gastrointestinal tract (mouth and esophagus) malignancies.

Excess

It may unmask gout and cause bony defects like genu valgum (knock-knee deformity).

Nickel

Nickel is a component of urease and nickel plasmin.
- *Dietary source:* Chocolates, fish and oatmeal.

Deficiency

- *Etiology:* Vitamin B_6 deficiency, kidney disease and liver disease.
- *Signs:* Range from urinary tract infections to severe allergic reactions, most often seen in the form of skin rashes. In very severe cases, paralysis alongside inflammation of the liver and lungs may occur.

Excess

Dermatitis, liver necrosis and lung cancer.

Vanadium

- *Functions:* Regulation of sodium and metabolism of glucose and lipids (insulin-like role).
- *Dietary sources:* Protein-rich foods (seafoods) and vegetables
- Deficiency:
  - *Etiology:* Malnutrition and PEM
  - *Sign:* Nutritional edema
- *Excess:* Manic depression.

Silicon

- *Function:* Silicon is important in cross linkage of collagen.
- Deficiency:
  - *Etiology:* TPN.
  - *Signs:* Defective bone growth and growth retardation.
- *Excess:* Fibrosis and granuloma of lung.

Arsenic

- *Function:* Arsenic is important in hair, skin and nail formation.
- *Source*: Water, foods from soil where arsenic has been used.
- *Deficiency:* Poor hair, skin and nail growth.
- *Excess:* Skin, central nervous system (CNS) and respiratory insult.

This is the most abundant mineral in the human body.

MACROMINERALS

Clinically important macrominerals include calcium, phosphorus, magnesium, sodium, potassium, and chloride.

Calcium

- *Functions:* Almost all (99%) of body calcium is in bones and teeth. The remaining 1% is involved in clotting cascade, nerve conduction, muscle stimulation, vitamin D metabolism and parathyroid function.
- *Metabolism:* Its metabolism is regulated by vitamin D, calcitonin and parathyroid hormone. Normal blood calcium level is 8-11 mg/dL. The ideal blood calcium and phosphorus product should be 40. In order that calcium performs its function well, adequate magnesium, phosphorus and vitamin A, C, D and E should be available in the body.
- *Absorption*: Whereas availability of fat facilitates its absorption from the gut, phytates (cereals) reduce its absorption.
- *Sources*: Milk dairy products and millets (say, ragi) and fruits.
- *Daily requirement:* 500-1000 mg/day. Requirement enhances at pre-pubertal growth spurt.

Deficiency

- *Etiology:* PEM, strict vegetarian diet, chronic diarrhea, malabsorption syndrome, calcium metabolism abnormalities and LBW.
- *Manifestations:* Tetany, muscle cramps, numbness, tingling, impaired growth, calcium-deficiency rickets, osteoporosis, arthralgia and palpitations.

Toxicity/Excess

Hypercalcemia which may manifest with anorexia, irritability, constipation, nausea, vomiting, soft-tissue swellings and neuropsychiatric symptoms. It may result from vitamin D excess, milk-alkali syndrome, prolonged immobilization, hyperparathyroidism, etc. Idiopathic hypercalcemia (William syndrome) is characterized by elfin facies and supravalvular aortic stenosis.

Magnesium

Next to potassium, it is the most abundant mineral cation in cells; more than 80% being in the bones and skeletal muscles.

- *Functions:* It is involved in:
  - Synthesis of fatty acids, proteins, cyclic adenosine monophosphate (AMP)
  - Oxidative phosphorylation
  - Autonomic control of heart.
- *Sources:* Plant foods (GLVs), bananas, legumes, whole grains/cereals, nuts and meat.
- *Daily requirements*:
  - First six months: 40–50 mg/day
  - Second six months: 60 mg/day
  - Later: 200–300 mg/day
- *Absorption:* GIT with renal tubular reabsorption regulating its balance.

Deficiency

- *Etiology:* These include PEM, diarrheal disease, malabsorption syndrome (MAS), losses through continuous suction or fistulas; chronic renal failure involving renal tubular reabsorption.
- *Manifestations*: Irritability, tetany, seizures, increased or decreased reflexes.
- *Treatment*:
  - Mild disease: Oral magnesium 6 mg (1 tablet); 2–3 times daily
  - Severe diseased: Oral magnesium 12 mg (2 tablets); 3–4 times daily
  - Acute severe hypomagnesemia: IV infusion of magnesium sulfate (50% solution), 25–50 mg/kg slowly 6 hourly × 2–3 doses. Dose in terms of elemental magnesium is 2.5–5 mg/kg. In renal insufficiency/impairment, dose needs a reduction.

Toxicity/Excess

Toxicity occurs with blood levels more than 5 mg/dL (normal level 1.5–3 mg/dL). Manifestations include respiratory depression, drowsiness and coma. Antidote is calcium which is antagonistic to magnesium.

Sodium

Human body contains 100 g of this very important constituent of body fluid and cells—50% each in extracellular compartment (ECC) and tissue cells and bones. Normal blood level is around 140 mEq/L. Excretion is in urine and sweat.

- *Functions:* Maintenance of osmotic balance; keeping cells in shape.
- *Dietary sources:* Add up to foods for imparting taste.
- *Daily requirement:* 2–3 mEq/kg/day.

Deficiency

- *Etiology:* Gastroenteritis, diarrhea, cholera, prolonged vomiting, excessive sweating, diuretic therapy, water intoxication, syndrome of inappropriate

secretion of antidiuretic hormone (ADH) (SIADH), Addison's disease and chronic kidney injury.
- *Clinical features:* Hyponatremic state.

Excess

Hypernatremia, occurring as a part of dyselectrolytemia in dehydration, prolonged therapy with steroids, etc. may manifest as thickened skin (sclerema-like), raised blood pressure, seizures, etc.

Potassium

This important component of body cell and fluids is mainly (90%) intracellular (in cells of tissues and RBCs). Total body content is 250 g. Excretion of surplus potassium is in urine. Normal blood level is 3.5–4.5 mEq/L.
- *Functions:* Assists in growth and development of tissue cells, regulates acid-base balance in cells, and contributes to glycogen synthesis cellular excitability of smooth muscles, skeletal, cardiac and nervous tissue and control of involuntary functions of the muscles.
- *Dietary sources:* Fruits, vegetables, whole bread, grain, dried skimmed milk, fish, meat, legumes and coffee.
- *Daily requirement:* 1–2 mEq/day.

Deficiency

- *Etiology:* Dehydration-associated hypokalemia in prolonged gastro-enteritis, diarrhea, vomiting; erratic intravenous (IV) fluid administration (without potassium); digitalis therapy and diabetic ketoacidosis.
- *Clinical features:* Abdominal distention and paralytic ileus.
- *Electrocardiography (ECG):* Flat T waves and U waves.

Excess

Ventricular fibrillation; ECG shows tall tented T waves.

IMPLICATIONS OF MICRONUTRIENT/MINERAL INTERACTIONS

- Useful interactions
  - Vitamin A is known for beneficial effect *via* enhancement of iron absorption.
  - Vitamin C too enhances iron absorption.
- Adverse interactions:
  - Zinc is known to cause copper deficiency by its depletion.
  - Zinc also competes with iron absorption.
  - High phosphorus interferes with calcium absorption. Infants fed on cow's milk stand fair chances of developing hypocalcemic tetany.

CONCLUSION

Micronutrients, also termed *trace elements* or *microminerals*, are needed only in minuscule amounts. These are considered the "magic wands" because of their ability to produce enzymes, hormones and other substances essential for proper growth and development. The consequences of their deficiency are critical. Of all micronutrients, deficiency of iron, iodine and vitamin A, most important in global public health terms, represents a major threat to the health and development of child populations, particularly in resource-limited regions.

> **KEY LEARNING POINTS**
> - *Micronutrients*, also termed trace elements or microminerals, are needed only in minute amounts (μg or mg/day rather than g/day) to perform various physiologic functions.
> - Less than 0.01% of human body is of human body is formed by them.
> - These are considered the "magic wands" because of their ability to produce enzymes, hormones and other substances essential for proper growth and development.
> - Deficiency of micronutrients causes critical health problems.
> - Iron, iodine and vitamin A are the most important micronutrients in global public health terms.

REFERENCES

1. Campbell M. Two types of minerals in food. Available at: http://healthyeating.sfgate.com/two-types-minerals-food-9640.html Accessed on: 27 January 2018.
2. Mehta MN, Mehta NJ. *Nutrition and Diet for Children Simplified*. New Delhi: Jaypee 2014.
3. Gupte S. Mironutrients/Trace Elements/Minerals. In: Gupte S (Ed). *The Short Textbook of Pediatrics*, 12th edn. New Delhi: Jaypee 2016:245-252.
4. Elizabeth K. Nutrition and Child Development, 4th edn. Hyderabad: Paras 2010.
5. Gupte S. Pediatric Nutrition, 2nd edn. New Delhi: Peepee 2012.
6. Diaz Jr, De Las cagigas A, Rodriguez R. Micronutrient deficiencies in developing and affluent countries. *Eur j Clin Nutr* 2003:57:s70-s72.
7. Bhaskaran P. Micronutrient malnutrition, infection and immunity: An overview. *Nutr Rev* 2002:60:S40-S45.
8. Bhatia J, Griffin I, Anderson D, Kler N, Domellof M. Requirement of iron, copper and zinc in preterm infants. *J Pediatr* 2013:162:S48-55.
9. Oken E, Duggan C. Update on micronutrients: iron and zinc. *Curr Opin Pediatr* 2002:14:350-353.

9   Iron Deficiency Anemia

VN Tripathi, Piyush Upadhyay, Rakhi Jain

ABSTRACT

Iron is an important nutrient for human body. It is the main component of hemoglobin in red blood cells (RBCs).

Iron deficiency is mostly nutritional and very common in children. It not only causes microcytic anemia but has other manifestations like neurodevelopmental and cognitive defects. These nonhematological defects fail to be reversed even after iron therapy. It can be easily diagnosed by laboratory test if blood hemoglobin, and serum ferritin levels among other investigations. Oral iron supplementation is the treatment widely recommended. Government of India has launched programs for iron folic acid supplementation to prevent iron deficiency anemia (IDA).

Keywords: Anemia, Congnitive defects, Hemoglobin, Iron supplementation, Iron-folic acid supplementation, Iron-deficiency anemia, Micronutrient, Neurodevelopmental defects, Nutrient, Serum ferritin.

INTRODUCTION

Iron is very important for the production of hemoglobin and hence for RBC production in bone marrow. Iron is also necessary to maintain healthy cells, skin, hair, and nails deficiency of iron in body due to any cause leads to iron deficiency anemia (IDA).

Iron store of body comprises of iron absorbed from food and through recycling of iron released after lysis of old RBCs. When red blood cells are no longer able to function (after about 120 days in circulation), they are reabsorbed by the spleen. Iron from these old cells can also be recycled by the body.

Iron deficiency anemia is the most common nutritional anemia in developing countries and still remains a common cause of anemia in children in developed countries as well.[1,2] IDA is not only a hematological disease but a multisystem disorder. Studies have shown that iron deficiency even

Table 1: Definition of anemia by hemoglobin value.[5]

Age	Hemoglobin Level
Infants 0.5–4.9 years	<11 g per dL (110 g per L)
Children 5.0–11.9 years	<11.5 g per dL (115 g per L)
Menstruating women	<12 g per dL (120 g per L)
Pregnant women	<11 g per dL (110 g per L)
Men	<13 g per dL (130 g per vL)

Table 2: Recommended dietary allowances (RDA) of iron.

Age	Male	Female
Birth to 6 months	0.27 mg*	0.27 mg*
7–12 months	11 mg	11 mg
1–3 years	7 mg	7 mg
4–8 years	10 mg	10 mg
9–13 years	8 mg	8 mg
14–18 years	11 mg	15 mg

*Adequate intake (AI)

without anemia has effects on cognitive and neurodevelopmental outcome of children which may be irreversible.[3,4]

SOURCES AND REQUIREMENT

Dietary iron comes from two sources heme and non-heme iron. Heme iron is present in meat, fish and poultry. It is better absorbed but intake is less. Major dietary iron is found in food of plant origin but its absorption depends on dietary factors. Pulses, green leafy vegetables, dates, nuts, jaggery, fish, meat are among the good sources of iron in the diet. Intake of viamin C along with food increases the absorption of dietary iron. Requirement of iron varies with age (Table 2).[6]

ETIOLOGY

Most iron in a neonate is circulating hemoglobin. As the hemoglobin concentration falls at 2-3 months of life, iron is recycled and this is sufficient for first 6-9 months of life in term babies. In preterm and low birth weight babies, these reserves get depleted earlier. Poor nutritional intake is one of the commonest cause of IDA in developing countries.[7] Blood loss due to pathology or menstrual loss in females is another important cause.

Cause of Iron Deficiency

1. Decreased intake/absorption
   - Delayed initiation of complementary feeding
   - Malnutrition/malabsorption/diet deficient in iron

- Chronic diarrhea
- Gastrointestinal surgery
2. Decreased iron stores
   - Preterm
   - Small for gestational age
3. Increased losses
   - Malaria
   - Hookworm
   - Peptic ulcer
   - Gastrointestinal bleed
   - Bleeding disorders
   - Repeated blood sampling
4. Increased demand
   - Prematurity
   - Small for date babies
   - Recovery from malnutrition
   - Growth spurt in adolescents

CLINICAL FEATURES

Hematological Effects

Mostly, it is asymptomatic discovered by routine screening at 12 months of age. Pallor appears when hemoglobin falls to <7–8 g/dL. As the decline is slow, subtle paleness of skin goes unnoticed by parents unless pointed out by a guest or relative.

Due to gradual decline in hemoglobin compensatory rise in 2, 3 diphosphoglycerate and shift of oxygen dissociation curve mask the symptoms and only mild irritability is present. When hemoglobin is <5 g/dL, anorexia, irritability, lethargy develop. Further fall in levels causes systolic flow murmur, tachycardia, increased cardiac output and cardiac failure.

Nonhematological Effects

- Koilonychia, glossitis, esophageal web.
- There are studies showing increased risk of seizures, breath holding spells in children and exacerbation of restless leg syndrome in adults.
- Pica, pagophagia (craving to eat ice).

Developmental and Neurophysiological Deficits in Iron Deficiency

Studies show iron deficiency affects brain metabolism, neurotransmitter function and myelination. This may lead to impaired neurocognitive function and developmental delay in infancy leading to cognitive defects during adulthood which may be irreversible. Motor development and coordination are reduced. There may be impaired language development, poor scholastic achievement, psychological and behavioral effects like insecurity, fatigue, poor attention span and decreased physical activity. These changes may not be reversed even after adequate iron therapy. Hence, the importance of prevention at apt time, early diagnosis and treatment.[8]

LABORATORY INVESTIGATIONS

Laboratory diagnosis of IDA can be done by analysis of Hb level and blood indices. Following are the indicators of iron deficiency:[9]
1. Hb <11g/dL (0.5-4 years)
2. MCV < 70 FL/RBC (6-24 months)
3. Serum feritin
   - <=5 years <12
   - >5 years <15
   In all age groups in presence of infection <30
4. Reti Hb content (CHr)
   - Children <27.5
   - Adult <28
5. Transferrin saturation <16%
6. Serum transferring receptor varies with assay, age and origin of patient
7. Erythrocyte zinc protoporphyrin level (ZPP)<= 5 years >70
   Children >5 years >80
8. Hepcidin usually<=10 ng/mL
9. Increased RDW (>14.5%)
10. Low serum iron (<75 mg/dL)
11. Increased TIBC (>470 µg/dL)

TREATMENT

Oral Therapy

- Oral administration of 3-6 mg/kg/day elemental iron in 3 div dose. Maximum dose 150-200 mg daily
- Ferrous sulfate provides 20% iron by weight given between meals. Iron therapy is associated with increased virulence of malaria and some gram negative bacteria. Iron overdose is shown to be associated with *Yersinia* infection.[10]
- In mild anemia, hemoglobin level is repeated at 4 weeks and an increase by 1-2 g/dL confirms diagnosis and response to treatment. In severe cases, reticulocytosis in 48-96 hours confirms diagnosis and hemoglobin rises by 0.1-0.4 g/dL.
- Treatment must be continued for 2-3 months after hemoglobin and red cell indices normalize, to replenish stores.[10]

Parenteral Iron Therapy

Indications

- Intolerance to oral iron
- Poor compliance
- Malabsorption
- Aggravation of gastrointestinal bleed by oral iron therapy

Commercially available iron preparations are:
- Iron-dextran complex
- Iron sucrose
- Iron ferric gluconate
- Ferric carboxymaltose injection

Iron dextran is a complex of ferric chloride and high molecular weight dextran. The dose is calculated as:

Iron (mg) = weight in kg × Hb deficit (g/dL) × 4

It is given by intravenous route. Anaphylaxis is the major adverse effect and could be life-threatening. Hence, it should always be given in hospital setting. Its use has decreased due to increased risk of anaphylaxis. Availability of ferric carboxymaltose that is less toxic, better tolerated and safer.

Oral therapy is preferred as it is easy, inexpensive, less toxic and equally efficacious.

Red cell transfusion is indicated in very severe cases when hemoglobin level is below 3–4 g/dL. Packed cell transfusion given slowly @ 2–3 mL/kg at a time.

The response to iron therapy can be assessed by the following parameters (Table 3).[10]

Box 1 lists the causes of poor response to oral iron therapy.

PREVENTION

Since defective nutrition is the most common cause of IDA, dietary modification is the best preventive strategy. Exclusive breastfeeding till 6 months of age followed by complementary feeding which is of apt quality and quantity is important for prevention of iron deficiency. Periodic deworming is another preventive measure in endemic areas.

Table 3: Response to therapy.

Time after iron administration	Response
12–24 hours	Replenishment of intracellular iron enzymes, subjective improvement, decreased irritability, increased appetite
36–48 hours	Initial bone marrow response, erythroid hyperplasia
48–72 hours	Reticulocytosis (peaks at 5–7 days)
4–30 days	Increased Hb level
1–3 months	Repletion of stores

Box 1: Causes of IDA not responding to oral iron.

- Poor compliance
- Incorrect dose or medication
- Malabsorption of administered iron
- Ongoing blood loss
- Concurrent infection, inflammation
- Concurrent B12 and folic acid (FA) deficiency
- Diagnosis other than IDA (Thalassemia and other microcytic anemias)

The American Academy of Pediatrics (AAP) recommends universal hemoglobin screening and evaluation of risk factors for iron deficiency anemia in all children at one year of age.[11] Risk factors include low birth weight, history of prematurity, exposure to lead, exclusive breastfeeding beyond four months of life, and weaning to whole milk and complementary foods without iron-fortified foods.[11]

Breastfed infants should be supplemented with 1 mg/kg per day of oral iron beginning at 4 months of age until appropriate iron-containing complementary foods are introduced. For partially breastfed infants, the proportion of human milk versus formula is uncertain. Therefore, beginning at 4 months of age, partially breastfed infants (more than half of their daily feedings as human milk) who are not receiving iron-containing complementary foods should also receive 1 mg/kg per day of supplemental iron.[11]

All preterm infants should have an iron intake of at least 2 mg/kg per day till 12 months of age.[11]

The Ministry of Health and Family Welfare (MOHFW) has revised the guidelines on IFA supplementation related to the National Nutritional Anemia Prophylaxis Program (NNAPP).[12]

- Children between 6 months to 60 months should be given 20 mg elemental iron and 100 μg folic acid per day.
- Children 6-10 year old should be provided 30 mg elemental iron and 250 μg folic acid per child for 100 days in a year.
- Fortification of food by newer products like double fortified salts/sprinkles/ultra rice and others need to be explored as an adjunct or alternate supplementation strategy.

The MOHFW, Government of India, developed the National Iron Plus Initiative (NIPI) guidelines for control of iron deficiency anemia in India in 2013. This initiative brought together existing programs for IFA supplementation for pregnant and lactating mother and children in the different age groups. This initiative reached following groups:[13]

- 6 months to 5 years (preschool children): Biweekly iron supplementation (1 mL of IFA syrup containing 20 mg of elemental iron and 100 μg of folic acid).
- Children studying in class I-V in government or government-aided schools or children who do not go to school (5-10 years of age): Weekly supplementation (tablet with 45 mg of elemental iron and 400 μg of folic acid).
- Adolescents (10-19 years of age): Weekly supplementation (tablet with 100 mg of elemental iron and 500 μg of folic acid).
- Pregnant and lactating women: 100 days of supplementation (tablet with 100 mg of elemental iron and 500 μg of folic acid).
- Women of reproductive age group: Weekly supplementation (tablet with 100 mg of elemental iron and 500 μg of folic acid).

CONCLUSION

Iron deficiency anemia (IDA) is most commonly nutritional. Iron deficiency also affects neurocognitive functions.

Prevention has a very important role as certain adverse effects of iron deficiency in earlier life may be irreversible. This can be avoided by timely screening, diagnosis and treatment.

> **KEY LEARNING POINTS**
> - Iron deficiency anemia is most commonly nutritional.
> - Persistence of ID affects childhood and adulthood.
> - Treatment is oral iron supplementation along with elimination of cause.
> - Preventive strategies include dietary modification, deworming, iron folic acid supplementation and food fortification.

REFERENCES

1. United Nations. *Fourth Report of the World Nutrition Situation.* Geneva: United Nations Administrative Committee on Coordination/Sub-Committee on Nutrition 2000.
2. Sherry B, Mei Z, Yip R. Continuation of the decline in prevalence of anemia in low-income infants and children in five states. *Pediatrics* 2001;107:677-682.
3. Lozoff B, Jimenez E, Smith JB. Double burden of iron deficiency in infancy and low socioeconomic status: a longitudinal analysis of cognitive test scores to age 19 years. *Arch Pediatr Adolesc Med* 2006;160:1108-1113.
4. Bruner AB, Joffe A, Duggan AK, Casella JF, Brandt J. Randomized study of cognitive effects of iron supplementation in non-anemic iron-deficient adolescent girls. *Lancet* 1996;348(9033):992-996.
5. US Preventive Services Task Force. Screening for iron deficiency anemia – including iron prophylaxis. In: *Guide to Clinical Preventive Services,* 2nd edn. Baltimore: Williams and Wilkins 1996:231-246.
6. Institute of Medicine. Food and Nutrition Board. *Dietary Reference Intakes for Vitamin A, Vitamin K, Arsenic, Boron, Chromium, Copper, Iodine, Iron, Manganese, Molybdenum, Nickel, Silicon, Vanadium, and Zinc: a Report of the Panel on Micronutrients.* Washington, DC: National Academy Press 2001.
7. Ray S, Chandra J, Bhattacharjee J, Sharma S, Agarwala A. Determinants of nutritional anemia in children less than five years age. *Int J Contemp Pediatr* 2016;3:403-408.
8. Yadav S, Chandra J. Iron deficiency:beyond anemia. *Indian J Pediatr* 2011;78:65-72.
9. Zimmerman MB, Hurrell RF. Nutritional Iron deficiency. *Lancet* 2007;370:511-520.
10. Lerner NB, Sills R. Iron deficiency anemia. In: Kliegman RM, Stanton BF, Geme III JW, Schor NF (Eds): *Nelson Textbook of Pediatrics,* 20th edn. Philadelphia: Elsevier 2016: pp.1655-1658.
11. Baker RD, Greer FR. Committee on Nutrition, American Academy of Pediatrics. Diagnosis and prevention of iron deficiency and iron-deficiency anemia in infants and young children (0–3 years of age). *Pediatrics* 2010;126:1040-1050.
12. Kumar A. National nutritional anmia control programin India. *Indian J Public Health.* 1999;43:3-5.
13. Umesh K, Bhadoria AS. National iron plus initiative guidelines for control of iron deficiency anemia in India. *Nat Med J* 2014;.27:27-29.

10
Neuropsychiatric Dysfunctions in Iron Deficiency Anemia

TM Ananda Kesavan

ABSTRACT

Iron deficiency is the most common micronutrient deficiency all over the world, manifesting with varieties of clinical picture including different types of neuropsychiatric manifestations. Iron deficiency as part of the differential diagnosis in these disorders is usually neglected. Some of the manifestations may become irreversible, if not treated in time. Hence, its early recognition, prevention and therapy are important.

Keywords: Attention-deficit hyperactivity disorder, Breath-holding spells, Cognition, Iron deficiency, Iron and brain, Neurological dysfunction.

INTRODUCTION

Iron is the one of the most abundant element in the earth. But iron deficiency (ID) is the most common micronutrient deficiency in the world! Nutritional anemia is a major public health problem in India and is primarily due to iron deficiency. The National Family Health Survey-3 (NFHS-3) data suggests that anemia is widely prevalent among all age groups, and is particularly high among the most vulnerable — nearly 58% among pregnant women, 50% among non-pregnant non-lactating women, 56% among adolescent girls (15-19 years), 30% among adolescent boys and around 80% among children under 3 years of age.[1]

Seven out of every 10 children aged 6-59 months in India are anemic—3% are severely anemic, 40% are moderately anemic, and 26% are mildly anemic. The prevalence of anemia ranges from 38% in Goa to 78% in Bihar. More than half of young children in 24 states have anemia, including 11 states where more than two-thirds of children are anemic. It is very sad to notice that the prevalence of anemia has actually increased from NFHS-2 to NFHS-3. The percentage of children with any anemia increased from 74.3% in NFHS-2 to 78.9% in NFHS-3. In the period between the two surveys, there was an increase in the prevalence of mild anemia (from 23% to 26%) and moderate anemia (from 46% to 49%).

Although the most common manifestation of iron deficiency is anemia, it is frequently associated with breath-holding spells, attention deficit hyperactive disorder, etc. The identification of iron deficiency as part of the differential diagnosis in these disorders is infrequent and, hence, remains untreated. The purpose of the current review is to highlight what is understood regarding ID and its underlying pathophysiology as it relates to the brain and the association of ID with common neurologic pediatric disease.

PATHOPHYSIOLOGY

The blood-brain barrier provides an effective regulatory point for iron movement from the plasma pool to the cerebral spinal fluid. The choroids plexus is also a likely source of iron movement into and out of the brain. Not all brain regions contain the same amount of iron.

Iron, transported by transferrin, enters brain endothelial cells via receptor-mediated endocytosis.[2] Once in the brain, the transportation of iron is poorly understood. Iron uptake during early postnatal development is rapid, leading to brain iron concentrations that are one half that of the adult rat (most investigations of brain iron have been performed in the rat model) by as early as the third week of life.[3] Iron uptake subsequently decreases with age. The iron attained by the developing brain becomes sequestered.

The distribution of brain iron changes with age, presumably as a result of the altering brain region requirements of iron at different neurodevelopmental stages.[4] Iron is distributed unevenly and is present in both gray and white matter.[5] It is most commonly located in oligodendrocytes of rat and human brains.[3] Iron-rich areas in the mature rat include the circumventricular regions and regions in which iron is associated with oligodendrocytes and the neuropil network (Box 1).

Iron-binding capability diminishes with age, suggesting that aged animals are unable to remove free iron that can lead to free radical production and cell death.[6] Free iron has been implicated in the pathophysiology of several brain diseases, including Parkinson's, Alzheimer's and multiple sclerosis.[7]

The biological basis of the behavioral and cognitive developmental delays observed in iron-deficient infants is not completely understood but possibilities include:
1. Decreased myelin formation
2. Alterations in brain-energy metabolism
3. Abnormalities in neurotransmitter metabolism.

Box 1: Iron-rich area in the brain.[5]

- Globus pallidus
- Ventral pallidum
- Substantia nigra reticulate
- Interpeduncular nucleus
- Cerebellar nuclei
- Facial nucleus
- Superior olive

Decreased Myelin Formation

Oligodendrocytes are the myelin-producing cells in the brain. Iron is required for myelin production, in that it is a cofactor for cholesterol and lipid biosynthesis.[2] Also oligodendrocytes have a high level of oxidative metabolism and therefore require iron for metabolic processes. In addition to myelin production, oligodendrocytes have the additional function of storing and mobilizing iron in the central nervous system.[2,8] Early exposure to ID during critical periods of brain development is believed to result in "irreversible" damage, resulting in clinical sequelae such as developmental delay.

Delayed myelination and hypomyelination have been demonstrated in rats with prenatal and lactational ID.[9] The ratio of sphingolipids were abnormal with nervonic acid synthesis decreased fourfold. The direct effect of decreased nervonic acid synthesis is the postulated mechanism by which ID delays myelination.

Alteration in Brain Energy Metabolism

Iron is directly or indirectly involved in various metabolic process in brain. A large number of enzymes are known to contain iron or require iron as a cofactor, including cytochrome oxidase, succinate dehydrogenase, aconitase, catalase, myeloperoxidase, cytochrome C reductase, ribonucleotide reductase, tyrosine hydroxylase, and xanthine oxidase. Consequently in ID, there are changes in nucleic acid biosynthesis, oxidative respiration and mitochondrial function, detoxification of metabolic byproducts, and catechol-amine metabolism.[3,4] Because iron is imperative to maintain normal organ function at a cellular level, it is not surprising that its deficiency results in a variety of clinical manifestations affecting most organ systems including nervous system (Table 1).

Neurochemical Effects

Iron dificiency affects neurotransmitters. The change in neurotransmitter activity has been a suggested mechanism resulting in the clinical abnormalities observed in ID (Table 2).

Table 1: Neurological manifestation of iron deficiency.

• Fatiguebility	• Cognitive impairment
• Anorexia	• Sensorineural hearing loss
• Reduced attention span	• Restless leg syndrome
• Irritability	• Febrile seizure
• Growth retardation (weight > height)	• Stroke
• Behavioral changes	• Breath-holding episodes
• Developmental delay	• Pseudotumor cerebri
• Learning disability (writing, mathematics)	• Cranial nerve palsies
• Poor scholastic performance	

Table 2: Neurochemical effect of iron deficiency.[10,11]

Neurochemical	Metabolic effect	Clinical effect	Reversibility
GABA	+/- GABA Decreased GAD, GABA-T	Impaired neurotransmitter regulation of hypothalamic-hypophyseal hormones	Irreversible in gestational iron deficiency
Dopamine	Decreased D2 receptor binding sites	Decreased motor activity and learning processes	Irreversible
Phenylalanine	Increased phenylalanine secondary to decreased phenylalanine like" effect hydroxylase activity	Decreased learning secondary to "PKU-like" effect	Reversible
Serotonin	Decreased 5-HT via decreased, tryptophan or tyrosine hydroxylase activity, Or Increased 5-HT via decreased degradation by aldehyde oxidase	Impairs neurodevelopment Or Increased drowsiness, decreased attention and learning due to serotonergic effect	Irreversible or Reversible

GABA: gamma aminobutyric acid; GAD: glutamate decarboxylase; D: Dopamine; 5-HT: 5-Hydroxy-tryptophan; PKU: phenylketonuria

NEUROLOGIC SEQUELAE OF IRON DEFICIENCY IN CHILDREN

Neurologic problems postulated to be associated with ID are described as follows:

Poor Cognitive Development

Cognitive performance and school achievement scores are low in children with low Hb.[12] Children with ID in early life demonstrate lower academic performance during their school years even after the anemia had been treated. When comparing to nonanemic children, ID children showed poor performance on tests assessing development, cognitive performance and in subjects like mathematics.[13] It is not reversible with an iron-replete diet.

A Cochrane review examined the impact of iron therapy in children less than three years with IDA.[14] Improvement was observed in mental and motor development, cognitive performance and language skills. Studies in developing countries have found a beneficial effect of long term treatment of anemic children.[15]

The children with moderately severe anemia in infancy had lower mental and motor scores in most areas compared with their non-anemic peers. It was suggested that prolonged severe iron deficiency in infancy is associated with poor developmental outcome at 5 years of age.[16] Unfortunately, no practice guidelines have been published on screening for ID or use of iron supplementation to prevent cognitive or behavioral defects.

Low iron exposure during lactational period results in irreversible brain ID despite adequate therapy. Early exposure to ID during critical periods of brain development is believed to result in "irreversible" damage, resulting in clinical sequelae such as delayed development.[17]

Walter et al.[18] studied a cohort of 196 subjects from infancy to 2-3/lakh/year of age. IDA infants had lower baseline mental and psychomotor scores that were not corrected after 3 months of iron therapy. Further analysis of the data suggested that prolonged iron deficiency and severe anemia in infancy result in irreversible developmental changes despite correction of anemia.

Lozoff[19] has looked further at behavior of ID infants. The study concluded that anemic infants are "functionally isolated" as a result of altered interaction with their physical and social environment. This in turn interferes with their natural development, resulting in motor and cognitive delay. Other authors have also noted similar observation.[20]

Pediatric Stroke

Pediatric stroke is uncommon, occurring in approximately 2-3/1 lakh/year. Stroke in association with ID has been reported in the pediatric and adult literature in a number of case reports.[21] Several mechanisms have been proposed (Box 2).

Breath Holding Spells

Breath holding spells (BHS) have been associated with ID and can occur in up to 27% of affected children.[24] Autonomic dysregulation resulting in vagally

Box 2: Proposed hypothesis to explain the association between iron deficiency and stroke.[22,23]

1. Thrombocytosis secondary to iron deficiency. Megakaryocytes and normoblasts are derived from a common committed progenitor cell, the CFU-GEMM. Thrombopoietin, the molecule that stimulates the growth of megakaryoytes and production of platelets, is structurally homologous to erythropoietin. The high levels of erythropoietin produced by iron deficiency anemia could cross react with megakaryocyte thrombopoetin receptors, modestly raising the platelet count.
2. Iron deficiency results in a hypercoagulable state. The microcytic poorly deformable red blood cells increase blood viscosity' and increase risk of venous thrombosis.
3. Some group of children also had cerebrovascular dilatation, which slows blood flow and further promotes thrombosis.
4. Anemic hypoxia may contribute to transient hemiplegia and cerebellar infarct. The anemic state is well tolerated until some infection (e.g. viral illness) increases metabolic demands that cannot be met in the face of anemia. Decreased iron-dependent enzymes necessary to metabolic processes may contribute to impaired energy metabolism and oxygen utilization

mediated cardiac arrest or bradycardia has been proposed, as have the effects of anemia on reducing oxygen carrying capacity. ID children also are known to be more irritable; presumably, this may increase the likelihood of an event. Treatment with iron supplementation has been shown to significantly reduce or eliminate the risk of recurrence.[24]

Benign Intracranial Hypertension

Iron deficiency as a cause of benign intracranial hypertension has been recognized years back.[23] It is most commonly seen in young females. Although the underlying mechanism is unknown it has been proposed that the tissue hypoxia leads to increased capillary permeability and development of brain edema or abnormalities in cerebrovascular hemodynamics that increase the cerebral blood flow, leading to increased intracranial pressure. Depletion of iron containing enzymes also may contribute to the development of cerebral edema. Benign hypertension due to ID is reversible with iron supplementation.[25]

Cranial Nerve Palsy

Another neurologic abnormality observed with IDA is bilateral cranial nerve VI palsy. This is supposed to be a consequence of increased intracranial pressure or focal pontine ischemia.

Hearing Problem

Auditory evoked brain stem response is found to be prolonged in ID children. It may be due to impaired myelin synthesis.[26] ID has also been hypothesized to be a cause of sensorineural hearing loss in the rat model. It is proposed that decreased iron-dependent enzyme activity in the cochlea, decreased spiral ganglion cells, and changes in stereocilia function result in hearing loss. Sun AH, et al. demonstrated that 10% of ID rats had moderate to profound sensorineural hearing loss.[27]

In humans, auditory brainstem-evoked response was measured in 5.5-6 month-old infants of which 29 had marginal iron deficiency.[26] Central conduction was delayed in the ID group.

Algarin demonstrated impaired visual evoked potential in ID children.[27]

Attention-deficit Hyperactivity Disorder

Attention-deficit hyperactivity disorder (ADHD) may be associated with ID. Serum ferritin levels were inversely correlated with the severity of ADHD. The children with the most severe iron deficiency were the most inattentive, impulsive, and hyperactive. Low iron stores may explain as much as 30% of ADHD severity.[28] Iron supplementation has been reported incidentally to decrease the cognitive deficiency in children with ADHD, decreasing the need for psychostimulants.

ADHD possibly modulated by the dopaminergic mesocortical pathways, and because patients with ADHD have increased dopamine transporter-binding potential and genetic polymorphisms in the dopamine receptor. It has been suggested that the symptoms of ADHD may be caused by dopamine dysfunction (children with ADHD benefit from dopamine stimulants). Because iron is a coenzyme of dopamine synthesis and iron deficiency alters dopamine receptor density and activity, brain iron stores may influence dopamine-dependent functions.

Restless Legs Syndrome

Iron deficiency in the central nervous system is known to cause motor impairment and periodic limb movement in the sleep. Restless legs syndrome (RLS) is frequently associated with low serum iron and a tendency toward low serum ferritin levels. Treatment with iron is associated with clinical improvement in most of these patients. Recent work shows that blood-brain barrier epithelial cells in persons with RLS have decreased iron stores, suggesting that there is insufficient availability of iron to meet the dynamic circadian iron requirements.[29]

Abnormal dopamine metabolism is a possible link between ID and each of these pathological conditions—BHS, RLS, and ADHD. Iron is a cofactor in catecholamine metabolism and in dopamine synthesis through tyrosine hydroxylase, the rate-limiting enzyme for catecholamine neurotransmitter synthesis.[30] Therefore, deficiency of iron would reduce dopamine synthesis and could exacerbate a variety of common clinical states.

Febrile Seizure

Children with febrile seizures were almost twice as likely to be iron deficient as those with febrile illness alone. The screening for ID should be considered in children presenting with febrile seizure.[31] In a study conducted by Daud, et al. also showed there is significant association between ID and febrile seizure.[32]

In a retrospective case control study of 361 children who presented to an emergency department with febrile seizures, compared to a control group of 390 children who presented with fever only, those with febrile seizures were almost twice as likely to be iron deficient.[33]

Reasons for this increased febrile seizure susceptibility are unclear. There is no established connection between dopaminergic systems and febrile seizures per se. Dopamine can modulate neuronal excitability in either direction-excitatory or inhibitory-depending on the specific neural circuit, cell type, and brain region.[34] The correlation between ID and febrile seizures might be secondary to a nonspecific alteration of cortical excitability, particularly in the setting of age-dependent fever, since there is no known predilection to seizures in iron deficient older individuals.

Other Neurological Manifestations

Iron is also critical for a many other biological functions including muscle metabolism, sleep regulation, heat production, catecholamine metabolism, immune function, pain perception, thermoregulation, circadian cycles, altered behavioral inhibition and abnormal responses to reward.[35,36]

CONCLUSION

Iron has important role in normal brain development, myelination, and neurotransmitter production. ID during gestation and lactation results in abnormalities in brain iron that are irreversible. So we have to prevent iron deficiency in women of childbearing age, during gestation, and throughout infancy and childhood.

Iron deficiency is rarely considered as a primary etiology in frequently observed pediatric neurologic disease, even though IDA is a very common problem in resource-poor countries like India. The developmental sequelae and other neurologic abnormalities caused by iron deficiency, are costly to society and devastating to those affected. With appropriate recognition and treatment the neurologic sequelae of iron deficiency are entirely preventable and reversible.

> **KEY LEARNING POINTS**
>
> - Iron deficiency may present with various neurological manifestations.
> - Identification of iron deficiency as part of the differential diagnosis in neurological disorders is uncommon and frequently goes untreated.
> - In conditions like cognitive impairment, breath holding spell and ADHD, underlying anemia should be corrected before costly treatment.
> - Iron deficiency anemia is a late manifestation of iron deficiency and neurological dysfunction may manifest earlier but go unrecognized.
> - Since neurological dysfunction due to chronic iron deficiency is often irreversible, so early recognition and prevention are important.
> - Strategies aimed at prevention of iron deficiency include taking food rich in iron, periodic deworming, iron supplementation in school and food fortification.

REFERENCES

1. *National Family Health Survey-3, India*: 2005-2006. Available at: http://rchiips.org/nfhs/nfhs3.shtml Accessed on: 19 January 2018.
2. Connor JR, Fine RE. Development of transferrin-positive oligodendrocytes in the rat central nervous system. *J Neurosci Res* 1987;17:51-59.
3. Dwork AJ, Lawler G, Zybert PA, et al. An autoradiographic study of the uptake and distribution of iron by the brain of the young rat. *Brain Res* 1990;518:31-39.
4. Beard JL. Iron deficiency and neural development: An update. *Arch Latinosam Nutr* 1999; 49:34S-39S.
5. Hill JM, Switzer RC. The regional distribution and cellular localization of iron in the rat brain. *Neuroscience* 1984;11:595-603.

6. Barkai AI, Durkin M, Dwork AJ, Nelson HD. Autoradiographic study of iron-binding sites in the rat brain: Distribution and relationship to aging. *J Neurosci Res* 1991;29:390-395.
7. Beard JL, Connor JD, Jones BC. Brain iron: Location and function. *Prog Food Nutr Sci* 1993;17:183-221.
8. Gerber MR, Connor JR. Do oligodendrocytes mediate iron regulation in the human brain? *Neurology* 1989;26:95-98.
9. Yu GSM, Steinkirchner TM, Rao GA, Larkin EC. Effect of prenatal iron deficiency on myelination in rat pups. *Am J Pathol* 1986;125:620-624.
10. Taneja V, Mishra K, Agarwal KN. Effect of early iron deficiency in rat on the gamma-aminobutyric acid shunt in brain. *J Neurochem* 1986;46:1670-1674.
11. Taneja V, Mishra KP, Agarwal KN. Effect of maternal iron deficiency on GABA shunt pathway of developing rat brain. *Indan J Exp Bio* 1990;28:466-469.
12. Sungthong R, Mo-suwan L, Chongsuvivatwong V. Effects of haemoglobin and serum ferritin on cognitive function in school children. *Asia Pac J Clin Nutr* 2002;11:117-121.
13. Halterman JS, Kaczorowski JM, Aligne CA, Auinger P, Szilagyi PG. Iron deficiency and cognitive achievement among school-aged children and adolescents in the United States. *Pediatrics* 2001;107:1381-1386.
14. Logan S, Martins S, Gilbert R. Iron therapy for improving psychomotor development and cognitive function in children under the age of three with iron deficiency anaemia. *Cochrane Database Syst Rev* 2001;(2):CD001444.
15. Lozoff B, Jimenez E, Wolf AW. Long-term developmental outcome of infants with iron deficiency. *N Engl J Med* 1991;325:687-694.
16. Stoltzfus RJ, Kvalsvig JD, Chwaya HM, et al. Effects of iron supplementation and anti-helmintic treatment on motor and language development of preschool children in Zanzibar: Double blind placebo controlled study. *BMJ* 2001;323:1389-1395
17. Lozoff B, Wolf AW, Jimenez E. Iron-deficiency anemia and infant development: Effects of extended oral iron therapy. *J Pediatr* 1996;129:382-389.
18. Walter T, De Andraca I, Chadud P, Perales CG. Iron deficiency anemia: Adverse effects on infant psychomotor development. *Pediatrics* 1989;84:7-17.
19. Lozoff B, Klein NK, Nelson EC, et al. Behavior of infants with iron-deficiency anemia. *Child Dev* 1998;69:24-36.
20. Deinard AS, List A, Lindgren B, Hunt JV, Chang PN. Cognitive deficits in iron-deficient and iron-deficient anemic children. *J Pediatr* 1986;108:681-689.
21. Belman AL, Rouque CT, Ancona R, et al. Cerebral venous thrombosis in a child with iron deficiency anemia and thrombocytosis. *Stroke* 1990;214-218.
22. Bruggers CS, Ware R, Altman AJ, et al. Reversible focal neurological deficits in severe iron deficiency anemia *J Pediatr* 1990;117:430.
23. Yager JY, Hartfield DS. Neurologic manifestations of iron deficiency in childhood. *Pediatr Neurol* 2002;27:85-89.
24. Daoud AS, Batieha A, Al-sheyyab M, et al. Effectiveness of iron therapy on breath-holding spells. *J Pediatr* 1997;130:547-556.
25. Tugal O, Jacobson R, Berezin S, et al. Recurrent benign intracranial hypertension due to iron deficiency anemia: Case report and review of literature. *Am J Pediatr hematol Oncol* 1994;16:266-272.
26. Roncagliolo M, Garrido M, Walter, et. al. Evidence of altered central nervous system development in infants with iron deficiency anemia at 6 month; Delayed maturation of auditory brainstem responses. *Am J Clin Nutr* 1998;68:683-689.

27. Sun AH, Wang ZM, Xiao SZ, Li ZJ, Zheng Z, et al. Sudden sensorineural hearing loss induced by experimental iron deficiency in rats. *ORL* 1992;54:246-250.
27. Algarin C, Peirano P, Garrido M, et al. Iron deficiency anemia in infancy: Long-lasting effects on auditory and visual system functioning. *Pediatr Res* 2003:53:217EE.
28. Eric K, Lecendreux MM, Isabelle A, Marie CM. Iron deficiency in children with attention-deficit/hyperactivity disorder. *Arch Pediatr Adolesc Med* 2004;158: 1113-1119.
29. Connor JR, Ponnuru P, Wang XS, et al. Profile of altered brain iron acquisition in restless legs syndrome, *Brain* 2011;134:959-968.
30. Walter T. Effect of iron-deficiency anaemia on cognitive skills in infancy and childhood. *Baillieres Clin Haem* 1994;7:815-27.
31. Alfredo, Renato S, Nicola I, et al. Iron deficiency anaemia and febrile convulsions: case-control study in children under 2 years. *BMJ* 1996;313:343.
32. Daoud AS, Batieha A, Abu-Ekteish F, Gharaibeh N, Ajlouni S. Iron status: a possible risk factor for the first febrile seizure. *Epilepsia* 2002;43:740-743.
33. Hartfield DS, Tan JY, Yager JY, et al. The association between iron deficiency and febrile seizures in childhood. *Clin Pediatr (Phila)* 2009;48:420-426.
34. Idjradinata P, Pollitt E. Reversal of developmental delays in iron-deficient anaemic infants treated with iron. *Lancet* 1993;341:1-4.
35. Lozoff B, Beard J, Connor J. Long-lasting neural and behavioral effects of iron deficiency in infancy. *Nutr Rev* 2006;34:43-59.
36. Beard JL. Iron biology in immune function, muscle metabolism and neuronal functioning. *J Nutr* 2001;131:568-579.

11. Zinc in Child Nutrition

Pushpendra Magon, Harmesh S Bains

ABSTRACT

Zinc is a micronutrient of utmost importance due to its established role in health and immunity. Being a part of several metalloenzymes, e.g. thymidine kinase, DNA polymerase, RNA polymerase, it plays a definite role in growth and differentiation and division of cells. Although severe zinc deficiency is unheard, mild-to-moderate deficiency is quite common. The potential danger of increased risk of diarrhea among zinc-deficient children prompted a global search for means to overcome deficiency like starting Zn-ORS etc. Even susceptibilities to pneumonia and malaria have been found more among moderately zinc-deficient children, thereby establishing its role in infection prevention and enhancing immunity.

Keywords: Diarrhea, Immunity, Infection, Infection prevention, Pneumonia, Zinc, Zinc deficiency, Zn-ORS.

INTRODUCTION

Zinc has been used for centuries as a healer. Initially it was used as an ointment of zinc oxide and later zinc carbonate (calamine lotion) became popular to treat sunburns and skin lesions. It is a key component of epidermis, hairs, eyes and tissues. It have been associated with spermatozoa. Its role as a membrane stabilizer and free radical scavengers, may be the key in reducing childhood illnesses and mortality thereby enhancing physical growth.

ROLE OF ZINC IN VARIOUS BODY ORGAN SYSTEMS (FIG. 1)

Zinc and Brain

Right from womb to the tomb, Zn is known to be necessary for cognition and thus supplementation during pregnancy and first 2 years of life becomes important as brain growth is at its peak during this period.[1] Zinc given to pregnant women before 26 weeks showed drastic fall in preterm birth in low income countries.[2] Zinc is vital nutrient for the brain in the synthesis of

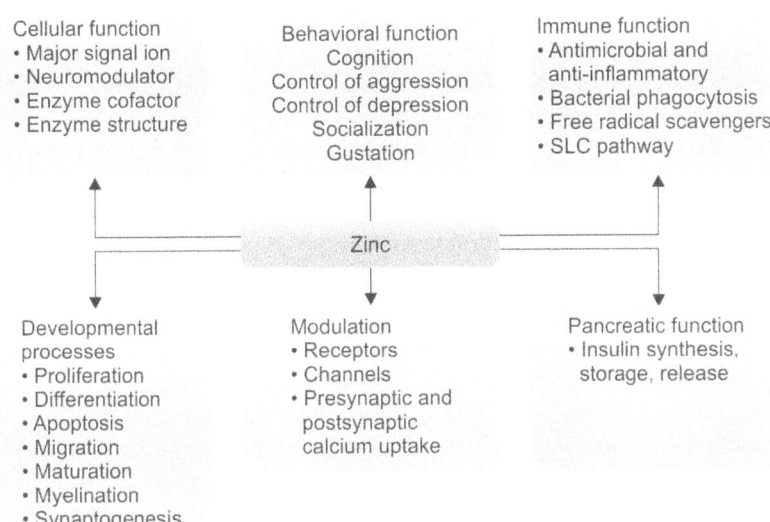

Fig. 1: Flow diagram showing zinc functions.

enzymes (RNA and DNA synthesis), being a cofactor and a catalyst.[3,4] Being a part of enzymes like hymidine kinase, DNA polymerase, RNA polymerase, it plays a definite role in growth and differentiation and division of cells. Scientists have found high levels of zinc in hippocampus, signifying its role in neurotransmission. A study conducted in infants administered with zinc/iron either alone or in combination definitely improve orientation. Absorption of zinc in small intestine through facilitated diffusion and transport via portal system attached to albumin and transferrin is almost similar to that of iron. Thus, there is competitive inhibition of each other. The levels of zinc are regulated by intestinal absorption and re-excretion, while the excess is excreted through the feces. Although supplementation appear to be a good strategy but it may lead to imbalance in copper levels as well. As it decreases the copper burden, it has been effectively used to treat Wilson disease[5] and even protect against liver injury in experimental animals.[6]

Zinc and Skin

Some genetic conditions like acrodermatitis enteropathica reveal that our body needs zinc for proper mucocutaneous differentiation, zinc uptake is a major defect in this condition.[7] Zinc uptake via intestine is a major defect. It presents as vesiculobullous dry scaly eczematous lesion in the perioral, perianal and acral area. Alopecia, conjunctivitis and photophobia may also be present.

Zinc and Infections

Frequent diarrhea and lower respiratory tract infections have been confirmed in various studies to be 4 times more common in zinc deficient children.[2,8]

Data collected showed decrease in diarrhea by 25% and significant reduction in hospitalization. Starting zinc in the national program Zn-ORS appears to be useful strategy in under five children. However, the evidence of impact on pneumonias, TB and malaria in under 5 children is insufficient.[9] A significant effect on energy was found in sickle cell patients.[10] Maternal zinc supplementation has been shown to decrease infant infections.[11] Secondly, routine zinc supplementation to low birth weight babies for one year has resulted in substantial reduction in mortality.[12]

Zinc, Stress and Wound Healing

Apart from stunting, stomatitis, irritability, slow wound healing and poor immunity are associated with zinc deficiency. Human milk contains zinc binding ligand which is not present in other milk and thus increase zinc bioavailability. Plasma zinc levels fall within hours of stress like surgery, trauma, inflammation, cancer and remains persistently low. Zinc deficient animals have impaired collagen synthesis and poor wound healing.[13]

Zinc and Hormones

Zinc has role in endocrine function. Zinc appears to influence insulin binding and degradation at the hepatocyte membrane. Some studies reveal impaired glucose tolerance associated with zinc deficiency.[14] Zinc deficiency lead to hypogonadism in males, taste abnormalities, delayed wound healing, growth, testicular function, prolactin release, thymopoetin (zinc dependent T cell maturation hormone).[15] There appears to be a complex relationship between zinc and type 1 diabetes as zinc plays a clear role in synthesis, storage and release of insulin.[14]

Zinc and Taste

Zinc has role in taste. A metalloproteins *gustin*, has been isolated from human saliva. It combines with taste buds and is essential for their optimal morphology and function.[16]

Zinc and Nephrotic Syndrome

Despite high levels of zinc intake, idiopathic nephrotic syndrome patients have zinc deficiency, which is most likely due to urinary zinc loss.[17]

Zinc and Cell Function

Zinc is a component of red blood cell enzyme (carbonic anhydrase) which is necessary for CO_2 exchange, while another zinc containing enzyme called carboxy peptidase, is necessary for hydrolysis of protein in the intestine. Deficiency of zinc is associated with disaggregation of RNA and increased ribonuclease activity[4] and ability to decrease adenyl cyclase and phosphodiesterase, thereby regulating cAMP and cGMP. It has been proposed that zinc protects from free radical oxidation.[18] Role of zinc in structural growth has been confirmed by meta-analysis of studies revealing its positive role in promotion of growth.

Zinc and Malnutrition

Serum zinc levels were found to be low in newly diagnosed and severely malnourished children with celiac disease.[19] However, plasma zinc levels cannot be used as a screening test to treat celiac disease with short stature.[20] Its association with malabsorption, chronic liver disease, diabetes and other chronic illnesses such as that zinc is vital for health.[5]

Zinc and Linear Growth

Linear growth has been shown to increase significantly following zinc supplementation especially after one year of age but some studies indicate that the increase occurs as long as zinc is continued.[21,22]

Zinc and Inflammatory Bowel Disease

Children with IBD show deficiency of zinc and selenium which act as free radical scavengers. Thereby low levels may contribute to continued inflammatory process.[18]

Dietary sources of zinc include meat, fish, cereals, almonds, watermelon seeds, pumpkin seeds, vegetables, etc.

Factors that decrease the absorption of zinc include: phytates, calcium, fiber, cellulose and phosphate.

CLINICAL FEATURES

Table 1 erlist the clinical features of zinc deficiency.

Table 1: Clinical features of zinc deficiency.

A	Acrodermatitis enteropathica Anorexia Acral dermatitis
B	Behavioral changes Blindness Birth defects like neural tube defects
C	Connective tissue defects like hypermobility of joints
D	Deficiencies like iron deficiency Dwarfism
E	Eczema Eye problems like glaucoma, cataract, nystagmus, photophobia, blepharitis
F	Fundal changes—retinal detachment
G	Growth disorders—short stature, delayed puberty
H	Hepatosplenomegaly Hyperkeratosis

DIAGNOSIS

a. Dietary history
b. Diarrhea history
c. Clinical features like dry scaly skin lesion, blepharitis, conjunctivitis, poor wound healing and diarrhea
d. Low zinc levels in plasma and hair.
   Reference values.
   0–10 years: 0.60–1.20 µg/mL
   >or = 11 years: 0.66–1.10 µg/mL

INTERPRETATION

Normal serum zinc is 0.66 to 1.10 µg/mL.

Burn patients with acrodermatitis may have zinc as low as 0.4 µg/mL; these patients respond quickly to zinc supplementation.

Normal daily requirement of zinc ranges between 3.5–5 mg/day.

MANAGEMENT

Recommended daily intake of zinc:
- Age < 4 years—3 mg/day
- 4–8 years—5 mg/day
- 9–13 years—8 mg/day

However, deficient states are treated with 0.5–1 mg/kg/day.

Malabsorption syndromes like celiac disease, liver disease, and children on ethambutol and vegetarians/vegans are at high risk of zinc deficiency. Doses >50 mg/kg may be rarely needed in acute deficiencies due to malnutrition. However >50 mg/kg dose may lead to nausea, abdominal discomfort and diarrhea. Doses >150 mg/kg may be toxic to the children.

Formulations available include zinc sulfate, zinc aspartate, zinc orotate, zinc gluconate, zinc oxide. However, zinc oxide has least absorption. In acrodrematitis enteropathica, doses are needed for life orally because zinc is required for enzymatic function. Parenteral zinc may be necessary only in prolonged parenteral nutrition or intestinal failure.

CONCLUSION

Zinc, a membrane stabilizer and free radical scavenger, has gained importance in human nutrition after 1960s. Sources of zinc include meat, fish, cereals, almonds, watermelon seeds, pumpkin seeds. Recommended daily intake of zinc: 3–8 mg/day depending upon age. Deficiency predisposes to dermatologic problems, respiratory problems, slow wound healing, poor immunity, persistent diarrhea, growth retardation. Children with IBD show deficiency of zinc. Deficient states are treated with 0.5–1 mg/kg/day of zinc.

> **KEY LEARNING POINTS**
>
> ¤ Zinc is a membrane stabilizer, free radical scavenger and vital nutrient for the brain.
> ¤ Zinc levels are regulated by intestinal absorption and re-excretion; excess is excreted through the feces.
> ¤ Supplementation appear to be a good strategy but it may lead to imbalance in copper.
> ¤ Zinc deficiency predisposes to disorders of mucocutaneous, frequent diarrhea, lower respiratory tract infections, slow wound healing and poor immunity, poor synthesis, storage and release of insulin, poor linear growth. Children with IBD show deficiency of zinc.
> ¤ Sources of zinc include meat, fish, cereals, almonds, watermelon seeds, pumpkin seeds.
> ¤ Recommended daily intake of zinc: 3–8 mg/day depending upon age.
> ¤ Deficient states are treated with 0.5–1 mg/kg/day.

REFERENCES

1. Black MM. The evidence linking zinc deficiency with children's cognitive and motor functioning. *J Nutr* 2003;133(suppl):1473S-1476S.
2. Sazawal S, Black RE, Bhan MK, Bhandari N, Sinha A, Jalla S. Zinc supplementation in young children with acute diarrhea in India. *N Eng J Med* 1995;338:839-844. [PubMed]
3. Prasad AS. Zinc and enzymes. In: Prasad AS (Ed): *Biochemistry of Zinc*. New York: Plenum Press 1993: 17-53.
4. Prasad AS. Zinc and gene expression. In: Prasad AS (Ed): *Biochemistry of Zinc*. New York: Plenum Press 1993: 55-76.
5. Prasad AS. Clinical spectrum of human zinc deficiency. In: Prasad AS (Ed): *Biochemistry of Zinc*. New York: Plenum Press 1993:219-258.
6. Stamoulis I, Kouraklis G, Theocharis S. Zinc and the liver: An active interaction. *Dig Dis Sci* 2007;52:1595-1612.
7. Ackland ML, Michalczyk A. Zinc deficiency and its inherited disorders—a review. *Genes Nutr* 2006;1:41-49.
8. Sandstead HH, Penland JG, Alcock NW, Dayal HH, Chen XC, Li JS, et al. Effects of repletion with zinc and other micronutrients on neuropsychologic performance and growth of Chinese children. *Am J Clin Nutr* 1998;68(2 suppl):S470-S475. [PubMed]
9. Haider BA, Bhutta ZA. The effect of therapeutic zinc supplementation among young children with selected infections: A review of the evidence. *Food Nutr Bull* 2009;30 (1 suppl):S41-S59.
10. Haider BA, Bhutta ZA. The effect of therapeutic zinc supplementation among young children with selected infections: a review of the evidence. *Food Nutr Bull* 2009;30(1 suppl):S41-S59.
11. Fischer Walker C, Black RE. Zinc and the risk for infectious disease. *Annu Rev Nutr* 2004;24:255-275.
12. Bhatnagar S, Natchu UC. Zinc in child health and disease. *Indian J Pediatr* 2004;71:991-995.
13. Scholl D, Langkamp-Henken B. Nutrient recommendations for wound healing. *J Intraven Nurs* 2001;24:124-132.
14. Chausmer AB. Zinc, insulin and diabetes. *J Am Coll Nut* 1998;17:109-115.

15. Prasad AS. Clinical, endocrinological and biochemical effects of zinc deficiency. *ClinEndocrinol Metab* 1985;14:567-589.
16. Yagi T, Asakawa A, Ueda H, et al. The role of zinc in the treatment of taste disorders. *Recent Pat Food Nutr Agric* 2013;5:44-51.
17. Perrone L, Gialanella G, Giordano V, et al. Impaired zinc metabolic status in children affected by idiopathic nephrotic syndrome. *Eur J Pediatr.* 1990;149:438-440.
18. Ojuawo A, Keith L. The serum concentrations of zinc, copper and selenium in children with inflammatory bowel disease. *Cent Afr J Med* 2002;48:116-119.
19. Singhal N, Alam S, Sherwani R, et al. Serum zinc levels in celiac disease. *Indian Pediatr* 2008;45:319-321.
20. Altuntas B, Filik B, Ensari A, et al. Can zinc deficiency be used as a marker for the diagnosis of celiac disease in Turkish children with short stature? *Pediatr Int* 2000;42:682-684.
21. Prasad AS. Zinc deficiency. *BMJ* 2003;326:409-410.
22. Sayeg Porto MA, Oliveira HP, Cunha AJ, et al. Linear growth and zinc supplementation in children with short stature. *J Pediatr Endocrinol Metab* 2000;13:1121-1128.

PART 4: NUTRITION IN DIFFERENT PEDIATRIC AGE GROUPS

12 Antenatal Nutrition: Effect on Fetal and Neonatal Outcome

Rashmi Dwivedi

ABSTRACT

Knowledge regarding optimum nutrition during antenatal period is of utmost importance. Together with genes, the main determinant of fetal growth is the availability of nutrients reaching the fetus through umbilical vein and through placenta. The nutrient composition in maternal blood depends on various maternal factors like diet during antenatal period, body composition, endocrine status, and metabolism. The importance of iron, folic acid, calcium, iodine and energy during antenatal period for maternal health and fetal development has been well documented. Adverse effects of their deficiency are also known. Other nutrients that have recently been studied for their effect on fetal and neonatal outcome are vitamins D, B_6 and B_{12}, and zinc. It has also been shown that not only the pre-pregnancy weight is important determinant of fetal growth and neonatal outcome but the BMI also is a predictor of fetal growth and neonatal outcome. As a pediatrician, we need to be aware about the various components for a healthy and balanced diet during antenatal period for positive fetal growth and development and a healthy newborn. Deficiencies of Iron, folic acid, iodine and B group of vitamins have long-term effect even beyond the neonatal period.

Keywords: Anemia, Antenatal nutrition, Balanced diet, Fetal growth, Gestational weight, Macronutrients, Micronutrients, Minerals, Nutrition, Trace elements, Vitamins.

INTRODUCTION

Nutrition during pregnancy (Fig. 1) plays a crucial role in influencing maternal, neonatal and child health and outcome in terms of maternal morbidity and mortality, fetal growth and development, LBW or premature delivery and stunting in childhood. To reach the minimal developmental goals (MDGs) target of 109 for stunting rates in children, improving the nutritional status of women is of crucial importance but has remained a low priority.[1]

The relationship of women's nutrition with birth outcomes and stunting rates in young children is well established. All 3 National Family Health Survey (NFHS) data and CES 2009 have shown that percentage of women with low BMI has remained almost stagnant in last two decades despite improvement in maternal health services.[2-4] According to NHFS 2 (1998-99)

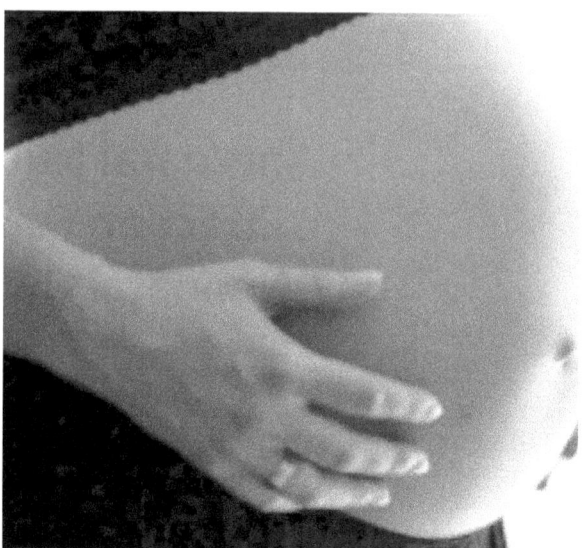

Fig. 1: Nutrition during pregnancy has a critical influence on the growth of the fetus as well as subsequent growth after birth.

and NHFS 3 (2006) data 13 Indian states have higher percentage of mothers with low BMI compared to national average of 35.6%.[3,4] The prevalence rates of under-nutrition was higher in rural areas compared to urban areas (40.6% v/s 25%). According to NHFS- 4 data proportion of women with BMI 18.5 kg/m² has reduced to 22.9% compared to 35.5% in NHFS-3.[5] It has also shown that rural women are more under nourished (26.7%) compared to urban (15.5%). According to UNICEF data also one third of women in reproductive age in India are undernourished with a BMI of <18.5 kg/m² whereas ideally it should be 20-23.[6] Maternal malnutrition/undernutrition leads to intrauterine growth restriction (IUGR) and low birthweight (LBW).[7] Timing of a nutritional insult impacts differently on the nature of adult disease by programming postnatal physiology indicating that early environment modified the genomic expression. Nutrition has its strongest regulatory effect during early life while growth hormone plays an important role during pregnancy.

PHYSIOLOGICAL CHANGES DURING PREGNANCY

Basal metabolic rate: Fetal growth and development increase the BMR by almost 5% during first trimester and 12% during second and third trimester. This increases the total energy requirement.

Gastrointestinal changes: This results in feeling of nausea, vomiting in early pregnancy and constipation in last trimester. Absorption of nutrients like vitamin B_{12}, iron and calcium increases in order to meet the increased maternal and fetal demands.

Changes in body fluids: Blood volume increases leading to lowered concentration of plasma proteins, hemoglobin and other blood constituents.

NUTRITION: COMPONENTS AND ROLE[8]

The prenatal diet should, therefore, include:
- **Macronutrients** (proteins, carbohydrate and fats)
- **Vitamins and minerals** to provide fuel for the body and helps in fetal growth and development.
- **Adequate fluids** for keeping them well hydrated as dehydration can lead to miscarriage and premature labor.
- **Fiber** is also important part of the diet as it helps to keep the bowels regular and prevents constipation.

Pregnancy leads to a modest increase in energy requirements. Additional 350 kcal/day on an average needs to be provided for women weighing 50 kg with sedentary lifestyle. Additional energy is required for:
1. Growth of fetus
2. Development of placenta and maternal tissues
3. To meet the increased BMR
4. To deposit fat which will be used for energy to support lactation and breastfeeding.

Carbohydrates should supply 40 to 50% of needed energy during pregnancy. Dietary carbohydrates are broken into glucose molecules. Rapid growth of fetus requires ample amount of energy in the form of glucose to be available.

Protein requirements also increase to:
1. Support growth of fetus.
2. Blood volume increase, protein is required for plasma.
3. Maternal tissues also require additional protein as they increase
4. For amniotic fluid formation
5. Provides basic building block necessary for the formation of enzymes, antibodies, muscle and collagen. Collagen is used as framework for skin, bones, blood vessels and other body tissues.

Additional 15 g is required during second and third trimester.

Lipids and fats, including sterols, phospholipids and triglycerides (which are primarily made up of fatty acids) are also basic building material for body tissue and integral to body functioning. They are essential for the formation of cell membranes and hormones. They are also source of calories. Around 20–35% of caloric requirement should be derived from fats.

Essential fathy acid (EFA): Linoleic acid (omega 6) and linolenic acid 9 (omega 3) are necessary for brain and visual development. They also play a key role as precursors of hormone-like *Eicosanoids* which acts as a signal for number of local reactions in body necessary for basic functioning such as muscle relaxation, blood vessel constriction, inflammatory response to injury and infection, etc.

Omega 3 fatty acid deficiency has also been linked to lower IQ scores in infants, lower visual acuity and increased risk of depression in adults. It is also suspected to be one potential reason for increased risk of cardiovascular disease. Adequate intake of EFA is 13 g/day of omega 6 and 1.4 g of omega 3, ensuring a ratio of not more than 5:1.

EFA has the following role in pregnancy:
1. Brain development in the fetus
2. Essential for visual development of the fetus
3. Prevents preterm labor
4. Reduces incidence of heart disease and related deaths in infants.

Choline a component of phospholipids is needed for lecithin synthesis which is an essential component of cell membrane and essential component of brain and nervous system, hence during fetal development it supports the function of brain and spinal cord. Choline is also necessary to make acetylcholine.

To meet the increase in energy requirements, the proportion of energy should be as follows: Fats—20-35%, proteins—15-20% and carbohydrates—40-50%. It has become clear in recent years that diet plays an important role not only during pregnancy but also during pre-pregnancy period (including adolescent and periconceptional period).

NUTRITION AND RELATION TO BODY COMPOSITION

Cetin and Cardellichio[9] have categorically stated that pre-gravidic weight is an important factor influencing fetal and pregnancy outcome.

BMI is one of the best indices for assessment of adult nutrition status. WHO classification of nutrition status based on BMI is as follows:[10]
- 25-29.9: Overweight
- >30: Obesity
- <19.8: Undernutrition

Maternal obesity is associated with increased risk for mother as well as newborn for pregnancy related complications like preeclampsia, gestational diabetes, cesarean section and macrosomia, etc. Obese women have lower insulin sensitivity. Hence, increased amount of substrates are available for placental transfer causing fetal overgrowth.

Maternal undernutrition is associated with increased risk of preterm labor, IUGR, LBW and maternal anemia.

Gestational weight gain is a strong predictor of infant outcomes at birth as it is directly associated with intrauterine growth. Very high or very low weight gains are associated with increased risks of preterm birth and infant deaths. In an attempt to optimize both maternal and neonatal outcomes in 2009, the *United States Institute of Medicine (IOM)* revised gestational weight gain guidelines based on BMI are as per Table 1.[1]

Table 1: Recommended weight gain in relation to BMI during pregnancy.

BMI (kg/m²)	Weight gain (kg)
<19.8 (low)	12.5–18
19.8–26 (normal)	11.5–16
>26–29 (high)	7–11.5 g
> 29 (obese)	5–9

Note: Calculations assume a weight gain of 0.5–2 kg in the first trimester.

MICRONUTRIENTS: ROLE IN ANTENATAL NUTRITION AND RECOMMENDED DIETARY ALLOWANCES

Macronutrients, i.e. carbohydrates, proteins and fats are source of calories or energy. These are so named as they are required in relatively large amounts for growth, development and repair.

Micronutrients, i.e. vitamins, some minerals and trace elements are needed in small quantities compared to macronutrients. They are crucial in order to maintain energy levels, metabolism, cellular function, physical and mental well-being. Micronutrients are fuel for protection just as macronutrients are fuel for growth and development and to support metabolic activities. Vitamins and minerals support every stage of maternal, placental and fetal interaction.

Micronutrients needing most attention in pregnancy and commonly provided as supplements are vitamins A, D, E, folate, B_{12}, B_6 and C, iron, zinc, iodine, copper and selenium. Moreover, other B-complex vitamins like niacin, riboflavin, thiamine are nearly always included though their exact metabolic roles are less well specified. UNICEF/WHO have identified 15 micronutrients for supplementation in pregnant women. These are: Folic acid—400 µg, Iron —30 mgm, Zinc—15 mg, Copper—2 mg, Selenium—65 µg, Vitamin A—800 µg, Vitamin D—200 IU, Vitamin E—10 mg, Vitamin C—70 mg, Vitamin B_1—1.4 mg, Vitamin B_2—1.4 mg, Vitamin B_6—1.9 mg, Vitamin B_{12}—2.6 µg, Niacin—18 mg, Iodine—150 µg.[12]

Iron and Folic Acid

In a study on "prevalence and consequences of anemia in pregnancy", Kalaivani[13] comments that prevalence of anemia in India is 65–75% which is amongst the highest in the world across all socioeconomic strata. According to NFHS-4 data, anemia in pregnant women age 15–49 years was found to be 50.3% as compared to 57.9% in NHFS-3.[5] WHO estimates that even among the South Asian countries, India has the highest prevalence of anemia, about half of global maternal deaths due to anemia occur in South Asian countries and India contributes to about 80%.[14] The most common factor responsible for this high prevalence is iron deficiency followed by folate deficiency. Recently contribution of vitamin B_{12} also has been highlighted.

Iron: Vital for fetal growth and development. It plays a key role as a cofactor for enzymes involved in oxidative-reduction reactions.
- Essential for normal neurodevelopment during fetal and early childhood development.
- Fetal iron stores are meant to last least until 6 months of age.
- Essential for maternal tissues including RBC mass.
- Maintain additional iron content of placenta.
- Compensate blood loss during delivery.

Folate: Available in its synthetic form as folic acid. It is used to manufacture neurotransmitters, neural tube closure and DNA synthesis in the cells.

Box 1 lists the consequences of maternal anemia.

Box 1: Consequences of maternal anemia.

- Decreased work capacity.
- Women with moderate anemia (<8 g/dL) have higher morbidity rates, more prone to infections and recovery from infections may be prolonged.
- Anemia in pregnancy also leads to low birth weight and premature delivery in neonates and is associated with high-risk of maternal mortality due to APH/PPH. It is also associated with increased risk of pregnancy induced hypertension and sepsis.

WHO suggested scheme for IFA supplementation in pregnant women is as follows:[16]

- Composition: 30–60 mg of elemental iron + 400 μg (0.4 mg) folic acid
- Frequency: One supplement/day
- Duration: Throughout pregnancy

A daily dose of 60 mg of elemental iron should be given in moderate to severe case of anemia. If anemia is diagnosed in clinical settings it should be treated with 120 mg of elemental iron till hemoglobin value reaches normal level.

Folic acid requirements are increased in pregnancy due to rapidly dividing cells and elevated urinary losses. To prevent neural tube defects folic acid needs to be started in periconceptional period as neural tube closes by 4th week of gestation, when pregnancy may not have been detected.

As per National Iron Plus Initiative for Anemia Control, pregnant and lactating women are given 100 mg of elemental iron and 500 μg of folic acid/day for 100 days starting after the first trimester, at 14–16 weeks gestation, to be repeated for 100 days postpartum.[17] The NFHS-4 survey shows that only 30.3% pregnant women consume IFA for 100 days or more with only 25.9% rural women taking the 100 days IFA compared to 40.8%.[5]

Table 2 summarizes the WHO and Government of India (GOI) recommendations.[16]

According to the UNICEF, one-third of women of reproductive age in India are undernourished with a BMI of <18.5 kg/m².

Vitamin B_{12}

Also called cyanocobalamine, vitamin B_{12} is essential for RBC production, manufacturing of genetic material and healthy functioning of nervous system. Its deficiency can result in anemia, neurologic damage, increased risk of birth

Table 2: Summary of recommendations by WHO and GOI.[16]

	Prophylaxis	Treatment
WHO	60 mg/day iron+ 400 μg folic acid till term	120 mg iron + 400 μg folic acid
GOI	100 mg/day iron+ 500 μg of folic acid for 6 months	Mild—2 IFA tablet/day for 100 days
		Moderate—IM iron therapy + oral folic acid

defects and and of preterm delivery. Since its dietary sources are animal, its deficiency is quite common in vegetarians.

Table 3 gives the RDA and role of other vitamins in antenatal period.

MINERALS AND OTHER VITAMINS

Calcium

In a multicentric trial conducted by the WHO in developing countries where calcium intake is low, shows significant reduction in the risk of severe gestational hypertension, eclampsia and neonatal mortality.[18] The risk of preterm delivery is also reduced significantly among younger woman (<20 years).

An Indian study has also shown beneficial effect of supplementation in reducing risk of preeclampsia, hypertension and preterm delivery. This study was carried out in nulliparous women with calcium intake less than 300 mg/day supplemented with 2 g/day.[19]

Considering the poor dietary calcium intake among pregnant and lactating women in India, high prevalence of hypertensive disorders in pregnancy and to maintain uniformity of dosage of maternal calcium supplementation across India, have emerged the *National Guideline and Calcium Supplementation* in 2014. Accordingly, all pregnant and lactating women should be informed and counseled to take calcium rich foods.[20] The recommendation is to take one glass of milk/one cup of curd everyday and include green leafy vegetables (GLVs) in diet.

The recommendation is for oral swallowable calcium tablets twice a day (total 1 g/day) from 14 weeks of pregnancy and continued up to 6 months postpartum. One tablet with morning/afternoon meal and second with evening/night meal. It has been cautioned that >800 mg calcium interferes with iron absorption. Hence, simultaneous administration should be avoided. Furthermore, calcium should not be taken on empty stomach as it causes gastritis.

Table 3: RDA and role of other vitamins in antenatal period.

Vitamin	RDA	Function
A	600 µg of retinol/day	Helps in boosting immunity, infection prevention, reduces morbidity and mortality
C	60 mg/day	Increases iron absorption, helps fetus to grow
B_6	2.5 mg/day	Helps fetal development and positive outcome
B_1 and B_2	+ 0.2 mg/day	With increase in total energy requirement, increase, so does the requirement of these vitamins also increase
Niacin	17 µg	
Riboflavin	1.6 µg	
Vitamin D	10 µg	
Vitamin E	10 µg	

Each calcium tablet should have 500 mg elemental calcium and 250 IU vitamin D3. The preferred calcium salt is calcium carbonate.

Phosphorus

During pregnancy, requirement of phosphorus is around 1,200 mg/day. The mother can easily get all the phosphorus she needs from a well-balanced diet (eventhough most prenatal vitamins do not contain phosphorus). A one cup of yogurt provides nearly half of the woman's phosphorus for the day. Deficiency manifestations include weakness, anemia, loss of appetite, and loss of bone mass.

Magnesium

Magnesium requirement in pregnancy is 320 mg daily. A cofactor in <300 enzymes in the body, its deficiency is associated with increased risk of miscarriage, fetal growth retardation, maternal hospitalization and preterm delivery.[21] Its deficiency has also been associated as a risk factor for gestational and type 2 diabetes. In neonates there is an increased risk of sudden infant death syndrome (SID).

Therapeutic IV magnesium is used to treat preeclampsia. It may also prevent leg cramps.

Vitamin D

Vitamin D deficiency in pregnant women is common (5-50%). Vitamin D is required for skeleton calcification in fetus which happens in last trimester. This increases the demand of calcium in pregnancy. Deficiency of vitamin D during pregnancy is linked to preeclampsia, Gestational diabetes mellitus, preterm labor and increased risk of C-Section. Vitamin D deficiency, defined as 25(OH)D levels <30 nmol/L is 60% in India.[22]

In full term infants maternal Vitamin D deficiency causes impaired fetal bone ossification and subtle fetal bone abnormalities like shorter knee-heel length, LBW and high-risk of SGA.

Defining vitamin D levels in pregnancy: Vitamin D researchers recommend that serum 25(OH)D concentration should be at least 30 ng/mL to provide optimal healthy outcomes. The correlation between vitamin D levels and intestinal absorption, maximal PTH suppression, bone fracture prevention and bone turnover has been established and indicate that levels >32 ng/mL are required. Vitamin D levels of >30 ng/mL may help to prevent asthma/recurrent wheeze in first 3 years of [23,24] low maternal vitamin D levels (10-32 ng/mL) is a significant predictor of NEC in preterms, correlating to bone loss and subclinical myopathy.[25] With levels <10 ng/mL there is increased risk of preeclampsia, calcium malabsorption, bone loss, poor weight gain, myopathy, higher parathyroid hormone, SGA, neonatal hypocalcemia and hypocalcemic seizures, infantile heart failure, enamel defects, large fontanels, rickets of infancy and reduced BMI.

Table 4: Varying recommendations on RDA of vitamin D in pregnancy.

Source	Recommendation
NICE Guidelines (UK)	400 IU
IOM	600 IU
Endocrine society	1500–2000 IU
Canadian Pediatric Society	2000 IU
American Congress of Obstetric and Gynecology	1000–2000 IU
ICMR	1200 IU

Table 4 lists the recommendations by various agencies on RDA for vitamin D in pregnancy.

Vitamin A

Prenatal vitamin A or beta-carotene supplementation or fortification may reduce maternal mortality in vitamin A deficient mothers, although an excessive intake has been shown to be teratogenic.[25,26] Adequate maternal vitamin A status is crucial for fetal lung development and maturation. Liver stores of retinol in human fetus shows a direct relation to progress in gestation and maternal retinol levels, hence supplementation after mid-pregnancy at physiological levels can improve the fetal stores and the risk of teratogenic effects. Insufficient vitamin A intake has also been associated with LBW.[2]

Dietary Antioxidants

Vitamins C and E, selenium, zinc and beta-carotene enhance the immune response and limit pathological aspects of cytokine mediated response.[28]

Poor maternal selenium status has been seen as a predisposing factor to development of preeclampsia. Selenium plays a critical role in regulating the antioxidant status through selenoproteins.

Poor maternal zinc status has been associated with poor pregnancy outcomes like fetal loss, congenital malformation, IUGR, reduced birth weight, prolonged labor and pre and post-term deliveries. It plays an important role in protein synthesis, cellular division and nucleic acid metabolism.

Oxidative stress during embryogenesis and in placenta can result in birth defects, early pregnancy failure, miscarriage and preeclampsia.[29] Dietary antioxidants seem to play a crucial role in regulating antioxidant status and prevent the adverse effect on maternal and fetal outcomes.

Iodine

Iodine is required to prevent the onset of subclinical hypothyroidism of mother and fetus during pregnancy. Maternal iodine deficiency is associated

Table 5: Dietary recommendations for women during pregnancy.

Food Group	Sources	Quantity	Total energy (Cals)	Protein (mg/day)
Group I	Rice, wheat, millets	300 mg(raw)	1035	20.4
	Oils, ghee, butter	30 g	279	0
	Jaggery/sugar	20 g	7.96	0.02
Group II	Milk/milk products	500 g	290	29.5
	Pulses/dried beans	60 g (raw)	208.8	14.7
	Nonveg	40 g	139.2	9.8
	Fish/eggs/meat	20 g	23.6	4.8
Group III	Fruits	200 g	169.5	1.65
	Vegetables	350 g	121	03
	GLV	150 g	48	3.65
	Other vegetables	120 g	22.2	1.08
	Roots and tubers	100 g	32	0.6

(*Source:* Indian Council of Medical Research. Dietary Guidelines for Indians- A Manual, 2nd edn. Hyderabad: National Institute of Nutrition; 2011)

with fetal hypothyroidism resulting in cretinism as thyroid hormone plays a critical role for normal brain development and maturation. Hypothyroidism developing in late pregnancy however does not result in severe neurological damage as in early pregnancy.[30] Higher levels of TSH were associated with a higher risk of having SGA or LBW babies. A RCT showed that a daily dose of 200 μg of iodine from 16th to 20th week of gestation in marginal iodine deficiency appeared to be effective in preventing gestational goiter without increasing the frequency of postpartum thyroiditis.

Dietary recommendations during pregnancy are given in Table 5.

Diet given is for pregnant woman weighing 50 kg and doing sedentary work (Table 6).

Special note:
1. Seasonal fruit may be included depending on availability and cost.
2. Nuts, such as cashew nuts, walnuts, almonds can help the mother meet her extra requirement for nutrients like folate, iron, calcium, MUFA and PUFA as well as providing fiber. They are nutrient dense and can be taken in moderation. A portion of energy from oils or cereals can be replaced with nuts.
3. Focus should be on eating nutrient dense foods, not empty calories which are devoid of nutrients.

Meal plan for pregnant woman is given in Table 6.
Extra allowances of nutrients during pregnancy are given in Table 7.

Table 6: Meal plan for pregnant woman weighing 50 kg and doing sedentary work.

Food group intake/day	Quantity/serving	Servings/day	Total
Cereals/grains	100 g	03	300 g raw
Pulses	30 g	02	60 g raw
Milk, milk products	250 mL	02	500 mL
GLV, roots, tubers, other vegetables	100–150 g	04	400 g
Fruits	100 g	02	200 g
Oils	30 mL	–	30 mL

Table 7: Extra allowances of nutrients during pregnancy (weight 55 kg).

Group	Energy (kcal/day)	Proteins (g/day)	Visible fat (g/day)	Calcium (mg/day)
Moderate work	2230	55.0	25	
Pregnancy	+350	+23	30	1200
Lactation	+600	+19	30	1200

Group	Riboflavin	Thiamine	Niacin	Pyridoxine	Ascorbic acid	Vitamin B_1 and B_2
Normal	1.3 mg/d	1.1 mg/d	14 mg/d	2.0 mg/d	40 mg/d	1.0 mg/d
Pregnancy	+0.3	+0.2	+2	2.5 mg/d	60 mg/d	1.2 mg/d
Lactation	+0.4	+0.3	+4	2.5 mg/d	80 mg/d	1.5 mg/d

Note: Density of ascorbic acid should at least be 20 mg /1000 kcal to increase iron absorption.
- Fiber: 40 g/2000 kcal
- Magnesium: 340 mg/day
- Selenium: 40 µg/day
- Iodine: 150 mg
- Vitamin E: 8–10 mg of tocopherol/day depending on type of oil used
- Zinc: 12 mg/day
- Vitamin A (retinol): 800 mg/day during pregnancy; 900 mg/day during lactation
- Beta-carotene: 6400 mg/day during pregnancy; 7600 mg/day during lactation
- Iron: 35 mg/day during pregnancy and 25 mg/day during lactation

(*Source:* Sesikaran B. Revised RDA for Indians. Report of Expert Group of ICMR. Hyderabad: National Institute of Nutrition, 2010)

CONCLUSION

Nutrition during pregnancy is an important determinant of maternal and fetal outcomes.

Nutritional deficiency has been linked to neonatal birth weight, development in utero, neurodevelopment and to adverse fetal and neonatal outcomes. Maternal undernutrition is associated with IUGR and LBW babies and preterm labor. Maternal obesity is associated with increased risk of preeclampsia, gestational diabetes, macrosomia and cesarean section. Omega-3 fatty acid deficiency has been linked to low IQ scores, low visual acuity and increased risk of cardiovascular disease and depression in adult life. Maternal anemia has been shown to have adverse effect on maternal and fetal health (Flowchart 1). Women with moderate anemia have higher

Flowchart 1: Maternal nutritional status: Cause and effect.

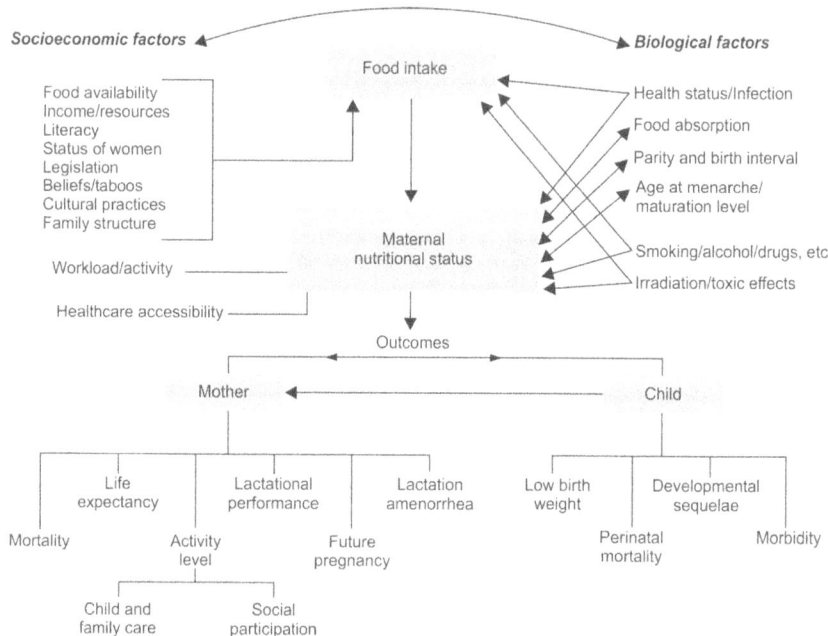

morbidity rates, more prone to infections and delayed recovery from infections. Mortality risk due to antepartum and postpartum hemorrhage, sepsis and pregnancy induced hypertension is high.

KEY LEARNING POINTS

- Both maternal undernutrition and obesity have adverse effects on fetal outcomes.
- Anemia, the most common nutritional deficiency in antenatal period carries with it the risk of premature delivery, SGA babies, and ante- and postpartum hemorrhage in mother.
- Prepregnancy BMI <18.5 is associated with poor fetal and maternal outcomes.
- Folic acid deficiency leads to neural tube defects and a combined deficiency of iron and folic acid can affect the intelligence level of the child.
- Iodine deficiency may cause neural tube defects and poor neurodevelopment.
- Vitamin D is associated with improper growth and development of bone and muscle mass as also with delayed dentition and anterior fontanels closure.
- A well-balanced diet from adolescent to antenatal period helps in reducing maternal and neonatal mortality and a healthy newborn.
- Many adult diseases like hypertension, cardiovascular problems, diabetes etc. are known to have their origin during fetal and neonatal period and to antenatal and neonatal nutrition.

REFERENCES

1. UNICEF India. Women Nutrition in India. Available at: http://unicef.in/Whatwedo/6/Women-Nutrition. Accessed on: 11 January 2018.
2. National Family Health Survey-1 Available at: *http://rchiips.org/nfhs/abt.html*. Accessed on: 12 January 2018.
3. National Family Health Survey-2. Available at: https://www.google.co.in/search?q=3.+National+Family+Health+Survey-2&rlz=1C1CHBD_en__764__764&oq=3.+National+Family+Health+Survey-2&aqs=chrome.69i57j0l2.2514j0j9&sourceid=chrome&ie=UTF-8 . Accessed on: 12 January 2018.
4. National Family Health Survey-3. Available at: http://rchiips.org/nfhs/nfhs3.shtml Accessed on: 27 December 2018.
5. National Family Health Survey-4, Available at: *http://rchiips.org/NHFS/pdf/NFHS4/India* Accessed on: 17 January 2018.
6. Government iof India/UNICEF. *Coverage Evaluation Survey 2009. All India Report, Govt: of India and & UNICEF*. Available at: http:/www.unicef.org.in/india/health. Accessed on: 17January 2018.
7. Mason JB, Saldana LS, Ramkrishnan U, et al. Opportunities for improving maternal nutrition and birthoutcomes: Synthesis of country experiences, Food Nutr Bul 2012;3 (2 Suppl 1): S104-S137.
8. Brown LS. Nutrition Requirements during pregnancy. London: Jones and Bartlett. Available at: https://publish.jblearning.com/index.php?mod=jbbrowse&act=book_details&id=402. Accessed on: 16 January 2018.
9. Cetin I, Cardechllichio M. Physiology of pregnancy. *Annals Nestle 2010; 68;7-15*
10. World Health Organization. Global database on BMI. Available at: www.who.int/bmi/index.jps?intropage. Accessed on 14 January 2018.
11. Institute of Medicine. Weight Gain During Pregnancy: Re-examining the Guidelines. Washington: National Academy Press 2009
12. Singh RB, Mishra S, et al. Micronutrient formulation for prevention of complication. *Sci Int* 2016;4:21-29.
13. Kalaivani K. Prevalence and consequences of anemia in pregnancy. *Indian J Med Res 130, 2009;* 130: *627-633*
14. World Health Organization Global Prevalence of Anemia. Geneva: WHO 2011
15. *Hemoglobin Concentration for Diagnosis of Anaemia and Assessment Of Severity.* Geneva: WHO 2011.
16. World Health Organisation. *Guideline: Daily Iron and Folic Acid Supplementation in Pregnant Women. Geneva: WHO 2012*
17. Governmernt of India. *National Iron plus initiative for Anemia Control:* NRHMP Guidelines. New Delhi: Adolescence Division, Ministry of Health and Family Welfare 2013.
18. Villar J Abdel-Aleem H, Merialdi M, Mathai M, Ali MM, et al. World Health Organisation randomised trial of calcium supplementation among low calcium intake pregnant women. *Am J ObstetGynecol* 2006;194:639-649.
19. Kumar A. Devi SG, Batra S, Singh C, Shukla DK. Calcium supplementation for prevention of pre-eclampsia. *Int J Gynecol Obstet* 2009;104:32-36
20. Government of India. *National Guideline on Calcium Supplementation*. New Delhi: Maternal Division, Ministry of Health and Family Welfare 2014
21. Markides M, Crowther CA (2002) Magnesium supplementation in pregnancy. *Cochrane Database Syst Rev* 2001;(4):CD000937.

22. Gernand AD, Schulze KJ, Stewart CP, West KP Jr, Christian P. Micronutrient deficiencies in pregnancy worldwide: health effects and prevention. *Nat Rev Endocrinol 2016;12:274-289*
23. Helene M, Wolsk MD, Benjamin J, et al. Vitamin D supplementation in pregnancy, prenatal 25(OH)D levels, race and subsequent asthma or recurrent wheeze in offspring. Secondary analysis from Vitamin D antenatal asthma reduction trial. *J Allerg* Clin *Immun* 2017 March 2009. https://www.google.co.in/search?q=prenatal+25(OH)D+levels%2C+race+and+subsequent+asthma+or+recurrent+wheeze+in+offspring.+Secondary+analysis+from+Vitamin+D+antenatal+asthma+reduction+trial.+J+Allerg+Clin+Immun+2017+March+09&rlz=1C1CHBD_en__764__764&oq=prenatal+25(OH)D+levels%2C+race+and+subsequent+asthma+or+recurrent+wheeze+in+offspring.+Secondary+analysis+from+Vitamin+D+antenatal+asthma+reduction+trial.+J+Allerg+Clin+Immun+2017+March+09&aqs=chrome..69i57.2573j0j9&sourceid=chrome&ie=UTF-8.
24. Litunjua AA, Carey VJ, Laranjo N, et al.: Effect of prenatal supplementation with vit d on asthma or recurrent wheeze in offspring by age 3years : The UDRAAT randomised clinical trial. *JAMA* 2016;315 362-370.
25. Rothman KJ, Moore LL, Singer MR. Teratogenicity of high vitamin A intake. N Engl J Med N Engl J Med 1995; 333:1369. Available at: http://www.nejm.org/doi/full/10.1056/NEJM199511233332101. Accessed on: 11 January 2018.
26. World Health Organization. *Global Prevalence Of Vitamin A Deficiency In Population at Risk 1995-2005. WHO Global Database on Vitamin A deficiency*. Geneva: WHO 2009.
27. Strobe IM. TinzJ, Biesalski HK. The importance of beta-carotene as a source of vitamin A with special reference to pregnant and breastfeeding women. *Eur J Nutr*. 2007;46 Suppl 1:I1-20.
28. Bendich A. Vitamin C, Vitamin E, Selenium & carotenoids. Washington DC .National Academy Press 2000.
29. Chappell LC, Seed PT, Briley AL, Kelly FJ, Lee R, et al. Effect of antioxidants on the occurrence of pre-eclampsia in women at increased risk.-A randomised control trial. *Lancet* 1999;354(9181):810-816.
30. World Health Organization/ Food Agriculture Oganization (WHO/FAO) *Vitamins And Mineral Requirements In Human Nutrition*. Geneva: WHO 2004. Available at: http://apps.who.int/iris/bitstream/10665/42716/1/9241546123.pdf). Accessed on 2 January 2018.

13 Infant and Young Child Feeding

Bhavana B Lakhkar

ABSTRACT

Appropriate nutrition is the right of every child. Malnutrition directly or indirectly is the cause in most under-5 deaths. Exclusive breastfeeding in first 6 months of life followed by complementary feeds with continued breastfeeding up to 2 years has been found to be the best intervention for reduction of mortality and morbidity in under fives. Breast milk is the best milk for children up to 2 years as nutritive elements in breast milk are tailor made for baby. Protective elements in breast milk protects baby from diarrhea, respiratory infections and other illnesses. Breast milk is also found to improve intelligence in children. It also is advantageous to mother. Technical aspects of breastfeeding are very important to understand as fallacies in it can lead to lactational failure due to lack of establishment of lactation. It is important to remember that in mother with HIV also, now exclusive breastfeeding is found to reduce mortality in children. Complimentary feeding is another important aspect of child nutrition. Unawareness on the part of mother may push the child towards malnutrition. After two years of age, food items should be selected very carefully as breast milk support is not there. Proper hygiene during feeding will also protect the child from infections and infestations. Growth monitoring in children up to 5 years is a reliable tool to detect malnutrition early. Immunization, nutrition and growth monitoring are the three important keys of efficient child care.

Keywords: Breastfeeding, Child care, Child nutrition, Complementary feeding, Food and child, Growth monitoring, Infant feeding, Lactation.

INTRODUCTION

Every infant and child has a right to get good nutrition according to the *Convention on the Rights of the Child*. The period during pregnancy and first 24 months of life (first 1,000 days of life) is called critical window of opportunity for prevention of malnutrition, as malnutrition is common between 3 and 24 months.[1]

Over 800,000 children's lives could be saved every year among children under 5 years, if all children between 0–23 months were optimally breastfed. The two strongest preventive measures reducing under five mortality are exclusive breastfeeding up to 6 months and complimentary feeding with breastfeeding up to one year age.[2]

India has 28% population below 15 years and out of which -80% are below 5 years. As per National Family Health Survey (NFHS)-4 around 38% of moderately stunted under five children reside in India. India has highest number of children with moderate wasting and 8% are severely wasted. This is because nutrition is one of the most neglected issues, not because food is not available but because people are ignorant about what to feed and how to feed their children. Only around 8.8% children between 6–23 months receive adequate diet.[1]

Malnutrition was found to be (directly or indirectly) the cause of 60% of under-5 deaths worldwide. More than 2/3rd of these were due to inappropriate feeding practices. Hence, it was obvious that inappropriate feeding practices and their consequences are found to be major obstacles to sustainable socioeconomic development and poverty reduction. Any efforts to accelerate economic development is not possible until optimal child growth and development is achieved through proper feeding practices.[1] India is making very slow progress in this direction hence was not able to race for millennium development goals.[3] Awareness about appropriate age specific feeding practices is very important.

COMPONENTS OF INFANT FEEDING

Infant and young child feeding has 3 important components:
a. **Feeding below 6 months:** Exclusive breastfeeding which means not even water or supplements during this period.
b. **Feeding between 6 months and 2 years:** Complimentary feeding starting after 6 completed months along with continuation of breastfeeding up to 2 years.
c. **Feeding between 2–5 years:** With or without breastfeeding. This is mainly feeding from family pot including all food groups.

FEEDING BELOW 6 MONTHS

Breast milk is the best initial food for the baby. It has been proved beyond doubt that survival is better in babies who received at least some breast milk. It is the most complete food which is tailor made for the baby. It is advantageous for baby as well as mother and is good in health or disease.

Advantages of Breast Milk to Baby

- It meets almost all nutritional needs of the baby. It has nutrients in amounts exactly needed by the baby.
- It has protective properties and protects against a large number of diseases (discussed in details below). Mortality and morbidity due to diarrhea and pneumonia are significantly less in breastfed babies.

- It helps in developing emotional bond between baby and mother, which eventually protects the baby against many behavioral and psychological illnesses.
- It improves survival and healthy development in children due to epidermal growth factors affecting brain.
- It protects baby against conditions like asthma, other allergies and lymphoma.
- It is protective against necrotizing enterocolitis (NEC) especially in preterm low birth weight babies.
- There is strong evidence that breastfeeding has modest positive effect on the intelligence of children[4]
- It provides some protection against overweight and obesity.[5]

Advantages to Mother
- It helps in uterine involution as during breastfeeding, oxytonin released from pitutary causes uterus to contract.
- Breastfeeding helps in control of uterine bleeding due to above action.
- The period of exclusive breastfeeding, can act as contraceptive method.
- It has been observed that ovarian and uterine malignancies are less common among mothers who breastfed their babies.
- It has been shown to reduce osteoporosis in mother.
- In mothers with diabetes, less insulin is required and control is better.
- Mothers who breastfeed their babies return to pre-pregnancy weight earlier.

Composition and Nutritive Value of Breast Milk

Composition of breast milk is dynamic. It changes with gestation (preterm milk and milk after term delivery), days after delivery (colostrums, transitional milk, mature milk), during feeding (foremilk and hindmilk). Composition also varies between different mothers and populations. It also changes if milk is stored in the fridge or is pasteurized.[6]

Colostrum: It is yellow color thick liquid secreted in first few days after the birth of baby. It mainly contains immunoglobin A, lactoferrin, protective leukocytes, and epidermal growth factors. Very less lactose and more immune factors are the specialty of colostrums so that it provides protection from diseases and acts as trophic feeds to prime the gut.

Transitional milk: Produced usually on 3rd day but can be delayed in mothers of preterm baby and obese mothers. It contains more lactose and less immunoglobulin. It has less sodium chloride and magnesium and more of potassium and calcium as compared to colostrums. As lactogenesis is established the amount of milk is substantial on third day.

Mature milk: Establishes by 2-4 weeks. After this, composition remains same except the differences between foremilk and hindmilk.

Foremilk: Initial milk in a particular feed. It is particularly low in fat hence is more watery.

Hindmilk: Last milk in a particular feed. It is rich in fat and provides satiety to the babies. It also contains a substance similar to benzodiazepines which is thought to be responsible for sound sleep in the baby after feed.

Nutrients in milk: Come from 3 sources, maternal diet, maternal stores and lactocytes (secretary cells in the breast). Composition remains constant even in maternal malnutrition except some vitamins and fatty acids. The composition of breast milk in comparison to cow's milk is depicted in Table 1.

Table 1: Nutrients in human (term and preterm) and cow's milk.[7,8]

S.No.	Nutrient	Mature milk	Preterm milk	Cow's milk	Remarks
1.	Proteins g/dL	0.9–1.2	1.9–2.2	3.5–4.5	Low protein provides less solute load on kidneys
2.	Casein: Whey proteins	60:40	60:40	80:20	Whey proteins—lactalbumin, lactoglobulin, lactoferrin
3.	Fats (g/dL)	3.3–3.6	4.4–4.8	3.4–4	Human milk—high content of palmitic and oleic acid, high in PUFA
4.	Lactose (g/dL)	6.7–7.8	7.5–7.6	3.5–4	Lactose is the main carbohydrate in milk. Oligosaccharide is non-nutritive
5.	Calories	65–70	70–75	65–70	
6.	Vitamin A (IU)/dL	240	240	140	
7.	Vitamin K (µg/L)	2		4	Low vitamin K in human milk—baby needs vitamin K at birth to prevent HDN
8.	Vitamin D (IU/L)	25		40–90	AAP recommends 400 IU of vitamin D starting early in life
9.	Vitamin C (mg/dL)	5.0	–	1.0	If baby is on cow's milk vitamin C supplementation is needed
10.	Iron (mg/100 mL)	0.03		0.05	Bioavailability of iron in human milk is highest of all foods
11.	Calcium (mg/dL)	33.0		118.0	High phosphorus content in cow's milk can lead to hypocalcemic convulsions in newborn
12.	Phosphorus (mg/dL)	14.0		93.0	
13.	Total ash (mg/dL)	0.2	0.2	0.7	Ash—mainly includes electrolytes. Less ash means less solute load on kidneys

(HDN: Hemorrhagic disease of newborn; PUFA: Polyunsaturated fatty acid; AAP: American Academy of Pediatrics)

Protective Elements in Breast Milk[9]

Breast milk contains a large amount of protective elements, protecting the baby from various diseases, hence mortality and morbidity is very low in these babies. Colostrum is especially rich in antibodies. Following is the list of protective elements in breast milk:

- **Secretory immunoglobulin IgA:** Protection against pathogenic organisms in gut. It has specific antigen targeted action.
- **Leukocytes, macrophages, T cells, lymphocytes:** These cells protect the baby from infections.
- **Cytokines and chemokines:** These agents help in bringing inflammatory cells to the site of infection.
- **Lysozymes:** Enzymes which directly kill the organisms.
- **Lactoferrin:** It is a whey protein and binds iron in the gut. Protects against organisms which need iron as growth factor, e.g. *E Coli*.
- **Bifidus factor:** Promotes growth of commensals and inhibits pathological organisms.
- **Bile salt lipase:** It provides protection against **Giardia**.
- **Human milk oligosaccharides:** It acts as prebiotic and promotes growth of commensals. It prevents attachment of pathogenic organism to gut.
- **Growth factors:** A large number of growth factors have been identified in breast milk.
  - **Epidermal growth factors:** It is critical to maturation and healing of intestinal mucosa and stimulates intestinal and enzymatic functions. It is highest in colostrum.
  - **Brain and glial cell line-derived neutrophic factor:** Controls peristalsis through intestinal nervous plexus.
  - **Insulin-like growth factor:** Most probably protects gut from oxidative stress.
  - **Vascular endothelial growth factor:** Role in reducing retinopathy of prematurity (ROP) has been suggested.
  - **Transforming growth factor:** Promotes epithelial cell growth.

Para-aminobenzoic acid (PABA): It is low in breast milk. It protects baby from malaria as parasite need it for growth.

Oligosaccharides: They act as prebiotics and promote growth of commensals in newborn gut. Prevents attachment of pathogenic bacteria.

Erythropoietin in breast milk not only prevents anemia in prematurity but also found to reduce necrotizing enterocolitis.[1]

Adiponectin and other metabolism regulating hormones (Ghrelin, Leptin): May have a role in regulating obesity in later life.[1]

Enzymes[6]

- **Acetylhydrolase:** Blocks action of platelet activating factor which is a strong pro-inflammatory agent. This factor is thought to prevent NEC in newborn.

- **Glutathione peroxidase:** Prevents lipid peroxidation and acts as antioxidant.
- **Nucleotidase:** Enhances antibody response to bacterial antigens.

Composition of Stored Milk

WHO and UNICEF have approved stored milk in banks in situations where mother's milk is not available.[10] Hence it becomes mandatory to know the effect of storing on the composition of milk. The composition changes with storing and heat treatment. Vitamin C is lost very early. Protective elements (bioactive components) lose their function, especially the ones made of proteins. Heat treatment is essential for decontamination but method used for it is also important. Boiling is most damaging. Pasteurization with thawing is also damaging specially for proteins. Flash heat technique is thought to be better.[1]

Modifications in Mothers' Milk

Major useful modification is through maternal immunization. It increases immunoglobulins in mothers' milk, specially shown with influenza vaccine.[6] Some dietary changes in mother like increasing DHA content in mother's milk enhanced secretion in breast milk.

Technical Aspects of Breastfeeding[9-11]

Techniques of breastfeeding become very important specially while dealing with primipara mothers. If proper technique is not known to mother, can lead to lactation failure.

Latching and Attachment

It is the way baby holds and suckles at the breast. If latching and attachment is not correct, can cause sore nipples in mother and failure on the part of baby to get adequate milk. Sore nipple further discourages mother to breastfeed.

Baby should hold whole or most of the areola, his tongue should be between breast and lower lip which should be everted. With this position baby will latch at areola and will be able to squeeze lacteal sinuses underneath (Fig. 1).

Position of mother: Feeding should be in sitting position and mother should sit with straight back, leaning will kink the ducts. She can take support of a pillow at the back (Fig. 2).

Usually feeding should be done in sitting position but if mother is tired or has undergone cesarean section can feed in side lying position. In this position baby and mother should face each other (Fig. 3).

Position of baby: Many choices can be given to mother for positions of baby while feeding.

1. **Cradle hold:** If feeding on left side, head is supported at left elbow and buttocks on the hand of same side (Fig. 4).
2. **Cross-cradle hold:** If feeding on left side, head of baby should be on right hand and buttocks on the right elbow (Fig. 5).

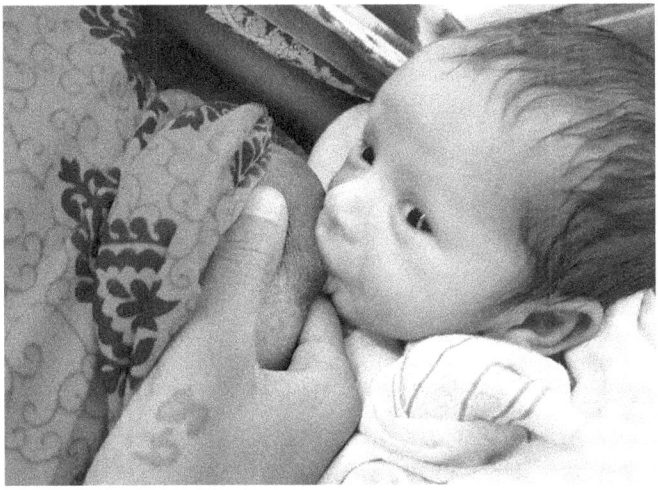

Fig. 1: Proper latching and attachment by newborn.

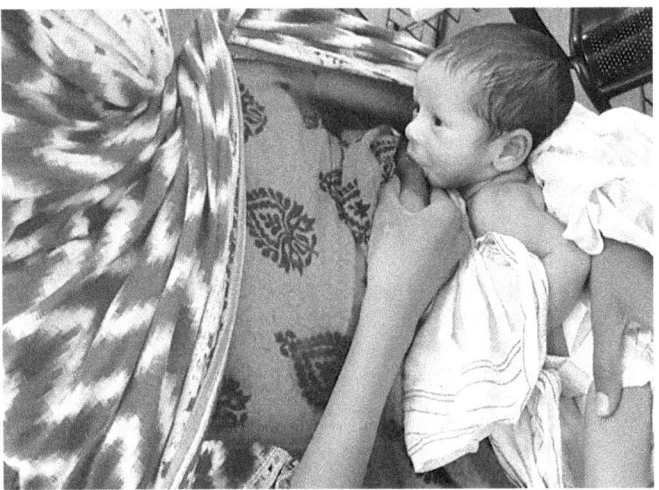

Fig. 2: Feeding position—sitting.

3. **Football hold:** The baby is tucked under mother's arm like a football. Lying along the side, the mother carries on the feeding. The mother may like to use pillows or cushions to help support the baby and her arms. The baby's head is in her hand , on the same side as the breast being used. The baby's upper body is supported by mother's arm. With that hand she can control the baby's head to bring the baby's mouth in quickly for a good latching of the breast. Her other hand reaches across to support and narrow her breast to facilitate proper feeding. In this position both twins can be fed at the same time (Fig. 6)

Offering the breast: Full breast should be offered to the baby. Mothers prefer to hold the breast by scissor hold (Fig. 7) which should be avoided. Mother should use C hold as shown in (Fig. 8).

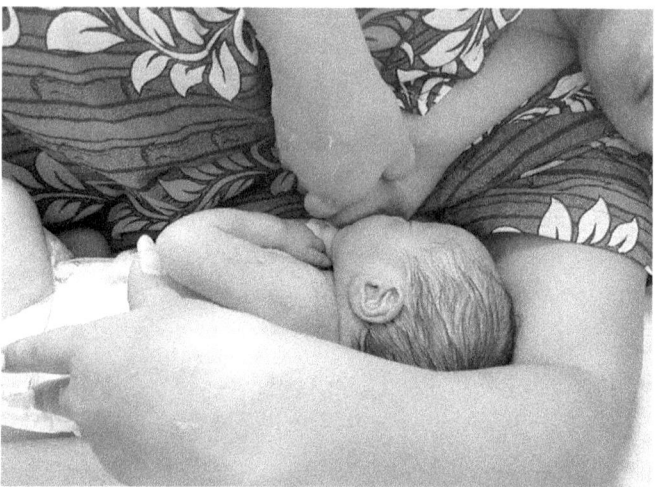

Fig. 3: Feeding in lying down position (side lying).

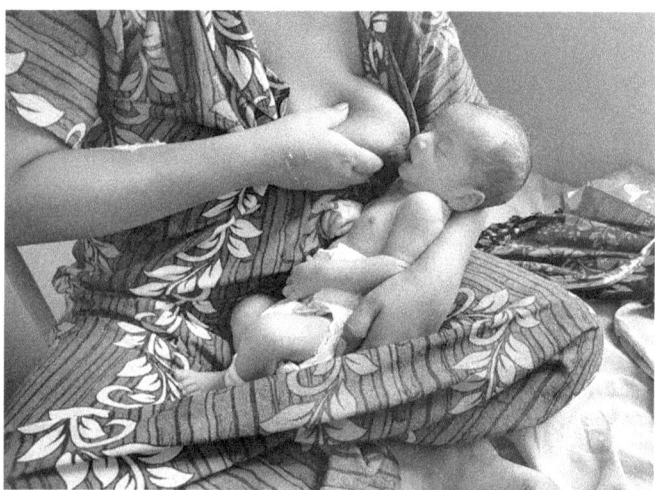

Fig. 4: Cradle hold.

Manual expression: Mothers when discharged from facility after delivery, should be well versed with manual expression of milk. This is very important for working mothers and it also gives some freedom to other mothers if they have to leave the baby and go for some work. The technique if performed well, is a painless procedure. If there is pain during manual expression the technique used is wrong.

Mother should hold breast with thumb above and index finger below the areola. She should push towards chest for 2 cm then she can press and start pumping milk. This way she can move around areola while expressing from

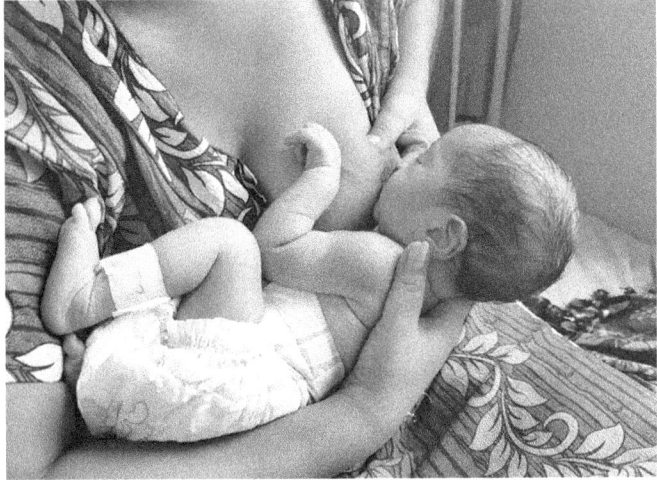

Fig. 5: Cross-cradle hold.

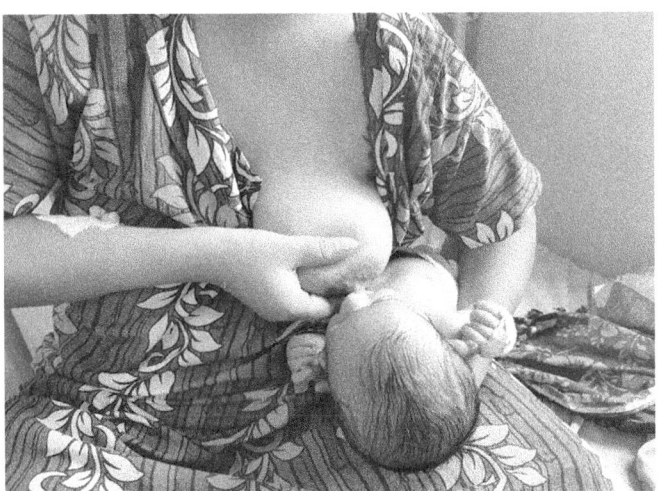

Fig. 6: Football hold.

different parts in the circle. Any amount of milk can be expressed with this method (Figs. 9A and B).

BABY-FRIENDLY TECHNIQUES

- Breastfeeding should be the only first feed given within an hour of birth. At this time baby's reflexes are active and suckling is better, it helps in early establishment of lactation. It also avoids prelacteal feeds which can be a source of infection and delays lactation.

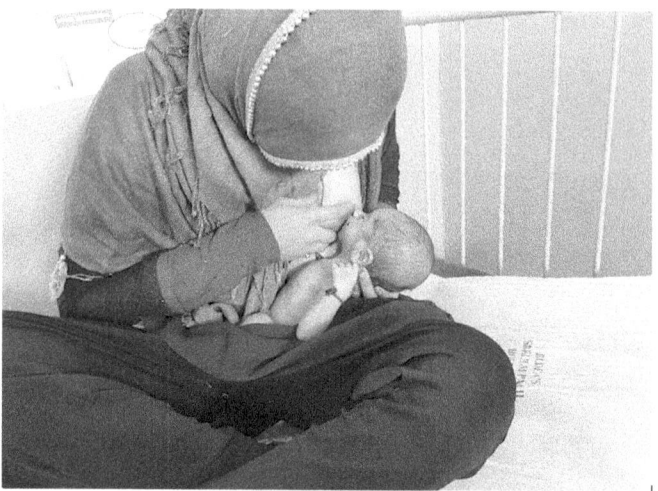

Fig. 7: Scissor hold (wrong technique).

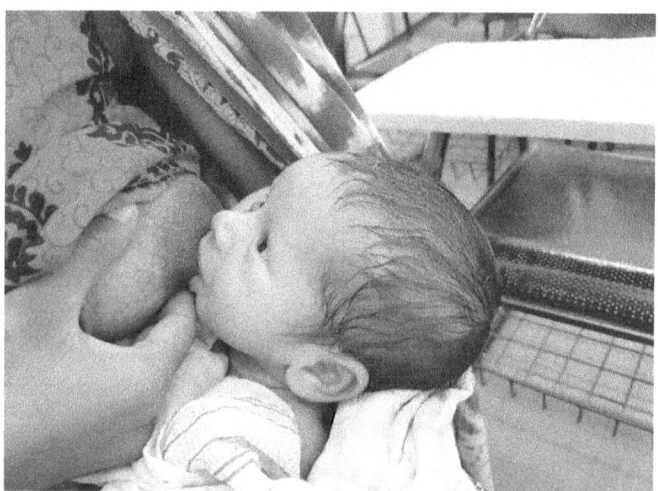

Fig. 8: C hold (correct technique).

- Responsive feeding: Baby should be fed on feeding cues.[10] Mother need not wait till baby cries for feed, she should respond to baby's cues like suckling sound, hand to mouth, rooting to whatever touches the cheek, etc.
- Mother should look at, caress and talk to the baby while feeding. This improves emotional bond between the mother and baby.
- Baby should be kept in mother's bed to promote skin to skin contact and helps keeping baby warm. Kangaroo mother care (Fig. 10) is very good to

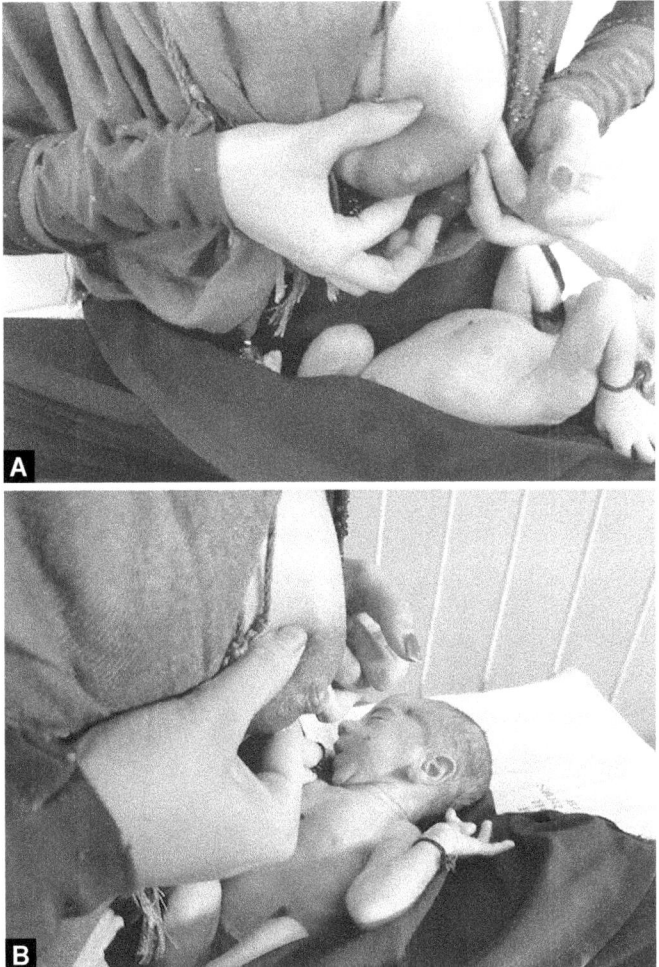

Figs. 9A and B: Manual expression of milk.

keep the baby warm. It is especially good for preterm and low birth weight babies in early establishment of lactation.

Feeding Reflexes

Feeding is a reflex process in early months of life and as mother and baby both are involved in feeding. There are 2 sets of feeding reflexes.

Maternal Reflexes

There are two maternal reflexes which initiate and maintain milk secretion till baby is breastfed (Fig. 11). Both reflexes are through pituitary gland.
1. **Prolactin reflex:** As baby suckles nipple the impulses travel to anterior pituitary. In response prolactin is secreted from anterior pituitary and acts

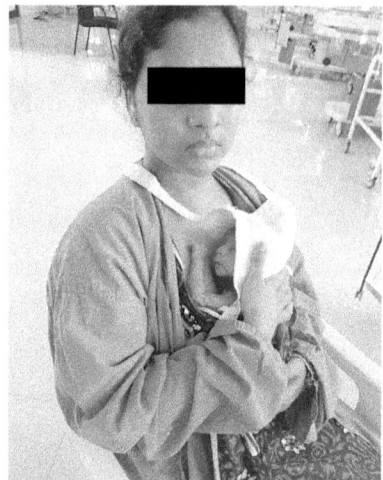

Fig. 10: Kangaroo mother care for low birth weight babies.

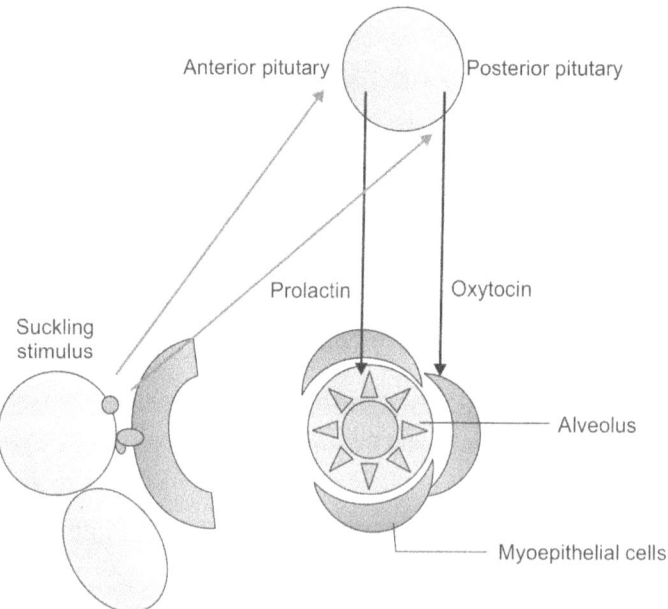

Fig. 11: Maternal feeding reflexes.

on secretary mammary cells to cause milk production (Fig. 11). Hence frequent suckling and breast emptying are important for milk formation.

2. **Oxytocin reflex:** This is also called *let-down reflex*. In this, reflex, on suckling that stimulates the nipple, the impulses reach posterior pituitary and lead to oxytocin secretion. Oxytocin acts on myoepithelial cells and helps in expelling milk from alveoli to lacteal sinus (Fig. 11). This reflex is very sensitive to emotional state of mother. If mother is emotionally

upset the milk ejection stops. It is facilitated by pleasant environment for mother. Hence, it is important for the family to provide happy environment to feeding mother. Oxytocin reflex is responsible for emotional bond between mother and baby. The signs indicative of successful oxytocin reflex are:
- Milk leaking from other breast when baby is fed on one breast
- Milk leaking from breast when mother thinks about baby lovingly
- Tingling sensation in breast when mother is about to feed
- Milk flow from breast when baby is suddenly removed from breast.

This reflex is indicative of milk adequacy also.

Neonatal Feeding Reflexes

There are 3 neonatal reflexes:
1. Rooting reflex—when nipple touches cheeks, baby turns towards it.
2. Sucking reflex—when nipple touches lips, baby starts suckling.
3. Swallowing reflex—when milk enters mouth, baby swallows.

Volume of Breast Milk and its Control

Milk production on first day is around 60-70 mL which gradually increases and reaches 400-600 mL by 4th week and around 700-800 mL by 4th month of life. Volume of milk secreted is tailored to the requirement of baby. Milk secretion is also controlled by a polypeptide present in breast milk, called feedback inhibitor of lactation (FIL). If milk is removed from breast, milk formation continues but if breast is not emptied, FIL collects and production stops. Sometimes if baby is suckled more on one breast, milk formation from other breast reduces, this phenomenon is also attributed to FIL. Whenever breast is regularly emptied milk production restarts (relactation).[6]

PROBLEMS DURING BREASTFEEDING[11-13]

Lactational Failure

Many times, mothers complain about inadequate milk and ask for other sources of milk it is called lactational failure. It is a rare occurrence and mostly the causes are:
- Poor technique while feeding
- Emotional problem in mother
- Poorly motivated mother
- Poor family support for mother.

Most of the time this problem can be managed by counseling the mother. Before managing lactational failure, we must assure the adequacy of milk. Following points can help in deciding the adequacy of milk:
- Baby passes urine frequently at least five times a day.
- Baby sleeps comfortably for 2-21/2 hours after feed.
- There is adequate weight gain in baby.

Relactation[14]

In case mother has discontinued feeding the baby and milk production has stopped, it can be restarted and is called relactation. Methods adopted for it are as follows:
- Frequent suckling and manual expression every 2 hours. As the breast is emptied milk production increases.
- Mother can be given drugs which promote prolactin secretion and increase milk production. Examples are metoclopramide and domperidone.
- **Drip drop technique:** In this method baby is allowed to suckle and a person drips milk from above the nipple.[13]
- **Infant milk supplementer:** An infant feeding tube is used as a supplementer. One end attached to breast so that tip is at nipple. Other end is open in a cup filled with expressed breast milk. When baby suckles breast he/she gets the milk. Sucking stimulus initiates prolactin and oxytocin reflexes.

Breast Problems

Sometimes there can be problems in the breast which can hinder the establishment of lactation. Following are common problems:

Breast Engorgement

Breast can become hard, painful and may become red (Fig. 12). Usual cause is inadequate suckling. Mostly seen when baby is not suckled due to illness or if baby is premature and unable to suck. Sometimes axillary tail also can be seen engorged (Fig. 12). It is managed by frequent suckling. Sometimes baby may not be able to hold the breast due to hardness, in this case some milk should be manually expressed and fed to the baby. When breast becomes soft, it is easy for baby to suckle.

Sore or Cracked Nipple

Usually occurs as a result of improper latching or attachment. Usually baby suckles directly on the nipple due to improper attachment leading to injury. It is a painful condition and demotivates mother for suckling the baby. This problem is easy to solve by educating mother about proper attachment. In case

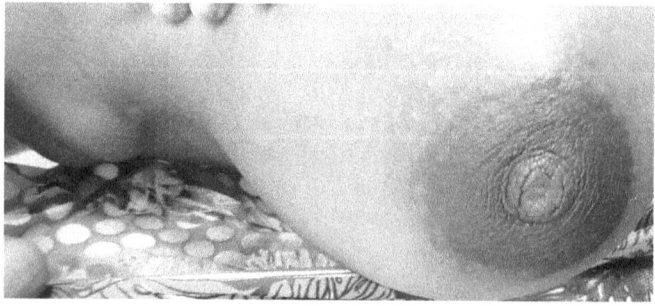

Fig. 12: Engorged breast with swollen axillary tail.

of sore or cracked nipple, breastfeeding should be continued and at the end, breast milk (hindmilk) should be applied to sore areas. No cream or ointment should be used.

Flat/Large Nipple
Size does not matter as baby suckles areola. There may be initial difficulty but within a day or 2 baby gets used to the size.

Inverted/Retracted Nipple
In this condition, there are adhesions at the base of nipple. If baby tries to suck the nipple it is pulled in. The treatment ideally should start in early pregnancy when mother can use inverted syringe method to pull the nipple out. Hoffman's technique is also simple and good where mother pulls breast tissue diagonally out from nipple, followed by rolling the nipple under the pulp of index finger.

Mastitis
In this condition, breast is inflamed and painful, mostly due to infection, mother may have fever. This condition usually follows engorgement, if not properly treated. A course of antibiotics and anti-inflammatory medications may be required. Breastfeeding can be continued for proper emptying of breast.

Breast Abscess
Usually occurs as a result of duct block. A part of breast is not emptied and collected milk gets infected. Usually occurs when mother prefers scissor hold, which clinks the ducts causing block. This condition also needs antibiotics and anti-inflammatory medications. In addition needs incision and drainage. Breast should be kept empty by expressing the milk. Baby can be fed on the other side. Even if baby is fed on the affected side there is no problem.

BREASTFEEDING IN SPECIAL SITUATIONS[10,11]

Premature or Low Birth Weight Baby
Breastfeeding remains the gold standard in these babies. Whether baby is fed directly or expressed breast milk is given, will depend upon the maturity of baby, and whether baby is stable or not. The aim is to start breast milk as early as possible. In babies between 30 and 32 weeks swallowing is invariably present but coordination of breathing and swallowing will not be proper. Hence, they may be initiated on tube feeds with oral stimulation (baby's own hand suckling) during tube feeds and then gradually, when suckling and better swallowing has developed can start on spoon or *palladai* feeding. Once sucking is better, nonnutritive breastfeeding can be started at least 2–3 times a day under supervision. Gradually babies can be shifted to direct breast-feeds with/or without expressed breast milk. Initial feeds can be as small as 5–10 mL/kg/day and are called trophic feeds. These feeds help in the growth of

intestine and colonization of gut with favorable organisms. These babies also need calcium and vitamin D from the age of 1–2 weeks and iron from the age of 1 month.[10] Kangaroo mother care (Fig. 10) should be initiated as soon as baby is stable. It helps in maintaining body temperature, helps in developing the bond between mother and baby and early establishment of lactation leading to good weight gain in baby.

Sick Mothers

If mother has psychological problems like postpartum psychosis, feeding may be a problem due to mother's condition as well as her drugs. Most babies can be fed with supervision. Most drug are safe but needs observation of baby. Most acute and chronic illnesses are not contraindications but need treatment of primary conditions. Some drugs in mother like antineoplastic drugs, immunosuppressive therapy may contraindicate breastfeeds.

Inborn Error of Metabolism and Galactosemia in Baby

Breast milk is safe in most inborn error of metabolism (IEM) conditions. Galactosemia is an absolute contraindication.

Adopted Baby and Induced Lactation[15]

Mothers' who have adopted babies can breastfeed their babies by inducing lactation. A nulliparous women who adopts a baby, can also breastfeed her baby, if she is motivated. Any or all of above methods can be used for it. Success ranges from total breastfeeding to token breastfeeding and is dependent upon mother's motivation.

Infant of HIV Positive Mother[10]

As per new recommendations exclusive breastfeeding should be the choice for first 6 months of baby's life. Mixed feeding should not be given. If mother chooses not to breastfeed, she should be told about the risk involved for baby due to no breastfeeding. As per WHO recommendations all pregnant and lactating mothers should receive antiretroviral therapy irrespective of CD4 count. Baby should receive nevirapine for 6 weeks if they are breastfeeding except, when mother is diagnosed at labor/postpartum period or infant is diagnosed after birth when they will receive navirapine for 12 weeks. If baby is positive at 6 weeks should receive complete antiretroviral therapy.

Baby-friendly Hospital Initiative

UNICEF and WHO together initiated baby-friendly hospital initative (BFHI) program in 1991 to promote and support breastfeeding. They have formulated 10 steps to ensure and promote successful lactation in any facility. The hospitals were assessed for these points and were labeled baby friendly, if they fulfilled required criteria.

These 10 steps are:
1. Every hospital should have written policy for breastfeeding which should be communicated to employees from time to time.
2. All the staff looking after feeding mothers should be trained in breastfeeding technique and re-training should continue regularly.
3. Mothers should be informed about breastfeeding during antenatal period.
4. Baby should be started on breastfeeds within an hour of birth.
5. Baby should be given exclusive breastfeeding for 6 months which means nothing except breast milk should be given. Not even water or any vitamin drops.
6. Every mother should be educated how to maintain lactation even if she is separated from baby. Technique of manual expression of milk should be taught to mother, which can be used if mother goes out for any work.
7. Encourage feeding on demand.
8. Baby should not be given any bottle-feeding, nipples, teats, pacifiers, etc.
9. Baby and mother should be kept in same room (rooming in) and same bed (bedding in) to promote skin to skin contact.
10. Facility should foster a lactation support group, mother should be able to contact them in case there is any problem about breastfeeding after discharge.

Expansion of this program is in the form of training, assessment and reassessment.

MILK OTHER THAN BREAST MILK WITH OR WITHOUT BOTTLE

In case breast milk is not available age appropriate formula can be used. If formula cannot be afforded by parents, cow's milk can be used. Use of bottle should be discouraged. Bottle use needs very eficient sterilization which becomes expensive and difficult for parents. Unsterile bottles are a source of infection and have been named as "baby killers".

If formula is to be used, it should be reconstituted as per companies' guidelines. The water used for reconstituting should be boiled and lukewarm. Most formulas provide a measure which should filled to brim and should be added to 30 mL of lukewarm water. Milk should be fed ad libitum (as much baby accepts).

Milk should be fed with a spoon and cup or a *palladai*. Baby should be in sitting position. If an educated affording mother/caretaker insists on bottle-feeding she should be explained about bottle hygiene. Bottle should be cleaned with soap and cold water using a bottle brush. The nipple and cap should also be cleaned. The bottle should be boiled for 8 minutes and nipple should be added in last 3-4 minutes. This process has to be repeated at each feed. If baby feeds eight times mother has to boil the bottle 8 times. Milk remaining in the bottle should be discarded. The bottle should be washed immediately after the feed.

FEEDING BETWEEN 6 MONTHS AND 2 YEARS[10-12]

This includes complementary feeds with breast milk continued up to 2 years of age.

Complementary Feeding

At the age of 6 completed months, breast milk may not be able to look after baby's nutritional needs. Hence it is complimented with semisolids. The term weaning should not be used as breast milk is still continued. Following are the characteristics of an ideal weaning food. Following points about complimentary foods should be kept in mind.

- **Consistency:** Should be soft semisolid food. Thickness is increased as the age advances. Around 10 months child can eat food without much alteration. In between coarseness of food is gradually increased.
- **Quantity:** It should be started with small amounts may be one to two spoonful once a day and gradually increased in amount. Initially child may spit the food as he/she is not used to it. Same food should be repeated till child starts accepting. At 1 year of age child should eat one-third or half of mothers' diet.
- **Food quality and selection:** Food is selected from the commonly used food items in the family. As stomach capacity is small, calorie dense weaning foods should be made. Ideally, there should be 8 to 1 cal/g of food. If calorie density is less calories can be increased by adding oil or ghee (5 g = 45 calories), by roasting the grains specially rice, by sprouting the grains specially legumes. During sprouting amylase is released which causes partial digestion and reduces food volume. Mixed food items from

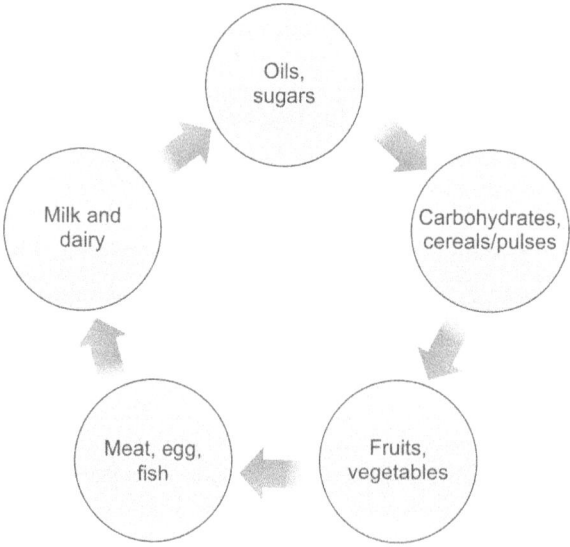

Fig. 13: Showing food groups in the relative proportion they should be used.

all food groups (Fig. 13) should be chosen to make a balanced feed for the baby. Cereal, pulse mixture in ratio of 2:1 along with green vegetables or other colored vegetables, jaggery and/or salt along with ghee/oil/butter are good combination.
- **Neophobia:** Initially, child may spit the food as he/she is not used to it. Same food should be repeated till child starts accepting it. Frequent changes due to rejection by the child is not advisable.
- **Frequency:** Initially (7th month) one feed is given, increased gradually to make 2-3 times a day. If required, in between one or two snacks which are nourishing and homemade can be given. At the age of 1 year baby should get 3 major meals with 2-3 snacks if needed.
- **Responsive feeding:** Child should be encouraged to eat by himself. Mother should stimulate the child by talking or playing with child. Spillage is expected and should be allowed. Forced feeding should be avoided.
- **Hygiene:** Hygiene is very important and mothers should be educated for the same. Handwashing should be practiced regularly by mother and child. Food should be in clean vessels given to the child in clean surroundings.

Following are some examples of good complementary foods:
- Rice + dal + green leafy vegetables + oil or ghee + jaggery/sugar+/- salt
- Mashed chapati + dal + green leafy vegetables+ oil or ghee + jaggery/sugar+/- salt
- Ragi powder + milk + jaggery (ragi eating areas)
- Khichadi + vegetables + ghee
- Payasam made of rice/wheat + dal + ghee + jaggery or sugar

These are all good nutritive complimentary food items. They are not expensive and do not need any extra item which has to be specially acquired.

FEEDING BETWEEN 2 AND 5 YEARS

At 2 years of age breastfeeding can be discontinued but if mother or baby wants, one or two feeds can be given. As breast milk, a major source of animal protein is not there, care should be taken to include animal protein through other milk, egg or any other animal food. Following points to be considered during feeding of these children which are as follows:
1. Food should be chosen from family pot. A balanced diet should include 55-60% calories from carbohydrate, 15% from proteins and rest 25-30% from fats. It should also provide all micronutrients in required amounts.
2. Variety of food from each group should be included (Fig. 13). Indian family food usually includes all the groups if chosen properly. The balance of calories are also good in Indian normal food as compared to western food.
3. Forced feeding, and rewards like chocolates, viewing TV should be avoided.

4. Self-feeding should be encouraged. Feeding should be encouraged when whole family is on the table.
5. Fortified items like iodinated salt, vitamin D, fortified oils, etc. should be used.
6. Micronutrients should be supplemented as required. Dewormig should be done regularly.
7. Junk foods, processed foods should be avoided.
8. Hand hygiene, food hygiene should be followed by mother and child both.
9. It is good to give at least 250 mL of milk daily. If child does not like milk, any changes like kheer or curd can be replaced to avoid forced feeding.
10. Usually 3–4 major meals and one to two snacks are sufficient.

GROWTH MONITORING AND TIMELY IMMUNIZATION AS PART OF INFANT AND YOUNG CHILD NUTRITION

All children below 5 years should be regularly monitored for growth using WHO growth charts. Any platue on the chart should be evaluated for the reason. Child should be immunized as per schedule to protect from preventable illnesses.

Mother's nutrition is also of utmost importance. Adequate nutrition in adolescence gives a good start to maternal nutrition. Mothers should be monitored for prepregnancy weight, and pregnancy weight gain which will affect birth weight of child. Low birth weight babies are prone for malnutrition. Postnatal weight gain also is important for lactating mothers. Diet of lactating mother specially vitamin and mineral content is very important to monitor.

In nutshell, infant and young child nutrition is important for adequate growth and development of child. Now when malnutrition is major health problem in India it is important to look after child's nutrition to bring down morbidity and mortality linked to nutrition. Breastfeeding exclusive up to 6 months and continued up to 2 years along with complimentary feeds is most useful measure for it. The period between 6 months to 2 years is vulnerable for child as new food is introduced and problems like infections, infestations, food allergies, food intolerance might crop up. Breast milk which is still substantial, protects the baby from these problems. After 2 years this support is not available hence malnutrition, specific deficiencies and infections are common during this period. Maternal counseling for hygiene, selection of food and amount of food is very important (Fig. 14).

CONCLUSION

Exclusive breastfeed should be given till at least up to months of age followed by complementary feeding and continued breastfeed up to 2 years of age. Advantages of breast milk are numerous including tailor-made composition for the baby, immense protective function against diarrhea, respiratory

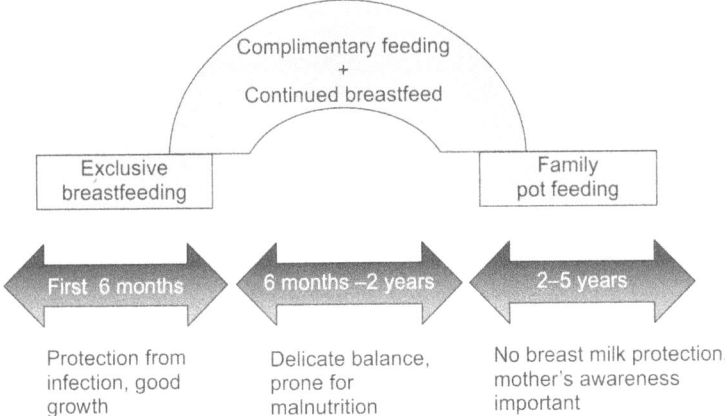

Fig. 14: Showing feeding in first 5 years of life and their implications.

infections and a large number of other diseases, support for emotional health and better intelligence in the child. Solid and semisolid food should be chosen from family pot and should include all food groups. Responsive and self-feeding should be encouraged and forced feeding should be discouraged. All the children should be monitored for growth during first 5 years. Good nutrition should run parallel with timely immunization, thereby reducing childhood morbidity and mortality.

KEY LEARNING POINTS

- Breastfeeding is the best feed for baby up to 2 years of age.
- Exclusive breastfeed should be given till 6 months of age followed by complimentary feeding and continued breastfeed up to 2 years of age.
- Breast milk is tailor-made for baby.
- Breast milk has immense protective function and protects baby from diarrhea, respiratory infections and a large number of other diseses.
- Breast milk is good for emotional health and has been shown to be associated with better intelligence in the child.
- Solid and semisolid food should be chosen from family pot and should include all food groups.
- Responsive and self-feeding should be encouraged and forced feeding should be discouraged.
- All the children should be monitored for growth during first 5 years.
- Good nutrition along with timely immunization reduces morbidity and mortality.

REFERENCES

1. Victora CG, de Onis M, Hallal PC, Blössner M, Shrimpton R. Worldwide timing of growth faltering: Revisiting implications for interventions. *Pediatrics.* 2010;125:e473-80. doi: 10.1542/peds.2009-1519.

2. World Health Organization. Infant and young child nutrition: Global strategy on infant and young child feeding. Report by secretariat, WHO 55th World Health Assembly, 16th April 2002. Available at: http://www.who.int/nutrition/publications/gs_infant_feeding_text_eng.pdf. Accessed on: 13 January 2018.
3. UNICEF. Improving Child Nutrition: The achievable imperative for global progress. New York: UNICEF 2013. Available at: *www.nicef.org/publications/index.html*. Accessed on: 13 January 2018.
4. Krammer MS, Aboud F, Mironova E, et al. Breastfeeding and child cognitive development; New evidence from a large randomized trial. *Arch Gen Psychiatry* 2008;65:578-584.
5. Kramer MS, Matush L, Vanilovich I, et al. Effect of prolong and exclusive breastfeeding on child height, weight, adiposity and blood pressure at age 6.5 years: Evidence from a large randomized trial. *Am J Clin Nutr* 2007;86:1717-1721.
6. Ballard O, Morrow AL. Human milk composition: Nutrients and Bioactive factors. *Pediatr Clin North Am* 2013;60:49-74.
7. Lawrence RA, Lawrence RM. Biochemistry of human milk. In: *Breastfeeding: A guide to Medical Profession*. 7th edn. Elsevier/Mosby 2011. Available at: http://doi.org/1016.B978-4377-0788-5,10025-2. Accessed on: 13 January 2018.
8. Wagner CL, Greer FR. Prevention of rickets and vitamin D deficiency in infants, children, and adolescents. *Pediatrics* 2008;122:5. Available at: http://pediatrics.Aappu blications. org/ content/ 122/5/1142. Accessed on: 14 January 2018.
9. Hamosh M. Bioactive factors in human milk. *Pediatr Clin North Am* 2001;48:69-86.
10. Tiwari S, Bharadva K, Yadav B, et al. Infant and young child feeding guidelines. *Indian Pediatr* 2016;53:703-713.
11. World Health Organization. WHO/UNICEF meeting on infant and young child feeding. *J Nurse Midwif* 2015;25:31-39.
12. Anand RK. Infant and young child feeding. In: Parthsarathi A (ed). *IAP Textbook of Pediatrics*, 6th edn. New Delhi: Jaypee 2016:136-152.
13. Infant and Young Child Feeding. Model chapter for textbooks for medical students and allied health professionals. Genva: WHO; 2009. Avaialble at: www.ncbi.nlm.nih.gov/books/BK148952. Accessed on: 11 January 2018.
14. Lakhkar BB, Shenoy VD, Bhaskaranand N. Relactation-Manipal experience. *Indian Pediatr* 1999;36:700-703.
15. Kinga AS, Sherry EA, Marc BR. Induced lactation and exclusive breast milk feeding of adopted premature twins. *J Hum Lact* 2010;26:309-313.

14 Adolescent Nutrition

Rashmi Dwivedi

ABSTRACT

Adolescents are defined by WHO as individuals between 10 and 19 years of age. Adolescents are future generation of any country. Hence, their nutritional needs are critical for the well being of society and productivity.

Adolescents make up roughly 20% of the total world population. In 1995, there were 914 million adolescents living in the developing world, that is, 85% of the total. Their number is expected to reach 1.13 billion by the year 2025.

Adolescence is a period of rapid growth: Up to 45% of skeletal growth takes place and 15 to 25% of adult height is achieved during adolescence. During the growth spurt of adolescence, up to 37% of total bone mass may be accumulated. Early adolescence period is marked by most rapid growth and development. Research evidence suggests that optimum nutrition during brief period of pre-pubertal growth spurt, some 18 to 24 months preceding menarche, results in catch-up growth from nutritional deficits suffered earlier in life. Adolescent populations in India and Bangladesh have shown deficiency in intake of all nutrients particularly iron, calcium, vitamin A and C. Adolescent nutrition is also important to prevent nutrition related diseases like, obesity, cardiovascular and other chronic disease. Addressing nutritional needs of adolescents can be an important step towards breaking the vicious cycle of inter-generational malnutrition and improve the nutritional behavior and lifestyle.

Keywords: Adolescent, Adolescent nutrition, Anemia, Balanced diet, Calcium, Catch-up growth, Growth, Micronutrients, Nutrition, Obesity, Rapid growth, Undernutrition

INTRODUCTION

According to the World Health Organization (WHO) and other agencies, adolescent population is on an increase and at a risk of erratic nutrition.[1-6] Globally, adolescent population is likely to increase from 1.2 billion to 1.3 billion in spite of forecast declines in fertility. It has been known that many children in low and middle income countries enter adolescence with a legacy of malnutrition from early childhood that is they are then stunted or anemic and often have other micronutrient deficiencies.[7] UNICEF has produced statistics based on analysis of 64 countries with available data indicating that nearly

50% of adolescent girls between 15 and 19 years in India are underweight and >25% of adolescent girls in other 10 countries were underweight.[8] Adolescent obesity is also on increase in developing world due to rapid transition to lipid rich diets and decrease in physical activity especially in urban areas leading to increase in chronic health issues during adolescent period and later in life.[9] An estimated 20–30% of adolescents and young adults are living with chronic disease especially diabetes.[10] An Indian study has shown higher risk of hypertension in these adolescents.[11]

Adolescence is also a critical period when health related behaviors regarding food, lifestyle habits and physical activity are formed. It is often considered a nutritionally vulnerable period because of its characteristic rapid physical and psychological changes. The growth in this period is under the influence of nutrition, genetic and hormonal factors.[12] Hormones mediating pubertal growth spurt are sex steroids and growth hormones, which are modulated to a great extent by nutritional factors.

It is also a period of rapid growth and an opportunity for catch-up growth.[13,14] Due to increased growth velocity, the adolescents have the highest energy and protein requirements compared to any other age group.[15,16] Similarly micronutrients requirements are also increased especially iron, calcium, zinc, and vitamin D.[1] Studies in India and Bangladesh have also shown deficiencies in the intake of all nutrients particularly iron, calcium, vitamin A and vitamin C.[5]

Obesity among adolescents is responsible for carrying weight related risks like cardiovascular diseases into adulthood. Anemia is the most common nutritional issue during adolescents and in females can also lead to maternal anemia and its adverse effects on fetal growth and development. Boys are as much prone to anemia as girls. There is a clear evidence of association between plasma serum levels of vitamin A and hemoglobin levels.[17] Nutrition is the key determinant for ensuring optimal health, normal growth and development as well as for preventing future chronic disease. Moreover psychosocial developmental changes in the form of autonomy, identity issues, body image concerns, experimentation and peer affiliation have a significant effect on dietary intake in adolescence.[18]

With the change in the socioeconomic milieu in India, there has been a change in lifestyle of the population which also includes "nutrition transition" from traditional whole grain diet to adopting modern processed diet.[18,19]

In our society where priorities have been based on morbidity and mortality rates, adolescents have been overlooked by health planners. Addressing the nutrition needs of adolescents could be an important step towards breaking the vicious cycle of intergenerational malnutrition, chronic diseases and poverty.

WHY ADOLESCENT NUTRITION?

There are a number of compelling reasons to focus on adolescent nutrition:[20]
1. Adolescent, population groupis increasing in numbers.
2. A marginalized and disempowered group.
3. A time of increased nutritional requirements.

4. It is a second window of opportunity to correct undernutrition in early years of life.[21]
5. To help adolescents to reach their optimal growth and development.
6. Opportunity to build up storage for future use.
7. To improve academics and physical performance.
8. Prevention of adult diseases related to cardiovascular system, endocrine system and other noncommunicable diseases.
9. Body image and psychological change have an impact on dietary habits.
10. Early marriage, teenage pregnancy make girls especially vulnerable and has implications for future generations.
11. **Economic implications:** Food insecurity among adolescents has also been linked to school absenteeism and low educational attainment.

Dietary intake with respect to adequate availability of food in terms of quantity and quality, ability to digest, absorb and utilize food and the social discriminations against girls can greatly affect the adequate nutrition. Health and nutritional education can help in achieving this goal.

ADOLESCENT GROWTH AND DEVELOPMENT

The three dimensions of growth during adolescence are physical growth, mental and emotional blooming and sexual development (Table 1). Growth spurt accounts for rapid increase in height and weight, changes in body proportion, fat deposition, development of sexual organs and secondary sexual characters.[22]

Table 1: Sex maturity index.

Variable	Early adolescence	Middle adolescence	Late adolescence
Age range	10–13 years	14–17 years	18–21 years
SMR	1–2	3–5	5
Physical changes	• Secondary sexual characteristics • Growth spurt	• Peak growth velocity, Menarche • Facial and body hair, Voice changes, acne	• Physical maturation slows • Increased lean body and muscle mass in males
Cognitive and moral	• Unable to perceive long-term outcome for current decisions • Follow rules to avoid punishment	• Abstract thoughts • May perceive future implications, but may not apply in decision making • Sense of vulnerability	• Future oriented with sense of perspective • Improved impulse control • Improved assessment of risk vs reward
Self concept	• Pre-occupied with changing body • Consciousness about appearance and attractiveness	• Concerns with attractiveness • Increasing introspection	• More stable body image • Attractiveness may still be of concern

Source: Parks EP, Shaikhkhalil A, Groleau V, Wendel D, Stallings VA. Feeding of infants, children and adolescents. In: Kliegman RM, Staton BF, St Geme III JW, Schor NF(Eds). *Nelsons Textbook of Pediatrics*, 20th edn. Philadelphia: Elsevier 2016.

SALIENT FEATURES[12]

- It is the growth hormone and sex hormone which plays a major role in growth spurt.
- Pubertal spurt begins at an average age of 12 years in girls and 14 years in boys. 25% adult height, and 40% adult bone mass is gained during this period.
- In girls:
  - Peak growth velocity occurs before attainment of menarche (stage 3)
  - Girls gain approximately 8.3 kg/year in early adolescence and 6.3 kg/year in late adolescence
  - LBM falls from 80% to 74%
  - Body fat increase from from 16% to 27%
  - During puberty females experience 44% increase in LBM and 20% of body fat mass each year.
- In boys:
  - Peak growth velocity during later stages (stages 4–5)
  - Fat decreases in males during adolescence to reach 12%
  - By age 18 years >90% of skeletal mass has been formed.
- Increase in body structure is paralleled by increase in blood volume and muscle mass.
- Neuromaturation is characterized by decrease in gray matter, increase in white matter, earlier maturation of amygdala and limbic structures which are involved in the experience of fear and emotions.[14]
- Psychosocial development includes separation from parents, increasing importance of peer groups, sexual awareness and interest and concerns regarding body image.

OBJECTIVES FOR ADOLESCENT NUTRITION

- Provide the necessary nutrients to meet the demands of physical and cognitive growth and development.
- Provide adequate stores for illness or pregnancy.
- Prevent adult onset of diseases related to nutrition, e.g. cardiovascular disease, diabetes, hypertension and cancer.
- Encourage healthy eating habits and lifestyle.

Inappropriate dietary intake during adolescence can have several consequences:
- Potentially retard physical growth, reduce intellectual capacity and delay sexual maturation.
- Affect risk for immediate health problems like iron deficiency, undernutrition, stunting, bone health, eating disorders and obesity.[23]
- Iron deficiency affects concentration. Learning and school performance.
- Can have long-term implications also, e.g. low calcium intake during adolescence leads to reduced bone density, increased risk of osteoporosis, etc.

- Overweight or obese adolescence have higher risk of diabetes as an adult and even affects the menstrual cycle. Increased fat intake carries a higher risk of heart disease.[24]
- Underweight and stunting in girls continues into adulthood and increases the obstetric risks.

COMMON NUTRITIONAL PROBLEMS IN ADOLESCENCE

According to the WHO, for adolescents, undernutrition, iron, folate, iodine, vitamin A and calcium deficiencies are of considerable importance.[25]

NUTRITION AND GROWTH FAILURE

Most of the Indians, especially rural and the urban poor fail to achieve the full endowed genetic potential for growth and intelligence. This is due to the suboptimum interaction of host factors with nutrition and environment. High prevalence of LBW babies and adolescent growth failure are indicators of social deprivation.

Growth failure is the net effect of influences like socioeconomic factors, poverty, illiteracy, childhood malnutrition, anemia, worm infestation and gender disparity. Beauty consciousness, adolescent dieting, alcohol, drug abuse, missing meals, fast food and cola culture, eating snacks and confectioneries, undesirable likes and dislikes for foods also add to the problem. Low protein, calcium and vitamin D intake results in low bone mineral density whereas undernutrition results in stunting, delayed puberty and sexual maturation.[18]

The vicious cycle of undernutrition and systemic disease is depicted in Flowchart 1.

Flowchart 1: The difficult-to-break vicious cycle of undernutrition and systemic disease.

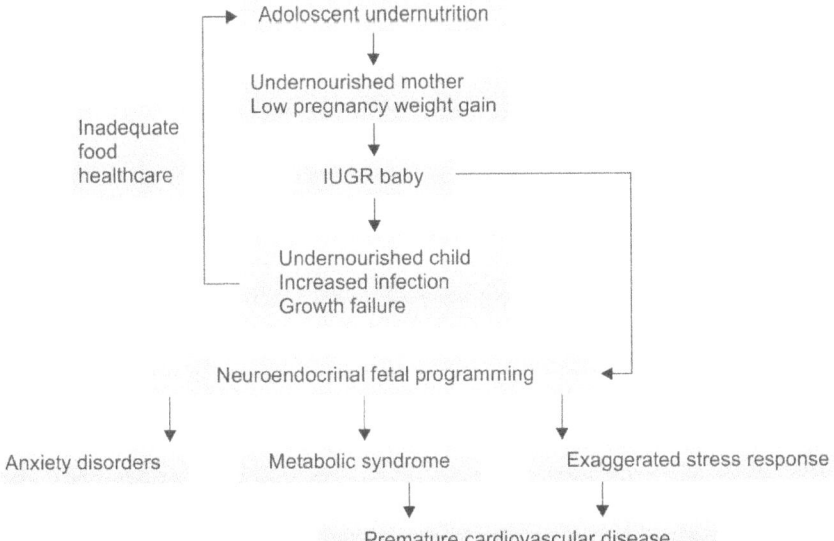

DIETARY RECOMMENDATIONS

Adolescent dietary recommendations include daily energy and nutrient requirements to maintain health and to support ongoing growth and development. Nutritional requirements in adolescence varies according to weight, age, sex, pubertal stage and physical activity level.[25]

Recommendation about different aspects dietary intake in adolescents are given in Tables 2 to 5.

Energy

Adolescent boys have a higher increase in height, weight and lean body mass compared to girls, their energy needs are greater. Nutritional requirement of an adolescent boy is equal to that of an adult sedentary male and that of an adolescent girl is more than of an adult sedentary female. Energy intake increases with increased levels of physical activity. Carbohydrates are major and immediate source of energy, complex carbohydrates are recommended.

Table 2: Recommended dietary allowances for adolescents.

Age (years)	Calories	Proteins (g)	Fats (g)	Calcium (mg)	Iron (mg)	Zinc (mg)	Magnesium (mg)
			Girls				
10-12	2010	40.4	35	800	27	9	160
13-15	2330	51.9	40	800	28	11	210
16-17	2440	55.5	35	800	26	12	235
			BOYS				
10-12	2190	39.9	35	800	21	9	120
13-15	2750	54.3	45	800	32	11	165
16-17	3020	61.5	50	800	28	12	195

Source: Recommended dietary allowances for Indian children. Guidelines, National Institute of Nutrition, ICMR, Hyderabad 2010.

Table 3: Recommended dietary allowance of vitamins for adolescent.

Age (years)	Retinol	Beta-carotene (mg)	Thiamine (mg)	Riboflavin (mg)	Niacin (mg)	Pyridoxine (mg)	Ascorbic acid (mg)	Folate (µg)	B12
				Girls					
10-12	600	4800	1.0	1.2	13	1.6	40	140	0.2-1.0
13-15	600	4800	1.2	1.4	14	2.0	40	150	0.2-1.0
16-17	600	4800	1.0	1.2	14	2.0	40	200	0.2-1.0
				Boys					
10-12	600	4800	1.1	1.3	15	1.6	40	140	0.2-1.0
13-15	600	4800	1.4	1.6	16	2.0	40	150	0.2-1.0
16-17	600	4800	1.5	1.8	17	2.0	40	200	0.2-1.0

Source: Recommended dietary allowances for Indian children. Guidelines, National Institute of Nutrition, ICMR, Hyderabad, 2010.

Table 4: Number of proportions constituting a balanced diet in adolescents.

Food group	Cereals and millets	Pulses	Milk and milk products	Roots and tubers	Green leafy vegetables	Other vegetables	Fruits	Sugar	Fat/oil
					Girls				
g/portion	30	30	100	100	100	100	100	5	5
Age									
10–12	8	2	5	1	1	2	1	6	7
13–15	11	2	5	1	1	2	1	5	8
16–18	11	2.5	5	2	1	2	1	5	7
					Boys				
Age									
10–12	10	2	5	1	1	2	1	6	7
13–15	14	2.5	5	1.5	1	2	1	4	9
16–18	15	3	5	2	1	2	1	6	10

(*Source:* Recommended dietary allowances for Indian children. Guidelines, National Institute of Nutrition, ICMR, Hyderabad 2010).

Table 5: Protein requirements in normal and special adolescents categories.

Group	Protein Requirements
Adolescent boys	0.29–0.32 g/kg/d
Adolescent girls	0.27–0.29 g/kg/d
Adolescent pregnancy: • 1st trimester • 2nd trimester • 3rd trimester	1 g/d 10 g/d 31 g/d
Adolescent lactation	19 g/d
High intensity athletes	1.2–1.8 g/kg

High sugar foods are not preferred. Sources include cereals, grains, fresh fruits and vegetables.

Proteins

Protein intake is low in adolescents. About 40–75% consume <50% of recommended dietary intake. Surveys from India show that boys consume foods of high nutrient value like milk, fruits and eggs.[26] Energy and protein needs correlate more closely with the growth pattern than with chronological age. The peak in protein and energy requirement coincides with the peak in growth of adolescents. If energy intake is limited, dietary protein may be used to meet energy needs and be unavailable for synthesis of new tissues or for tissue repair. This may result in diminished growth rate and muscle mass despite an apparent adequate protein intake.

Sources include pulses, lentils, soybean, dairy products and animal foods.
Table 5 lists protein requirement in normal and special categories.

Fats

Fats are source of essential fatty acids. Unsaturated fats recommended as saturated fats increase cholesterol. Cottonseed, corn, *til*, soybean, sunflower oils are recommended which contains 50% PUFA.

Calcium

Growing children and adolescents require more calcium. Though recommended dietary allowances for calcium are about 600–800 mg/day, it is desirable to give higher quantities of calcium for adolescents to achieve high peak bone mass. To achieve optimal peak bone mass, it is recommended to consume calcium rich foods like milk and milk products, millet (Ragi), *til*, etc. Poor dietary intake will result in long-term risk of osteoporosis. Along with calcium adequate vitamin D, parathyroid hormone and doing weight bearing exercises are essential to maintain the bone mineral density. Contraceptive use, alcohol abuse, and excessive soft drink consumption in adolescence impairs calcium absorption.[25]

Iron

Iron needs are increased in adolescents as there is higher production of myoglobin and hemoglobin due to an increase in lean muscle tissue and red cell mass.

In boys, there is sharp increase in needs of iron from approximately 10 to 15 mg/day. In girls, iron is also required to cover monthly menstrual losses of approx 30–40 mL. The mean requirement for iron reaches a maximum of approx 15 mg/day at peak growth but settles to approximately 13 mg to 15 mg/day because of the need to replace menstrual losses. *Diet rich* in iron includes green leafy vegetables, legumes, dry fruits, meat, fish, poultry. Poor dietary intake results in anemia that impairs growth and cognition and leads to fatigue and increased risk of infections.[17,20] (Flowchart 2)

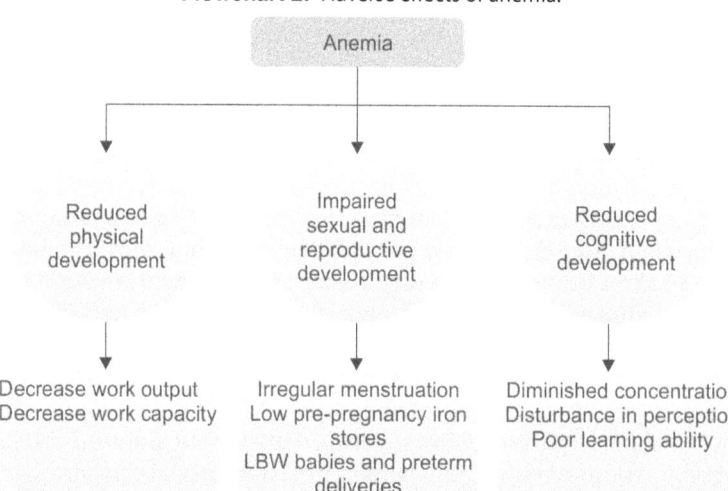

Flowchart 2: Adverse effects of anemia.

Zinc

It has an important role in protein synthesis, general growth and maintenance of tissues. Dietary sources include meat, dairy products, nuts and whole grains. Inadequate intake results in growth failure, delayed sexual maturation, loss of taste and appetite and mental lethargy.[20]

Iodine

It is important in adolescence for two reasons. These are high growth velocity and increased iodine requirements in pregnancy. As a large number of girls get married early and bear children during adolescence, there requirements for iodine increases to provide for their own growth as well as for the needs of the fetus.[20]

Vitamin A

It is essential for growth and development, normal vision, expression of selected genes and reproduction. Even minor or subclinical vitamin A deficiency may have adverse effect on bone growth and sexual maturation of adolescent. Serum retinol binding protein concentrations have been shown to increase throughout puberty indicating that vitamin A is needed for adolescent development.[17]

Vitamin B Group

Higher energy demands increase needs of thiamine, riboflavin and niacin for the release of energy from carbohydrates. B_{12} and folate are required for formation of RBC. B_6 is required for heme synthesis and for synthesis and metabolism of amino acids. With increasing evidence of the role of folic acid in the prevention of birth defects, all adolescent girls of childbearing age should be encouraged to consume recommended amount of folic acid (4 mg). Higher intake of folate has also been linked to better academic performance according to a Swedish study.[24] Vitamin C and E are needed in increased amount for new cell growth.[20] Vitamin C is required for synthesis of collagen, carnitine and neurotransmitters. It is also highly effective antioxidant and has a role in increasing absorption of nonheme iron.[25]

NUTRITONAL STATUS OF ADOLESCENTS

Adequate nutrition of any individual is determined by two factors. The first is the adequate availability of food items in terms of quality and quantity which depends on socioeconomic status, food practices, cultural traditions and allocation of food. The second factor is the ability to digest, absorb and utilize the food.[20]

Observations of nutritional status of Indian adolescents as per National Family Heath Survey-3 are summarized in Table 6.

Table 6: National Family Health Survey-3 observations on nutritional status of Indian adolescents.

Nutrition status (BMI)	Undernutrition (<18.5)	Normal	Overnutrition (>25)
Female	46.8%	50.8%	2.4%
Male	58.1%	40.2%	1.7%

(*Source:* National Family Health Survey-3 (2005-2006) Available at: chiips.org/nfhs/nfhs3.shtm. Accessed on: 20 January 2018).

Figure 1 presents the proportion of adolescents with energy and protein intake below 50% of RDA in India.

Figure 2 presents the proportion of adolescents with iron and vitamin intake below 50% of RDA in India.

BARRIERS TO BALANCED NUTRITION IN ADOLESCENCE

Policymaking
- Adolescent friendly health services
- National Nutritional Programs
- Legislation
- Media regulation.

Community Level
- School: Nutrition, education, play area
- Socioeconomic status: Food availability, accessibility, cultural norms, neighborhood, fast food joints.

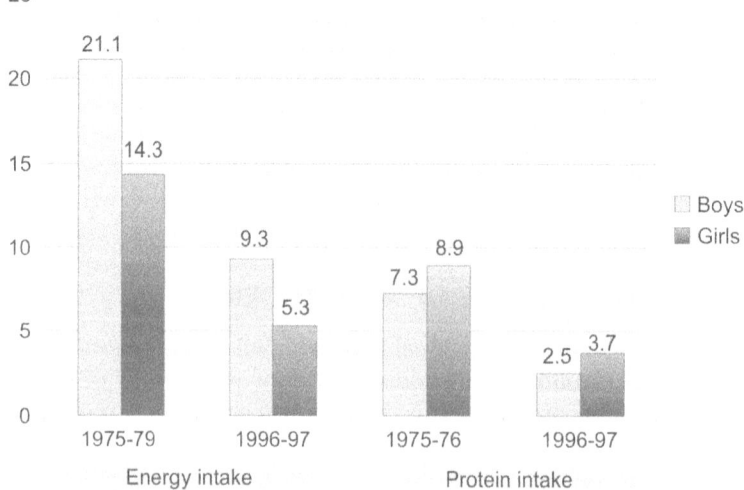

Fig. 1: Proportion of adolescents with energy and protein intake below 50% of RDA (India)[20].
(*Source:* National Nutrition Monitoring Bureau. Available at: nnmbindia.org/nnmbreport 2001-web.pdf Accessed on: 21 January 2018).

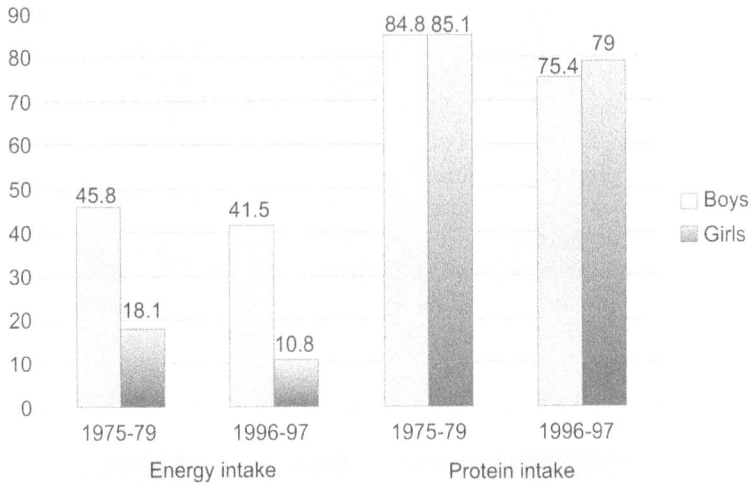

Fig. 2: Proportion of adolescents with iron and vitamin intake below 50% of RDA (India)[20]. (*Source:* National Nutrition Monitoring Bureau Available at: nnmbindia.org/nnmbreport2001-web.pdf. Accessed on 21 January 2018).

Interpersonal Level
- Family: Parenting, meals, role model
- Health professionals:
  - Peers: Attitude, behavior.

Individual Level
- Physiological factors
- Psychosocial factors.

EATING BEHAVIOR

Some important facets of eating behavior in adolescents that need attention are as follows:[12]
1. Missing meals: Missing breakfast, aptly termed the "brain's food" may even affect classroom performance.
2. Instant foods/fast foods/junk foods: *Instant foods* are those which undergo special processing designed to dissolve or to disperse particles more rapidly in a liquid than the untreated product. For instance, instant noodles, soup powders, cornflakes fall under this category. Although all instant foods need not be unhealthy in terms of high calorie or salt contents, there are concerns about the presence of certain additives like monosodium glutamate which may also add up to the overall sodium intake from the foods.

Fast foods are foods already made or cooked to order within minutes for consumption like noodles, burgers, fried fish, milk shakes, chips, salads, pizzas, sandwiches, etc. Storage, handling and microbiological contamination are the major concerns. Further, these are calorie dense foods.

Street foods comprises of a wide range of ready-to-eat foods and beverages prepared and/or sold by vendors and hawkers especially on streets and other public places. Idli, wada, dosa, chat items, etc. are examples of street foods. They may be contaminated with pathogenic organisms unless hygienically prepared.

Junk foods are those containing little or no proteins, vitamins or minerals but are rich in salt, sugar, fats and are high in energy (calories). Some examples are chocolates, artificially flavored aerated drinks, potato chips, ice creams, french fries, etc.

Frequent consumption of unhealthy processed food increases calorie intake without providing any protein, vitamins and minerals. Apart from being non-nutritious, processed foods also contain food additives. Food additives consumed beyond permissible limits may have adverse effects on health.

3. Alcohol consumption.
4. Distinctive likes and dislikes for food like aversion to roots and tubers, steamed food items.
5. Low intake of some nutrients especially micronutrients.
6. *Adolescent dieters:* Special dieting is resorted to remain slim. In contrast, some want to become tall and muscular. Psychological disorders like anorexia nervosa, bulimia nervosa. Acne vulgaris is another problem that necessitates dieting.

OVERALL STRATEGY FOR NUTRITION INTERVENTION IN ADOLESCENTS

Box 1 lists the overall strategy for nutrition intervention in adolescents. By altering dietary behaviors, nutrition interventions during adolescence have the potential of affecting children at that time and later in life. Though the majority of interventions implemented in the teen years are addressed in

---

Box 1: Nutrition interventions for adolescents.

- **Nutrition promotion**
  - Healthy eating
  - Breastfeeding
  - Physical activity
  - Self-esteem
- **Prevention management**
  - Micronutrient malnutrition
- **Clinical case management**
  - Diabetes
  - HIV/AIDS
  - Malaria
  - Infestations

schools, there is need for other intervention sites, such as libraries, after-school play grounds, summer camps, community centers, etc. Most programs with successful outcomes are likely to be behavior-based with modification as and when needed.

CONCLUSION

Adolescence, an important period of life characterized by rapid growth and development is a nutritionally vulnerable period as the requirement for various nutrients is increased. The most common nutrition-related issues during this period is anemia, under nutrition, chronic energy deficiency, eating disorders and besity.

Nutrition during adolescence should include nutrients required to meet the demands of physical as well as cognitive growth and development and also provide stores of energy for illness and pregnancy and prevent adult onset of nutrition related diseases like diabetes, hypertension, cardiovascular problems, osteoporosis etc. Iron, iodine, calcium, folate, zinc, vitamin A, and vitamin C are important micronutrients required for prevention of anemia, improving bone mass and mineral density, for immune function and for overall growth and development.

KEY LEARNING POINTS

- Adolescence is a period of most rapid growth and development having increased requirement for macro- and micronutrients.
- Nutrient requirements are increased two-to-five folds during peak height velocity as they are required to meet the growth demands and also for physiological functions.
- Macro- and micronutrients along with minerals demand and increased to provide for energy requirements, cellular increase and for biochemical functions.
- Requirement of some nutrients in adolescence is as high as or higher than any age group. Vitamin A, Thiamine, Riboflavin, Niacin, Folic acid, vitamin B_{12}, vitamin C and Iodine requirements reach levels required by adults.
- Hormones mediating pubertal growth spurt are sex steroids and growth hormones which are modulated to a great extent by nutritional factors.
- Nutrition is also related to body image and psychological well-being.
- Since adolescents are in a stage of gaining independent identity, this is the period to influence them to develop healthy eating habits and lifestyle and help them to become healthy adults.
- A well balanced diet containing all the four food groups should be advocated through nutrition counseling.
- Focusing on adolescent nutrition improves the nutrition status of the adolescents, help in having well nourished mother deliver healthy newborn, reduce maternal and neonatal mortality and morbidity, improve work efficiency through physical well-being and improve productivity.
- Prevention of anemia, undernutrition and obesity in adolescence ensures a safeguard from adult health problems like cardiovascular disease, hypertension, diabetes etc. in long-term and improve academic performance in adolescent.

REFERENCES

1. UNICEF. Adolescence: An age of Opportunity. In: *The State of the World's Children 2011.* New York: UNICEF 2011.
2. Rees JM, Christine MT. Nutritional influence on physical growth and behaviour in adolescence. In: Adams G (ed): *Biology of Adolescent Behaviour and Development.* California: Sage 1989.
3. Key JD, Key LL Jr. Calcium needs of adolescents: Current opinion. *Pedia J* 1994;6: 379-382.
4. Spear B. Adolescent growth and development. In: Rickort V (Ed): *Adolescent Nutrition : Assessment and Management.* New York; Chapman and Hall 1996:1-24.
5. World Health Organization. *Adolescent Nutrition Review in SEAR.* New Delhi: WHO 2006.
6. Gupte S, Sahni AK. Adolescent medicine. In: Gupte S (Ed): *The Short Textbook of Pediatrics,* 12th edn. New Delhi: Jaypee 2016:116-129.
7. White EW. Micronutrient requirements at different ages. *Bull Nutr* 2017;2:102-108.
8. UNICEF. *Progress for Children. A Report Card on Adolescents.* New York: UNICEF 2012.
9. Schneider D. *International Trends in Adolescent Nutrition.* New Brunswich: Department of Urban Studies and Community Health , Edward J.Bloustem School of Planning and Public Policy ,Rutgers University 2015.
10. FAO/ WHO. *Diet, Nutrition and Prevention of Chronic Diseases. Joint FAO/WHO Expert Consultation. WHO Technical Report Series No 916.*Geneva; WHO. 2003.
11. Chahar PS. Physiological basis of growth and development among Children and adolescent in relation to physical activity. *Am J Sports Sci Med* 2014;2:17-22. DOI:10.12691/asjssm-2-5-A-5.
12. Elizabeth KE. *Nutrition and Child Development,* 5th edn. Hyderabad: Paras 2015.
13. Golden MM. Is complete catch up growth possible foe stunted malnourished children? *Eur J Clin Nutri* 1994; 48 suppl 1:558-570.
14. Gabard-Durnam LJ, Flamney J, Goff B, et al.The development of human amygdala functional connectivity at rest from 4 to 23 years –A cross-sectional study. *2014;95:193-197.doi:10.1016/j.neuroimage.2014.03.038*
15. BA Woodruff BA, Duffield A, Blanck A, et al. *Prevalence of low body mass index and specific micronutrients deficiencies in adolescents 10-19 years of age in Bhutanese refugee Camps, Nepal.* Atlanta: Center for Disease Control & Prevention 1999.
16. Stang J, Story M. *Guidelines for Adolescent Nutrition Services.* Minneapolis: Center for Leadership, Education and Training in Maternal and Child Nutrition, Division of Epidemiology and. Community Health, School of Public Health, University of Minnesota 2005.
17. Michaelsson, Vahlquist A, Juhlin L, Melbin T, Bratt L. Zinc and Vitamin A; Serum concentration of Zinc and retinol binding protein (RBP) in healthy adolescent *Scand J Clin Lab Invest* 1947;36:827-832.
18. Robinson A, Kaul AK. Adolescence in Europe and SE Asia. *Eur Chr Adolesc Med* 2017;7:234-239.
19. Shettty P. Nutrition transition and its health outcomes. *Indian J Pediatr* 2013;80:Suppl S21-S27.
20. World Health Organization. *Adolescent Nutrition: A Review of the Situation in Selected South East Asian Countries.* Geneva: WHO 2005.
21. Gopalan C. Growth of affluent Indian girls during adolescence. In: *National Formulary for India,* Scientific Paper No.10. New Delhi:NFI 1986:22-23 .

22. Parks EP, Shaikhkhalil A, Groleau V, Wendel D, Stallings VA. Feeding of infants, children and adolescents. In: Kliegman RM, Staton BF, St Geme III JW, Schor NF (Eds): *Nelsons Textbook of Pediatrics*, 20th edn. Philadelphia: Elsevier 2016.
23. Gabard-Durnam LJ, Flamney J, Goff B, et al. The development of human amygdala functional connectivity at rest from 4 to 23 years: A cross–sectional study 2014;.95:193-207.*doi:10.1016/j.neuroimage.2014.03.038*
24. Nilson TK, Yngve A, Bothger AK. Hurtig Wennlof, Sjostorm. Min High Folate intake is related to better acaedemic achievement in Swedish adolescent. *Pediatric 2011;128(2)l,e,358-365.*
25. Maggini S, Weinzlaff S, Horning D. Essential Role of Vitamin C and Zinc in Child immunity and Health. *J Int Med Res* 2010;38:386-414.
26. Kodali P, Kopparty S, Vallabhuni R, Kalapela GR. Midday meal programme and adolescents: An epidemiological study in Hyderabad, India. *J Pharma Prac Commun Med* 2016;2: 6-20.

PART 5: UNDERNUTRITION AND OBESITY

15 Protein-Energy Malnutrition: Overview

Suraj Gupte, Utpal Kant Singh

ABSTRACT

The global problem of child malnutrition is a matter of deep concern. Its adverse effects are on the survival, health performance and progress of population groups. The effects are of the highest order in the resource-limited countries such as India.

In the recent decades, the incidence of severe malnutrition has gradually fallen though only to an unsatisfactory level. According to the National Family Healthy Survey-4 (NFHS-4), stunting is around 38%, wasting 21%, severe wasting 7.5% and underweight 35%. The undernourished survivors are likely to suffer from consequences such as poor quality of life, low cognitive development and learning skills over and above other handicaps. Nutritional anemias and other micronutrient and vitamin deficiencies also contribute to significant morbidity and, at times, mortality directly or indirectly.

Whereas treatment of mild-moderate malnutrition is by and large home-based, severe acute malnutrition is best treated employing the World Health Organization guidelines of 10 steps, starting with resuscitative and stabilizing measures followed by nutritional rehabilitation and follow-up.

Too rapid and aggressive dietary therapy, invariably with carbohydrate-rich foodstuffs needs to be avoided as a safeguard against feeding syndrome.

Likewise, very high protein intake during nutritional rehabilitation should be discouraged to prevent the occurrence of nutritional recovery syndrome (Gomez syndrome) and other adverse phenomena that become a roadblock in attaining the goal of satisfactory recovery.

Keywords: Gopalan's hypothesis, Kahan syndrome, Kwashiorkor, Malnutrition, Marasmus, Mid-upper arm circumference, Nutritional rehabilitation, Nutritional recovery syndrome, Prevention, Ready to use therapeutic food (RUTF), Severe acute malnutrition, Stunting, Wasting.

INTRODUCTION

According to the World Health Organization (WHO), malnutrition is a ***global problem***, having adverse effects on the survival, health performance and progress of population groups. The effects are of the highest order in the resource-limited countries, such as India.

In India, over the recent decades, the incidence of severe malnutrition as also low birth weight (LBW) infants has gradually fallen though only to an unsatisfactory level.[1-4] According to the National Family Healthy Survey-4 (NFHS-4), stunting is around 38%, wasting 21%, severe wasting 7.5% and underweight 35%. These substandard survivors are likely to suffer from consequences such as poor quality of life (QoL), low cognitive development and learning skills over and above other handicaps.

CERTAIN DEFINITIONS

- The term, *protein-energy malnutrition (PEM)* implies undernutrition predominantly of energy and protein.
- *Undernutrition* means a state of poor nutritional status as a result of inadequate intake, malabsorption or excessive loss of nutrients.
- *Overnutrition* denotes excessive intake of nutrients as in exogenous obesity.
- The term, malnutrition has under its umbrella both undernutrition and overnutrition.
- *Underweight* means low weight for age; it is a combined indicator of both acute and chronic undernutriton.
- *Wasting* indicates low weight for height as a consequence of recent/acute undernutrition.
- *Stunting* means low height for age. It is an indicator of chronic undernutrition.

PREVALENCE

South Asia (India, Pakistan, Bangladesh, and Nepal) is known for the highest prevalence of underweight children. In India, prevalence of undernutrition, is higher in rural than in urban population. At present, despite improving economy, prevalence of child malnutrion continues to show only marginal decline with the country harbouring the largest number of malnourished children in the word.[5-10] However, the incidence of severe malnutrition in the form of kwashiorkor, marasus and marasmic-kwashiorkor has considerably fallen with the central stage getting occupied by stunting, underweight and wasting.

Table 1 presents the comparative prevalence of underweight, wasting and stunting in India in 2006–2007 and 2015–2016 as per the National Family Heath Survey-3 and 4, respectively. So far 4 such surveys have been conducted, namely NFHS-1 1992–1993, NFHS-1998-99, NFHS-3 2005–2006, and NFHS 2015-16.

Table 1: Prevalence of salient indices of undernutrition in India.

Indicator	NFHS-3 (2005–2006)	NFHS-4 (2015–2016)
Underweight	43%	36%
Wasting	20%	21%
Stunting	48%	38%

(NFHS: National Family Health Survey).

ECOLOGY OF MALNUTRITION

Ecology of malnutrition is complex It is customary to consider it as:
- **Primary:** It is primarily due to dietary deficiency.
- **Secondary:** It is due to systemic, diseases such as tuberculosis or malabsorption.

In a considerable proportion of cases, both the factors may be operative. Even children with the so-called *isolated PEM* without any superimposed infection or infestation do demonstrate some degree of absorptive defect which further aggravates the state of undernutrition.

Bad Economy (Food Insecurity)

Poor socioeconomic status of the family contributes a lot to the development of malnutrition in the developing regions. With very low income, it is a tough task to provide nutritious diet to the children. It is estimated that, among the downtrodden, hardly 10% of the money is spent on foods obtained from animal sources, i.e. egg, milk, curd and meat, etc. With the further pressure on the meager income from increasing requirements, including clothing and entertainment, during modern times, still more curtailment of expenditure on food results.

Ignorance

Food insecurity may not always be the cause of primary undernutrition. Despite availability of food, the child may develop undernutrition as a consequence of factors, such as ignorance, erratic feeding practices, irrational beliefs and superstitions and poor access to health facility, etc.

Faulty Food Habits and Feeding

Many deep-rooted beliefs, customs, practices, superstitions, food taboos and ignorance join hands to cause malnutrition. Many families frown at the idea that semisolids should be introduced early enough, when the infant is about 6 months old. They wish to wait until the infant begins to approach the first birthday for a date from the priest to start semisolid food at a ceremony called *annaparasana*. By this time the infant is perhaps already anemic and having some degree of PEM.

Decline in the good practice of breastfeeding just because ignorant mothers wish to ape the sophisticated city women leading to the widespread practice of artificial feeding, providing diluted and most probably, dirty formula, is today contributing considerably to malnutrition.

Great reliance on milk, which may be awfully diluted, continues to dominate the scene even in educated and well to do families. We have seen mothers complaining that their toddlers are failing to thrive (FTT). On enquiry, it is revealed that these children have been almost entirely on milk and virtually no solids.

Most parents would withhold all foods other than diluted milk once the child has some illness like diarrhea, measles, or abdominal pain—a practice which is bound to deteriorate child's nutritional status.

Yet another limiting factor in adequate nutrition is the belief that certain foods are not given to the baby just because they are said to be *hot* or *cold* in nature.

Medical Reasons

Infections and disorders, such as diarrhea, malaria or measles may prove major contributory factors in the development of malnutrition, indirectly or directly. Besides the deliberate restriction of food by the parents, child's intake may be reduced due to reduced appetite. At the same time, they may result more catabolism to produce the heat energy lost during a febrile episode.

Intestinal parasitic infestations may either deprive the host of nutrients or lead to malnutrition by reducing appetite, causing diarrhea, or by producing absorptive defect.

Large Families

Nutritional status is adversely affected by the large size of the family. It has been convincingly demonstrated that malnutrition is much higher among children of birth order fourth and higher than in the first three children of a sibling ship. When there are too many children, the family has to do with whatever food it can manage. The brunt of the suffering falls on the preschool children and on the mother.

Closely-spaced Families

There is an evidence that when pregnancies occur rapidly, perhaps every year, or every other year, incidence of malnutrition is much higher. Ideally, there should be at least 3 years of gap between the two pregnancies.

Working Mother

It is a common observation that a higher proportion of the mothers of malnourished children are daily laborers who find little time to take care of child's feeding and rearing. More often than not, mothering is done by an elder sibling.

Bad Start

A LBW infant starts life with a handicap. He is difficult to feed and is vulnerable to infections. Born usually to a malnourished mother, such an infant has a high morbidity and mortality. The significantly LBW (VLBW, ELBV) babies who manage to survive usually have poor growth as compared to normal ones.

Secondary Malnutrition

The causes are diseases, such as intestinal malabsorption (say celiac disease, tropical sprue, cystic fibrosis, etc.) tuberculosis, intestinal parasitic infestations, diabetes, galactosemia and other metabolic disorders. Mismanagement of diarrhea with starvation therapy or hypocaloric diet (still a common practice in developing countries) is an important cause of malnutrition.

PATHOPHYSIOLOGY

Virtually all organs are affected in malnutrition (Box 1).

> **Box 1:** Adverse effect of malnutrition on systems/organs.
>
> **Central nervous system (CNS):** Retarded brain growth (microcephaly), cerebral atrophy; auditory brainstem and visual evoked potential abnormalities; dendritic arbonization and dendritic spine abnormalities
> **Gastrointestinal intestines (GIT):** Smooth tongue because of flattening of papillae; mucosa atrophic and shiny; small intestinal villous atrophy of variable magnitude depending on severity of malnutrition; reduced disaccharides level in brush border; rectal prolapsed
> **Liver:** Fatty in edematous malnutrition (kwashiorkor and marasmic kwashiorkor); shrunk in marasmus
> **Pancreas:** Predominant involvement of exocrine pancreas leading to extraintestinal steatorrhea; reduced insulin level; reduced glucagon production
> **Endocrines:** Adrenals atrophied; thyroid involution and fibrosis; high growth hormone level
> **Lymphoreticular system:** Lymphocytic depletion; thymus involution.

PROTEIN-ENERGY MALNUTRITION: A SPECTRUM

The term, PEM, refers to a class of clinical conditions that may result from varying degree of protein lack and energy (calorie) inadequacy. The term has been adopted because it is now widely agreed that the major limiting factors in the diet of children, particularly in the resource-limited countries, are energy and proteins, usually more of the former. Deficiency of proteins is usually not primary and isolated. Almost always it appears to be due to poor intake of food (energy) as such. There is an evidence that if child's energy is taken care of, it will be difficult for him to have significant protein deficiency. Else, if his energy consumption is poor, whatever proteins he takes are likely to be consumed to provide energy rather than to build the tissues.

Among the various factors that influence the clinical manifestations of PEM figures:
- Magnitude of deprivation, its duration, relative inadequacy of different principles of food
- Accompanying infection or some other disease.

Broadly speaking, two major clinical syndromes, kwashiorkor and nutritional marasmus, are widely recognized.
1. *Kwashiorkor* is said to result from gross deficiency of proteins though energy deficiency is also present.
2. *Nutritional marasmus*, on the other hand, results from gross deficiency of energy though protein deficiency also accompanies.

Thus, it is clear that there is deficiency of both, proteins and energy, in both the states. The predominance of the deficiency determines whether it is going to be kwashiorkor or nutritional marasmus.

Many malnourished children show overlap in the clinical picture, demonstrating features of both the deficiency states at a time. It is often quite appropriate to label them as marasmic kwashiorkor. But, the aforesaid severe form of PEM constitutes only a tip of the widespread problem of malnutrition (Fig. 1). A vast majority of the children suffering from mild-to-moderate forms of it remain hidden in the community for one or another reason. The two types of this subclinical malnutrition are—(1) nutritional dwarfing (stunting) and (2) prekwashiorkor.

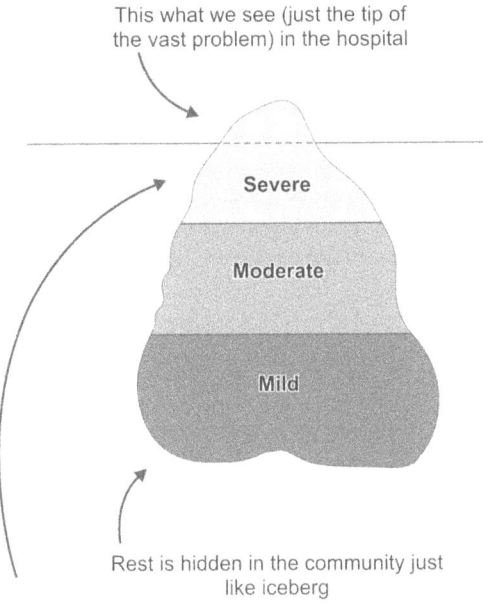

Fig. 1: Malnutrition (tip of iceberg).

All these form of PEM, in actuality, constitute a continuous spectrum of the manifestations of malnutrition. Growth failure and poor tissue repair (due to protein lack) and energy shortage (due to calorie deficiency) are common to all forms.

EVOLUTION OF PEM[11-14]

Dietary Hypothesis
According to the widely accepted dietetic hypothesis, kwashiorkor is predominantly a protein deficiency and marasmus an energy deficiency. Of course, both proteins and energy lack exist in both the syndromes. This hypothesis has a good deal of support from studies in the laboratory animals as well as work on human beings.

Adaptation Hypothesis
The noted nutritionist, Gopalan, has claimed that dietary background of children suffering from kwashiorkor and marasmus may well be the same. According to his postulation, the so called *adaptation hypothesis*, marasmus is an extreme degree of adaptation to prolonged inadequacy of proteins and energy in the diet. Kwashiorkor is a stage of adaptation failure or dysadaptation which may follow two situations:
1. Continued prolongation of the stress of malnutrition.
2. Sudden precipitation or aggravation by a fulminant infection such, as measles, pertussis, bronchopneumonia or acute diarrheal episode.

Gopalan feels that whereas nutritional marasmus may be the result of extreme degree of adaptation and kwashiorkor is the result of dysadaptation, relatively mild effect of adaptation may be responsible for nutritional dwarfing. Since, according to Gopalan's hypothesis, kwashiorkor follows occurrence of dysadaptation in a marasmic child, most of the cases are likely to show features of both, i.e. marasmic kwashiorkor.

Aflatoxin Contamination Hypothesis

More recently, it has been postulated that aflatoxin contamination of food may well be an important factor in the causation of kwashiorkor.

Golden's Hypothesis of Free Radicals

According to Golden's hypothesis of free radical damage, kwashiorkor results from overproduction of free radicals (because of infection, toxins, iron, etc.) and breakdown of protective mechanism (provided by vitamin A and E, carotene, zinc, copper, selenium and manganese, etc.).

Jelliffe's Hypothesis of Interactions and Sequelae

According to Jelliffe, kwashiorkor is an intrinsically nutritional disorder with vulnerability to other factors, some identified and some unidentified. It is the cumulative result of a mixture of interactions and sequelae of dietary imbalances and/or deficiency, infections, parasitosis, emotional trauma from maternal deprivation due to abrupt weaning from breasts, toxins like aflatoxin or ochratoxin.

PEM AND DISTURBANCES OF METABOLISM

Many like to designate PEM as a *metabolic disorder*. This is quite understandable if we recall that the disease is characterized by profound disturbances of water and electrolytes, minerals, protein, fat, carbohydrate and energy metabolism.

Water, Electrolytes and Minerals

- *Total body water:* Total body water is increased in PEM, irrespective of whether it is of kwashiorkor or marasmic type. A positive correlation exists between the magnitude of rise in body water and the extent of weight loss. Thus, lowest values are found in kwashiorkor and the highest in marasmus. Whether the alteration is secondary to increased cellular mass which constitutes the active protoplasm of the body and reduction in the adipose tissue is not clearly understood. A noteworthy point is that despite increased body water, a malnourished child is thirsty. This paradoxical observation is ascribed to the defective thirst mechanism in PEM.
- *Potassium:* There is a definite reduction in the total body potassium by as much as 25%. Though all organs are depleted of potassium, the musculature suffers the most followed by the brain. Potassium depletion is more marked in cases of PEM with diarrheal disease. In kwashiorkor, it is significant even in the absence of diarrhea. Whether potassium depletion results from

gastrointestinal losses through the gut or from defects in specific enzymes (that have a role in carbohydrate metabolism), or both, is not clear. Potassium deficiency may be existing despite absence of any clinical manifestations of dehydration and/or hypokalemia.

A very high frequency of pyelonephritis and acute renal failure is encountered in cases of severe malnutrition whose potassium depletion has not been attended to. Of course, the contributory role of concomitant dehydration and infection cannot be denied.

- *Sodium:* Unlike potassium depletion, sodium is retained by the body. Sodium retention is primarily extracellular though muscle, skin, brain and viscera, too are affected. Intracellular sodium retention and potassium deficit may change the function of important enzymes in carbohydrate metabolism and oxidative phosphorylation.
- *Magnesium:* Its depletion in PEM is now well established. This deficiency may cause grave disturbances, including neurologic signs, such as twitching, tremors and convulsions.
- *Phosphorus:* Both forms of phosphorus (organic as well as inorganic) are decreased in the muscles of malnourished children. Adequate nutritional correction leads to increase in both the forms. The exact significance of this observation, particularly from a clinical angle, remains obscure.
- *Calcium:* Its depletion is a common feature of PEM, more so when the assessment is based on blood levels. However, clinical evidence of tetany is infrequent.
- *Iron:* Iron deficiency anemia is a common feature of PEM. It is, however, complicated by other deficiencies involving folic acid, vitamin B_{12}, vitamin E and probably some other vitamins.
- *Copper:* Low levels of copper in serum, hair and liver of subjects suffering from PEM have been documented. There may also be low levels of ceruloplasmin which plays the role of a link in copper and iron metabolism.
- *Chromium:* Its deficiency has been blamed for the impaired glucose tolerance in malnourished children. There is an evidence that it may contribute to poor growth of the child during the earlier stage of nutritional rehabilitation. Chromium therapy may accelerate growth in marasmic infants.
- *Zinc:* Low serum as well as muscle and liver zinc values exist in PEM. Zinc deficiency may play an important role in the etiology of the syndrome of growth retardation with short stature, hypogonadism, hepatosplenomegaly and anemia in boys. The supplementation of zinc to such boys results in a dramatic improvement. Sometime within 3 weeks of initiating treatment, significant gain in weight and acceleration of sexual maturity are achieved. Zinc deficiency is also associated with infantile tremor syndrome and diarrheal disease.

Protein and Amino Acids

Total serum protein level is always reduced, principally due to hypoalbuminemia which is remarkable in kwashiorkor. The level of β-globulins is also reduced.

α and γ-globulin levels are variable in absolute terms; it is invariably high in relation to other serum protein fractions.

There is a remarkable reduction in the total body protein. Its turnover, unlike that of albumin, may be high rather than low. Significant reduction in plasma amino acids occur in kwashiorkor. Valine, leucine, isoleucine and tyrosine are the ones most affected. There is a rise in amino acid recycling in kwashiorkor. This mechanism, together with low urea synthesis, increased ammonia and urea nitrogen utilization for protein synthesis contributes to increased nitrogen economy in protein deficiency.

Lipids

There is a reduction in fat absorption from the gut. Also, there is increase in fecal fat (steatorrhea) even when diet is free from fat. Free bile acids are increased whereas there is a decrease in the concentration of conjugated bile acids. The latter are supposed to be essential for dissolution of lipids in the lumen of the gut and their eventual absorption.

The transport of fat from liver to tissues as low density lipoproteins is considerably reduced though transport from gut to liver is not much altered. Various factors that may contribute to the fatty liver of kwashiorkor are increased fat transport from tissues to liver, reduced synthesis of β-lipoproteins, increased liver lipogenesis, and probably reduced level of essential fatty acids.

Carbohydrates and Energy

Hypoglycemia occurs frequently and may prove fatal in a proportion of cases. Glucose absorption is impaired due to deficiency of disaccharides enzymes in the intestinal mucosa. Handling of intravenously administered glucose and galactose is abnormal. Circulating insulin levels are low. The levels fail to respond to stimulation with glucose or arginine.

Disaccharide intolerance is a common transient phenomenon. Hence, it is advisable to avoid large loads of lactose containing foodstuffs during early part of management of PEM. Levels of growth hormone are high, but of somatostatin low. Basal metabolic rate (BMR) is reduced. Thyroid function, too, is low.

PEM AND INFECTION

There is a considerable evidence supporting the definite association between malnutrition and infection.[14] Malnutrition is the most common immunodeficiency in pediatric practice and breaksdown the host resistance by and large in all segments (Figs. 2 and 3). The most consistent abnormality is impairment in cell-mediated immunity (CMI). The implications of this observation are:
- Bacterial infections which count on CMI for host's defense against them, are very severe in children suffering from PEM.
- Secondly, children with PEM are difficult to sensitize by repeated antigens.
- Even the delayed hypersensitivity reactions that recall previous sensitization are also delayed.

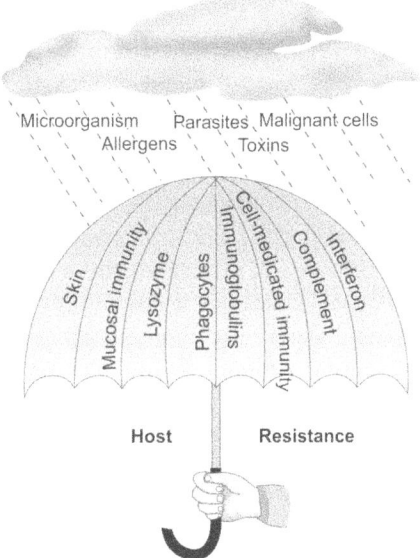

Fig. 2: Resistance in a healthy, well-nourished child provides protection against adverse influences and insults.

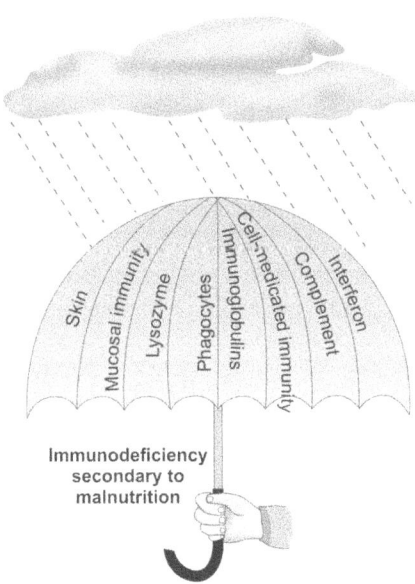

Fig. 3: Immunodeficiency secondary to malnutrition. Note the widespread breakdown in host resistance involving almost all organ and systems.

There is evidence that iron deficiency anemia has an adverse effect on the cellular immune response. The underlying mechanisms include:
- Lymphopenia
- Reduced number of T-lymphocytes in the peripheral blood
- Impaired response to mitogen and antigens
- Decreased lymphokine production
- Serum inhibition.

It has been demonstrated that levamisole improves the ability of lymphocytes to proliferate in vitro in response to phytomitogens and increases the number of rosetting T-lymphocytes. However, the effect on lymphocyte stimulation response is less than that achieved by nutritional supplementation both at 2 and 4 week intervals after initiation of therapy. When given together with nutritional rehabilitation, levamisole administration is associated with an increase in cell-mediated response in vivo and in vitro. The change is observed earlier than a significant gain in weight.

Interrelationship between PEM and infection is summarized in Box 2.

PEM AND DIARRHEA

Diarrhea is a common accompaniment of the clinical picture of overt PEM. Its prevalence is 5–7 times more and its severity 3–4 times greater in malnourished children as compared to normal children. In the not-so-distant past, recurrent diarrhea in malnourished children was generally ascribed to superimposed infections and infestations. No doubt, malnourished patients are particularly susceptible to infection because of the impaired cellular immunity which is an important adverse sequel of malnutrition per se.

- It was earlier suggested that, besides bacterial and parasitic contamination of the gut, gastrointestinal candidiasis may contribute to the common occurrence of diarrhea in malnutrition. The investigations from Indonesia and Australia lend support to this hypothesis.
- PEM may per se cause striking morphological as well as functional damage to the small intestinal mucosa leading to malabsorption.

Box 2: Interrelationship between PEM and infection.

Causes of malnutrition leading to infection
- Micronutrient deficiency—iron, zinc, copper and selenium
- Vitamin deficiency—vitamin A, C, E, B_6 and folate
- Impaired CMI, phagocytic function and complement system
- Reduced cytokine production
- Reduced concentration of IgA, IgM and IgG.

Cause of infection leading to malnutrition
- Reduced intake of food, especially micronutrients
- Enhanced catabolic losses
- Reduced absorption of nutrients
- Metabolic inefficiency because of micronutrient deficiency.

(CMI: cell-mediated immunity; PEM: protein-energy malnutrition; Ig: immunoglobulin)

Box 3: Factors contributing to diarrhea in PEM.

- Superimposed gastrointestinal infection—bacterial, parasitic, fungal
- Villous atrophy causing malabsorption
- Disaccharidase deficiency in brush border, causing transient lactose intolerance and osmotic diarrhea
- Iron deficiency anemia causing exudative enteropathy
- Pancreatic insult causing digestive disturbances, steatorrhea and diarrhea

- Transitory secondary disaccharides deficiency causing lactose intolerance and osmotic diarrhea has also been observed in significant proportion of cases. The earlier reports suggesting existence of some monosaccharide malabsorption have now been substantiated.
- Moreover, it is to be noted that iron deficiency is a common occurrence in PEM. Since there is evidence that iron deficiency may itself contribute to an exudative enteropathy in childhood, the role of such anemia in etiology of diarrhea of malnutrition seems to be convincingly established.
- A recent study has documented significant decline in histamine augmented maximum acid output as also presence of chronic gastritis and gastric mucosal atrophy in per oral gastric biopsies in marasmic children.
- Finally, there is evidence that PEM may give rise to pancreatic atrophy and decreased enzyme secretion, resulting in digestive disturbance and diarrhea. Thus, it becomes obvious that diarrhea in malnutrition is of multifactorial etiology (Box 3).

PEM AND FAMILY PLANNING

In developing countries, women (often malnourished) begin to produce children at a much younger age. They continue doing so quite frequently with poor spacing. Result is in the form of too many births. What is still more disturbing is that they continue doing so as long as they are not old enough.

This phenomenon leads to impaired nutritional status of both the mother and her babies, many of whom may be born after intrauterine growth retardation has already affected their bodies and perhaps brains. Such infants start life with a distinct disadvantage. They are also candidates for high morbidity and mortality. Undoubtedly many of such deaths could be prevented. The biostatisticians call such deaths as excessive *reproductive wastage*.

The question arises, *Why do women reproduce at such a high pace in developing world?* The reason is simple. Unless parents can be assured that the children they have are going to survive into adulthood, they will be unwilling to consider limiting their reproductive activities. It has, therefore, been argued that nutrition and general health activities should be coordinated to provide major support for maintaining health and promoting survival of infants and children.

A strong plea is made for promoting the traditional breastfeeding with suckling done throughout the 24 hours each day. This practice is not only a safeguard against malnutrition, but it also has an effect on ovulation and birth spacing.

PEM AND ENDOCRINE STATUS

Cortisol

Contrary to earlier studies, now it has been convincingly shown that serum cortisol levels in gross PEM are high, suggesting hyperfunction of the adrenal cortex. Factors, such as infection and hypoglycemia are said to contribute to this observation. High cortisol levels mediate the following useful functions:
- Augmentation of lipolysis
- Enhancement of muscle protein catabolism
- Promotion of liver protein synthesis.

Somatomedins

Serum levels of insulin-like growth factor (IGF-1 and 2) are low due to one or more of the following factors:
- Low protein and/or energy supply in diet
- Lack of essential amino acids
- Low insulin/cortisol ratio.

Low somatomedins levels mediate the useful function of reducing energy and oxygen utilization by retarding growth.

Insulin

Impaired serum insulin levels are found in kwashiorkor and marasmic kwashiorkor, but not in marasmus due to:
- High energy low protein ratio in diet
- Low body potassium
- Deficient insulinotropic factors and insulin transport by the damaged pancreas.

Growth Hormone

Growth hormone levels are high in PEM, reflecting increased secretion rather than impaired clearance. The causative factors include:
- Low somatomedin levels
- Hypoalbuminemia and low amino acid levels
- Low serum tyrosine level.

The useful functions mediated by the above observations include:
- Facilitation of the process of lipolysis
- Boosting of glucogenesis
- Decrease in catabolism of albumin.

Glucagon

Glucagon levels are high whereas insulin levels are low in PEM leading to low insulin/glucagon ratio. The following useful functions may be mediated:
- Reduction in glucose uptake by muscles and adipose tissue, sparing heart and brain
- Increased muscle protein catabolism
- Increased lipolysis and fatty acid supply to peripheral tissues.

Thyroxin

Contrary to earlier observations, thyroid hormone production is either normal or high in kwashiorkor, but normal or low in marasmus.

PEM AND CARDIAC FUNCTION

Gross malnutrition is known to considerably reduce the weight and the size of the heart. This is ascribed to atrophy of the cardiac muscle. On the functional front, cardiac output is reduced in keeping with the severity of weight loss. There is prolongation of the systemic recirculation time, appearance time, bradycardia and reduced peripheral blood flow. Congestive cardiac failure (CCF) may occur. Electrocardiography (ECG) shows nonspecific changes. Radiology shows reduction in heart size. Not only does malnutrition per se affect cardiac function, but other factors, such as accompanying severe anemia, reduced oxygen consumption and hypothyroid state too contribute to it.

PEM AND RENAL FUNCTION

PEM causes reversible impairment of renal function as manifested by:
- Reduction in glomerular filtration and renal plasma flow, especially when there is accompany gastroenteritis.
- Aminoaciduria, phosphaturia and inefficient excretion of acid load from disturbed tubular function.
- Urine is acidic due to increased excretion of hydrogen ions to conserve potassium.

PEM AND DRUG DISPOSITION

It is now well established that nutritional status of a child has significant effect on the bioprocesses involved in disposition of various drugs in the body. As a result, bioavailability of the drug(s) for therapeutic purposes is influenced, often warranting alteration in dose and frequency of administration. The exact observations concerning different drugs in various studies, however, are far from uniform.

VARIOUS CLASSIFICATIONS OF PEM

Based on Clinical Features

Syndromal Classification
- Kwashiorkor
- Marasmus
- Marasmic kwashiorkor
- Prekwashiorkor
- Stunting
- Underweight
- Invisible PEM.

Based on Weight for Age

Gomez Classification

- **First degree:** Weight between 90% and 75% of expected for age
- **Second degree:** Weight between 75% and 60% of expected for age
- **Third degree:** Weight below 60% of expected.

Wellcome or International Classification

- **Weight between 80% and 60% of expected for age with edema:** Kwashiorkor
- **Weight between 80% and 60% of expected for age without edema:** Undernutrition
- **Weight below 60% of expected with edema:** Marasmic kwashiorkor
- **Weight below 60% of expected without edema:** Marasmus.

Indian Academy of Pediatrics (IAP) Classification

- **First degree:** Weight between 80% and 70% of expected for age
- **Second degree:** Weight between 70% and 60% of expected for age
- **Third degree:** Weight between 60% and 50% of expected for age
- **Fourth degree:** Weight below 50% of expected in case the child has demonstrable pitting edema, the letter "K" is placed in front of the evaluated grade.

Jelliffe Classification

- **First degree:** Weight between 90% and 80% of expected for age
- **Second degree:** Weight between 80% and 70% of expected for age
- **Third degree:** Weight between 70% and 60% of expected for age
- **Fourth degree:** Weight below 60% of expected.

All these classifications recommended Harvard standard as the reference standard (now obsolete). WHO 2006-2007 reference standards are the current recommendation.

Based on Weight for Height

Waterlow Classification

- **Weight more than 90% of expected for height:** Normal
- **Weight 80–90% of expected for height:** I degree
- **Weight 70–80% of expected for height:** II degree
- **Weight less than 70% of expected for height:** III degree.

MacLaren Classification

- **Weight more than 90% of expected for height:** Normal
- **Weight 85–90%:** Mild (I degree)
- **Weight 5–85%:** Moderate (II degree)
- **Weight less than 75%:** Severe (III degree).

Based on Height for Age
Waterlow Classification
- **Normal:** 98%
- **Mild:** 95-90%
- **Moderate:** 85-90%
- **Severe:** Less than 85%.

Based on Weight for Height and Height for Age
Waterlow Classification
- **Acute:** Weight for height—low, height for age (normal, wasted not stunted)
- **Acute/chronic:** Weight for height—low, height for age low (wasted and stunted)
- **Nutritional dwarfing:** Weight for height—normal, height for age low (stunted but not wasted).

Application of both the indices (as in Waterlow classification) is, therefore, of greater value than application of one.

WHO Classification
The WHO classification of PEM is given in Table 2 and shown in Figure 4.

Table 2: WHO classification of PEM.

Criteria	Moderate PEM	Severe PEM
Symmetrical edema	No	Yes
Weight for height (index of wasting)	70–79% of expected (wasting)	Less than 70% of expected (severe wasting)
Height for age (index of stunting)	85–89% of expected (stunting)	Less than 85% of expected (severe stunting)

(PEM: protein-energy malnutrition; WHO: World Health Organization).

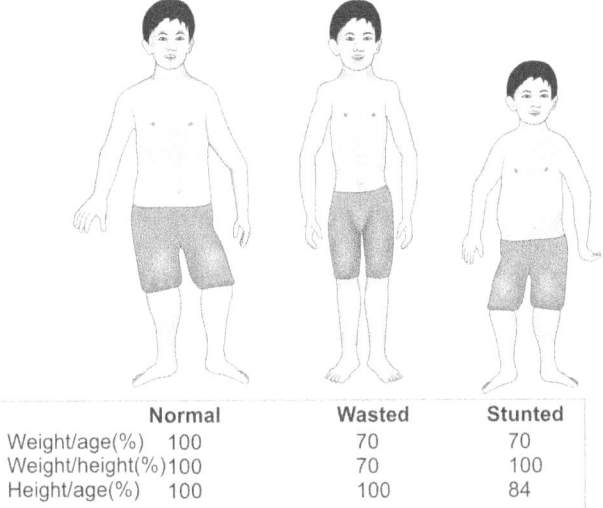

	Normal	Wasted	Stunted
Weight/age(%)	100	70	70
Weight/height(%)	100	70	100
Height/age(%)	100	100	84

Fig. 4: Normal wasted and stunted children. Weight for age is low in both wasted child and stunted child. But weight for height is not affected in the stunted child.

Based on MUAC

Arnold Classification
- **Mild:** MUAC between 12.5 cm and 13.5 cm
- **Moderate:** MUAC between 11.5 cm and 12.5 cm
- **Severe:** MUAC under 11.5 cm.

Based on Skinfold Thickness
- **Mild:** 80-90% of expected for age (8-9 mm)
- **Moderate:** 60-80% of expected for age (6-8 mm)
- **Severe:** Less than 60% of expected for age (less than 6 mm).

Based on BMI (kg/m^2)
- **Mild (underweight):** 15-18.5
- **Moderate:** 13-15
- **Severe:** Less than 13
- **Normal:** 18.5-22
- **Overweight:** 22-25
  Unlike adults, in children 25-30 is considered obesity
- **More than 30:** Moribund obesity.

- Weight for height $= \dfrac{\text{Actual weight}}{\text{Weight of normal child of the same age}} \times 100$

- Height for age $= \dfrac{\text{Actual height}}{\text{Height of normal child of the same age}} \times 100$

- Currently, reference norms for comparison are WHO (2006-2007) standards.

SPECIAL FEATURES OF CLINICAL SYNDROMES

Kwashiorkor (Edematous Malnutrition, Malignant Malnutrition)

The earliest description of kwashiorkor in the English medical literature was made in 1933 by Cicely Williams, a noted British physician. That time she did not really know how to christen the disease. Later, in 1935, she introduced the term *kwashiorkor*, the local name for the disease in Ghana. It was said to mean the *red boy*, because of the characteristic pigmentary changes. In 1950, the term was more aptly interpreted to apply to the mystique of the disease that affected the deprived child due to the arrival of yet another.

Clinical Features (Figs. 5 to 7)

The disease is chiefly encountered in infants and children in the preschool age group. A vast majority of the cases are in 1-4 years age group. No age is, however, exempt. Occasionally, it may be seen in infants aged few months, in adolescents and even in adults. A classical case of kwashiorkor is following:

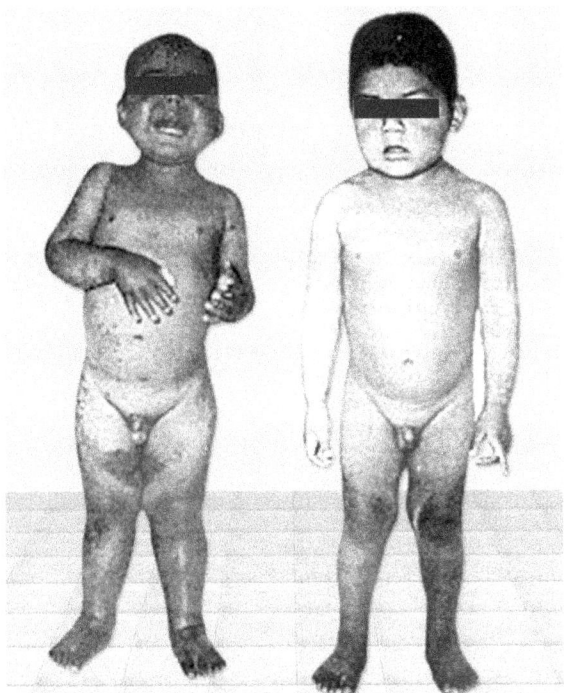

Fig. 5: Kwashiorkor. Note the classical features including growth retardation, remarkable muscle wasting with some retention of subcutaneous adiposity and nutritional edema and psychomotor changes. Protuberant abdomen seen in these two children are frequently present.

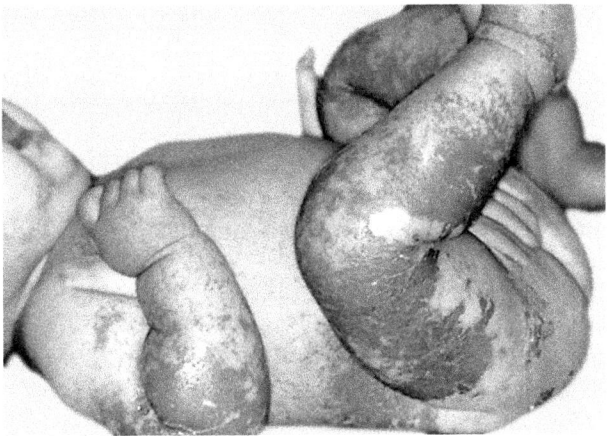

Fig. 6: Kwashiorkor. Note massive edema and flaky-paint dermatosis.

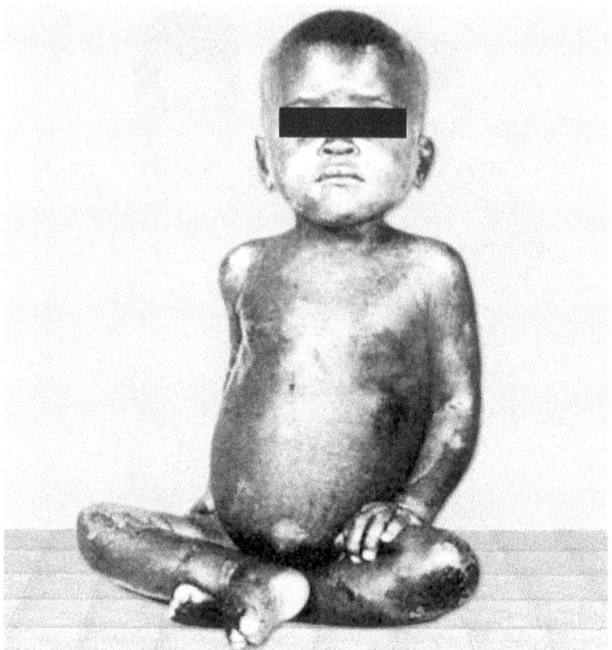

Fig. 7: Kwashiorkor. Note the flaky-paint dermatosis and essential features (growth retardation, edema, muscle wasting with retention of some subcutaneous adiposity and psychomotor change) in this 24-month-old boy weighing only 8 kg (including weight of edema fluid).

Table 3: Rading of kwashiorkor.

Grades	Characteristics
1	Pedal edema
2	+ Puffiness of face
3	+ Edema of chest wall and back
4	+ Ascites

Note: Grading of kwashiorkor based on edema is not the same as grading of edema as such.

- Dull, apathetic and miserable, evincing hardly any interest in the surroundings
- His growth is stunted
- Marked muscle wasting with some retention of subcutaneous fat
- He has pitting edema over the legs and feet and perhaps over certain other parts of the body (Table 3).

There may be diarrhea, skin and hair changes, anemia and vitamin deficiency signs. Liver is, as a rule, enlarged due to fatty change.

Though this is the picture of full-blown kwashiorkor, it may be noted that only four signs (growth failure, muscle wasting with retention of some subcutaneous fat, mental apathy and hypoalbuminemic edema not of cardiac, renal or hepatic origin) taken together are sufficient by themselves to label a case as kwashiorkor.

The remaining elements may individually or collectively accompany the essential features depending on the severity of the disease, dietary pattern and regional variations.

Biochemical Changes
These are striking:
- Serum proteins are always low, the maximum reduction being that of the albumin fraction; the globulins may often be found relatively elevated.
- Anemia is usually moderate to severe and may be of variable morphology though iron deficiency is a common denominator in most cases.
- Low serum enzymes (esterase, amylase, lipase, choline-sterase and alkaline phosphatase), serum cholesterol, glucose, urea, certain vitamins, potassium and magnesium occur. The activity of pancreatic enzymes is considerably reduced.
- Total body potassium is diminished.
- Imbalance of plasma amino acids and amines aciduria are common findings.
- Impaired cellular immunity is present.

Diagnosis
Dietetic enquiry reveals deficient intake of proteins and calories, the protein lack being more predominant over a prolonged period. Occurrence of an added stress like measles, whooping cough, diarrhea or bronchopneumonia often precipitates the overt picture leading to the development of pitting edema. Diagnostic criteria may be divided into two major subdivisions—(1) essential and (2) nonessential.

Essential Features (Minimal Diagnostic Criteria)
- Growth retardation as evidenced by low weight and low height.
- Muscle wasting with retention of some subcutaneous fat.
- Psychomotor change as evidenced by mental apathy in the form of silent listless inertness, lack of interest in the surroundings.
- Hypoalbuminemic pitting edema, at least over the pretibial region. Serum albumin should be less than 2.5 g/dL and cardiac, hepatic, renal and angioneurotic causes of edema should be ruled out. These essential features are to be considered the minimal diagnostic criteria for kwashiorkor.

Nonessential Features
These are variable features and may or may not be present in each and every case.
- *Hair changes (Figs. 8 and 9)* in the form of hypochromotrichia (light-colored hair), sparseness (areas of alopecia), change in texture (coarseness, silkiness) and easy pluckability. Alternate bands of light and dark color have earned the name flag sign which signifies periods of inadequate nutrition, adequate nutrition and again inadequate nutrition over a prolonged period. This fascinating sign is only occasionally encountered.
- *Skin changes* include light-colored skin, but the most classical dermatosis consists of areas of hyperpigmentation intervened by areas of raw red skin caused by shedding of the superficial skin flakes. This has been called *flaky-paint dermatosis*. Another similarly characteristic skin lesion of kwashiorkor

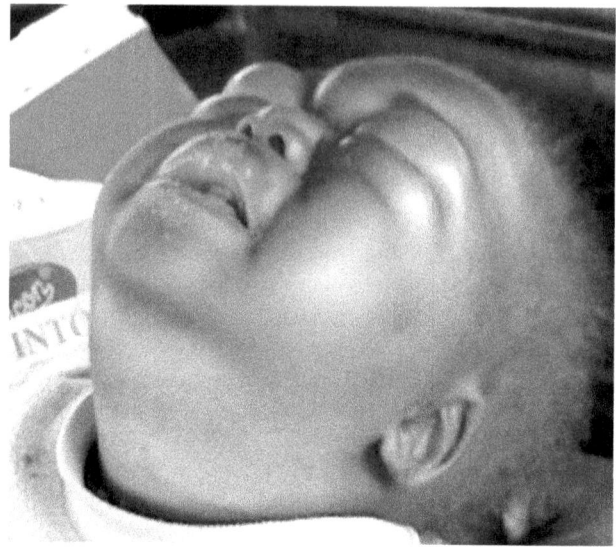

Fig. 8: Kwashiorkor. Note the characteristic mental apathy, moon facies with periorbital edema and sparse light-colored hair.

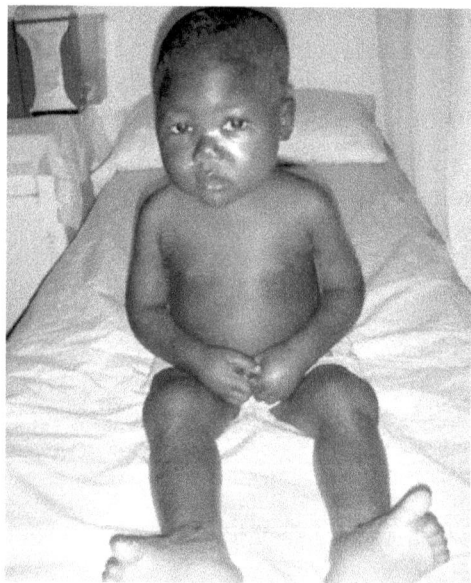

Fig. 9: Kwashiorkor. Note the psychomotor changes, light-colored sparse scalp hair, moon facies, periorbital edema, and pedal edema.

is crazy-pavement dermatosis. Reticular pigmentation, mosaic dermatosis and pellagra-like lesions over the exposed parts (usually dorsal surfaces) may also be encountered (Figs. 10 to 13).

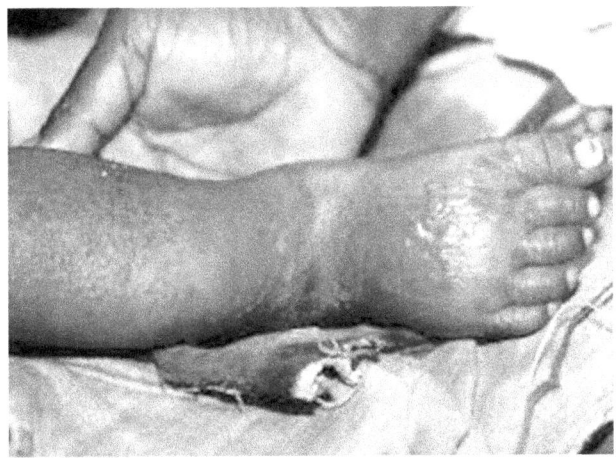

Fig. 10: Kwashiorkor showing massive edema over feet and legs as also mosaic dermatosis. This is the same child as in Figure 8.

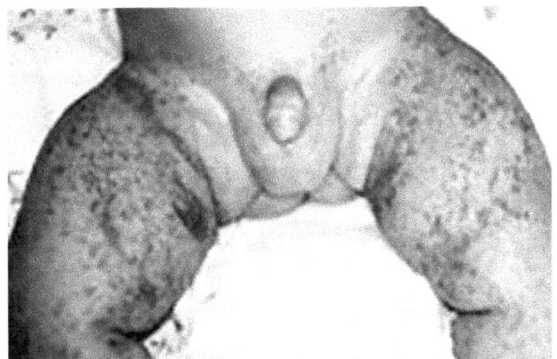

Fig. 11: Kwashiorkor. Note the classical flaky-pain dermatosis and massive edema. Absence of hair changes reflects acute nature of the ailment.

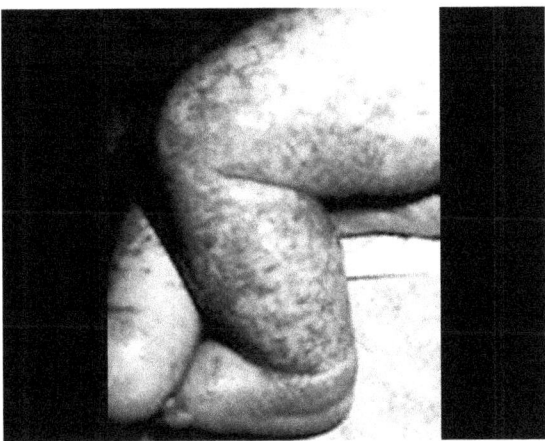

Fig. 12: Kwashiorkor in a toddler. Note the classical skin lesions and massive edema.

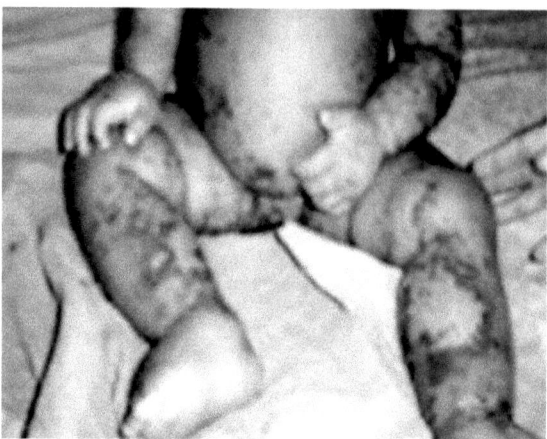

Fig. 13: Kwashiorkor. Typical crazy-pavement dermatosis and gross edema.

Besides the aforesaid dermatosis, kwashiorkor children may suffer from indolent sores and ulcers besides superadded skin infections like pyodermas and scabies.

- *Gastrointestinal manifestations* include diarrhea, vomiting and anorexia. In spite of edema, the child may develop dehydration. Diarrhea may be due to quite a few factors, including superadded infections and infestations and effect of malnutrition per se as already discussed.
- *Mineral and vitamin deficiencies* are common. Anemia is usually present and is moderate to severe in intensity. It is frequently iron deficiency type though dimorphic and even pure megaloblastic morphology may be encountered. There is evidence that PEM may per se cause anemia. Accompanying factors, such as intestinal parasitic infestations and systemic infections may also play a contributory role. Other mineral deficiencies are those of potassium and magnesium.

  Deficiency of vitamin A is frequent and may lead to serious problem of keratomalacia and irreversible blindness. Deficiencies of vitamin B-complex, C, D and E may also complicate the picture.
- *Hepatomegaly*, quite often fairly remarkable (liver may touch the umbilicus), is invariably present. The consistency is usually soft, the edge rounded and the surface smooth.
- *Superadded infections* (say, tuberculosis, bronchopneumonia, enteritis, measles, pyodermas, etc.) and intestinal parasitic infestations (*Lamblia giardia, Entamoeba histolytica*, roundworm, hookworm, threadworm, *Hymenolepsis nana*, etc.) are common. Infection by gram-negative organisms (usually enteritis and septicemia and occasionally urinary tract infection) is most troublesome to manage in such patients.
- *Clubbing* may be encountered in a proportion of the children with kwashiorkor as a result of the accompanying steatorrhea.
- *Nonspecific ECG changes* may be found in a small proportion of the cases. A significant cardiac involvement is seldom seen.

Box 4: Grading of kwashiorkor.

- *Grade I:* Pedal edema
- *Grade II:* Facial puffiness
- *Grade III:* Paraspinal and chest edema
- *Grade IV:* Ascites/anasarca.

When kwashiorkor occurs in its full-blown picture, it is termed *florid kwashiorkor*. Box 4 shows grading of kwashiorkor in terms of severity.

Marasmus (Nonedematous Malnutrition with Severe Wasting)

Though kwashiorkor has received far greater attention from the researchers, nutritional marasmus is encountered more frequently in several parts of the world particularly in north India. At times, the condition is referred to as *atresia* or *infantile atrophy*.

Clinical Features (Figs. 14 to 16)

Nutritional marasmus occurs usually in subjects less than 3 years of age; the peak incidence is seen during the first year of life. The disease may be encountered in later childhood.

A characteristic feature of the clinical picture is remarkable wasting of both muscles and subcutaneous fat. The face is wizened and shriveled—just as in the case of a monkey. In the early stages, the child is irritable, hungry and craves for food. However, in the later stages, he may become miserable and apathetic, refusing to take anything. Edema is conspicuous by its absence. Significant hair changes, dermatosis and marked fatty liver are also absent. As in kwashiorkor, diarrhea, mineral and vitamin deficiencies, superadded infections and parasitic infestation are commonly seen. Table 4 provides Achar's grading of nutritional marasmus.

Biochemical Changes

These are slight until marasmus is of very advanced degree. The reason is that the amino acids liberated from child's own tissues make possible a continuing synthesis of serum enzymes, albumin and other essential metabolites.
- Anemia is mild to moderate and may be of any morphologic type though iron deficiency anemia undoubtedly dominates the picture.
- Electrolyte disturbances may occur in the presence of diarrhea and vomiting.
- Blood urea is usually normal.
- Blood sugar slightly raised.
- Duodenal enzymes show little or no reduction.

Diagnosis

Dietetic history suggests inadequacy of both proteins and calories (carbohydrates) in child's intake in the recent past. The predominant lack is of calories. Diagnostic criteria may be essential and nonessential features as follows:

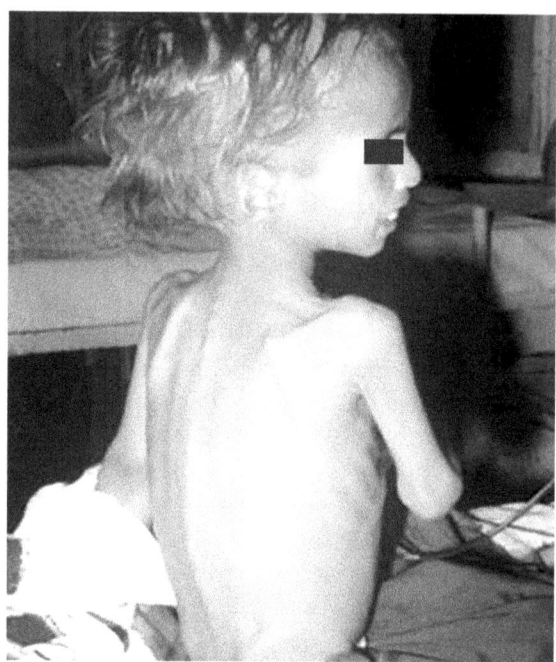

Fig. 14: Marasmus. Note the remarkable wasting of both muscles and subcutaneous adiposity. The child had been on only highly diluted formula.

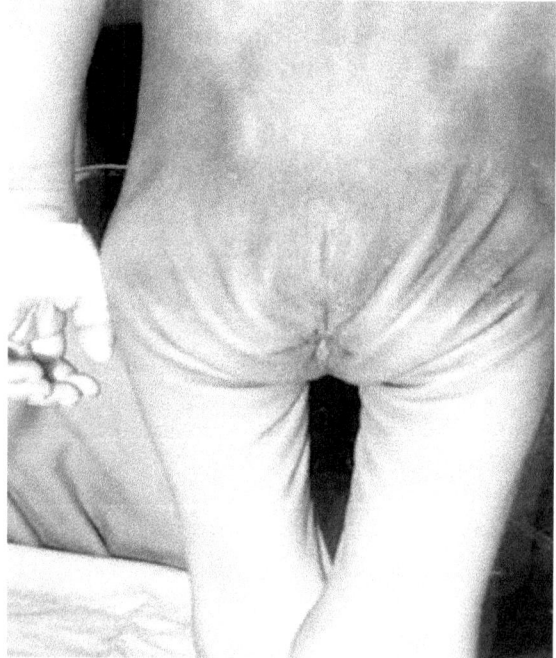

Fig. 15: Marasmus. Note remarkable wasting over gluteal region. This is the same marasmic child as in Figure 14.

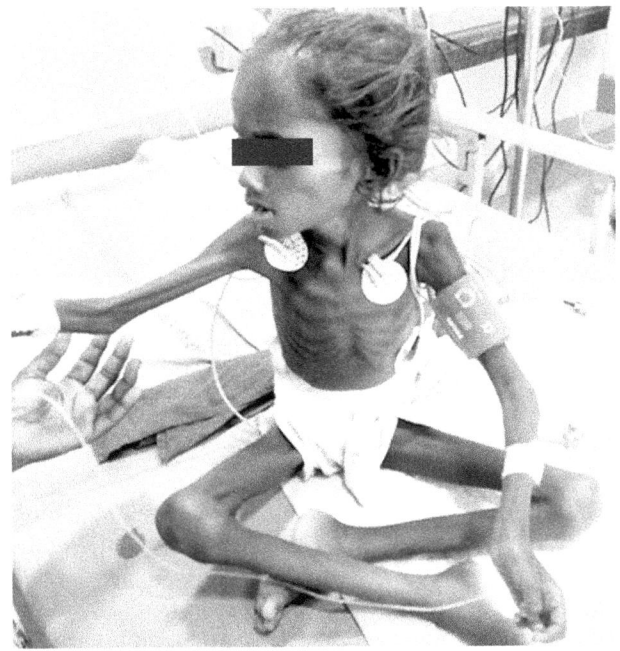

Fig. 16: Marasmus. This is an example of PEM secondary to tuberculosis.

Table 4: Achar's grading of nutritional marasmus.

Grades	Characteristics
1	Loss of fat from axilla/groin
2	Loss of fat from abdominal wall and gluteal region
3	Loss of fat from chest wall and back (paraspinal region)
4	Loss of buccal pad of fat (which consists of fatty acids); it takes longer time to disappear

Essential features (minimal diagnostic criteria)
- Growth retardation as evidenced by marked loss of weight and subnormal height/length.
- Gross muscle as well as subcutaneous fat wasting.
- Absence of edema.

Nonessential features
- *Hair changes* are usually not present.
- *Classical dermatosis* of kwashiorkor is not seen. However, indolent sores and ulcers as also superadded skin infections occur very frequently.
- *Gastrointestinal manifestations* like diarrhea and vomiting occur as in kwashiorkor. A marasmic child is, however, hungry rather than anorexic, though he may develop anorexia once marasmus has advanced to extreme degree.

- *Mineral and vitamin deficiencies* occur fairly commonly. Anemia is usually mild to moderate and may be of varied morphology. Potassium and magnesium deficiencies occur in patients with diarrhea and vomiting. Vitamin deficiencies occur relatively less often compared to kwashiorkor.
- Liver is rather shrunk which is in sharp contrast to the fatty, enlarged liver of kwashiorkor.
- *Superadded infections and infestations* are nearly as common as in kwashiorkor.
- *Psychomotor change* is usually in the form of irritability rather than listlessness. Advanced cases may, however, become apathetic as is seen in kwashiorkor.
- *Clubbing* may be seen in a proportion of marasmic children. It seems to be related to the accompanying steatorrhea.

Marasmic Kwashiorkor

Marasmic kwashiorkor refers to cases demonstrating a combination of features of kwashiorkor and marasmus. Presence of edema is essential for this diagnosis (Fig. 17). For instance, an established case of nutritional marasmus may be mistakenly initiated on a diet consisting of lots of calories, but very little proteins. Such a child is a candidate for developing hypoproteinemia and clinical edema. Remaining features of kwashiorkor may or may not be present.

Pre-kwashiorkor

Prekwashiorkor refers to a child who has quite poor nutritional status and certain other features of kwashiorkor, such as hair changes minus edema. Such a child,

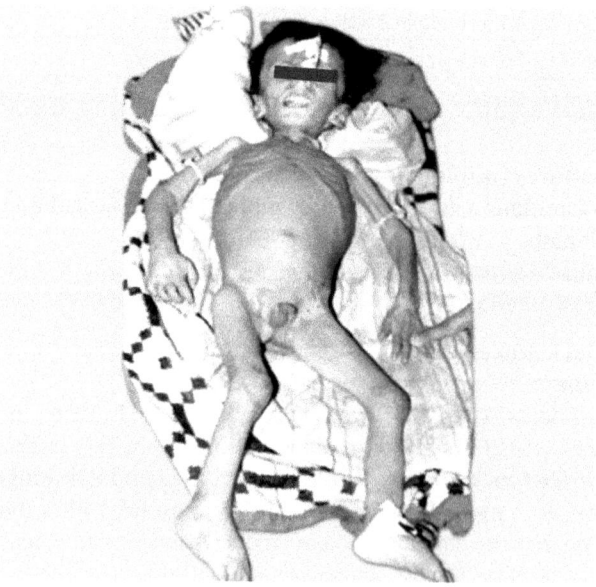

Fig. 17: Marasmic kwashiorkor. Note remarkable wasting with pedal edema.

unless taken care of at this very stage, may develop edema and other features of full-blown kwashiorkor. A comparison of important features of marasmus and kwashiorkor is presented in Table 5.

Table 5: Kwashiorkor versus Marasmus—comparison of important features.

Feature	Marasmus	Kwashiorkor	Special comment
Age	First 3 years; usually less than 1 year	1–5 years	No age is a bar in both cases
Essential features			
Growth failure/retardation	Yes Severe (weight less than 60% of expected for age)	Yes Moderate (weight more than 60% of expected for age)	Growth retardation is evidenced by low weight and low length/height
Muscle wasting	Remarkable (skin-bone appearance)	Less remarkable	In kwashiorkor, muscle wasting though severe is somewhat masked by edema
Subcutaneous fat wasting	Remarkable	Some subcutaneous adiposity retained	
Psychomotor change	Irritable, alert	Listless, apathetic, disinterested in surroundings	
Edema	Absent	Hallmark	In marasmic kwashiorkor, edema is present
Nonessential (variable) features			
Classical hair changes	Absent	Usually sparse, light-colored, easily-pluckable and brittle; infrequently flag sign	
Typical dermatosis	Absent	Often present	In marasmus, classical dermatosis (say flaky paint, crazy pavement) is absent. Other skin conditions, such as pyoderma, impetigo or scabies may be present in both kwashiorkor and marasmus
Diarrhea	Yes	Yes	Villous atrophy leading to malabsorption, among other factors contributes considerably to development of diarrhea in both. Magnitude of steatorrhea is far more in kwashiorkor than in marasmus.
Appetite	Initially good	Anorexic	Eventually with worsening of condition, marasmic child also becomes anorexic

Contd...

Contd...

Feature	Marasmus	Kwashiorkor	Special comment
Anemia	Mild to moderate	Moderate to severe	
Superimposed infection(s)	Frequent	Common	
Serum proteins	Low	Very low, albumin less than 2.5 g%	
Liver	Shrunk	Enlarged due to fatty change	
Clubbing	Sometime present	Sometime present	Chronic steatorrhea and/or coexisting tuberculosis may be responsible for clubbing
Electrocardiogram (ECG)	Low voltage	Low voltage	
Response to treatment	Early	Slow	

Nutritional Stunting

If PEM starts fairly early in life and goes on and on over a number of years without causing overt picture of kwashiorkor or marasmus, child's height as well as weight may be significantly low for his age. This is what has been termed ***nutritional dwarfing*** or ***stunting***.

Let this be understood through this illustrative case. A healthy looking child appearing aged 6 years is brought to a physician for a trivial medical problem. His height is 101 cm and weight 16 kg. Naturally, the physician forms an impression that the nutritional status of the child including height and weight is good enough for the age of 4 years. Right at this stage, the mother reveals that the actual age of the child is 7 years. This indeed surprises the physician. The fact is that this child is quite stunted (height only 101 cm instead of expected about 115 cm) and underweight (weight only 16 kg instead of expected about 22 kg) for his actual age.

Nutritional dwarfing is a common problem in developing countries, but cases are not as frequently detected. It seems to be a kind of adaptation to poor diet (not as grave as to cause frank kwashiorkor or nutritional marasmus) over a prolonged period. These children are generally less active and less lively. They are more prone to diarrhea, pneumonia, tuberculosis or other infections prevalent in the region.

COMPLICATIONS OF PEM

Serious complications of PEM are summarized in Table 6.

Table 6: Serious complications of advanced PEM.

Complication	Remarks
Superadded infections	Both overt and hidden: Septicemia, pneumonia, diarrhea, pyoderma, scabies, UTI, tuberculosis
Dehydration and dyslectrolytemia	Usually complicating accompanying diarrhea, often with lactose intolerance
Hypothermia	An unattended rectal temperature of less than 35°C may prove fatal, causing SIDS
Hypoglycemia	It contributes to poor response to nutritional therapy and carries a poor prognosis
CCF	It is usually precipitated by excessive intake of sodium and fluid or severe anemia. Since cardiac size is invariably small in PEM, even a normal sized heart in X-ray should arouse suspicion of CCF
Anemia	Moderate to severe anemia may result from malnutrition as such or factors, such as superadded infection(s), contributing to development of CCF
Bleeding	DIC may complicate the clinical picture (Fig. 18)
SIDS	Sudden death 4–7 days after admission. Usually, the cause remains unclear

(UTI: urinary tract infections; CCF: congestive cardiac failure; SIDS: sudden infant death syndrome; PEM: protein-energy malnutrition; DIC: disseminated intravascular coagulation).

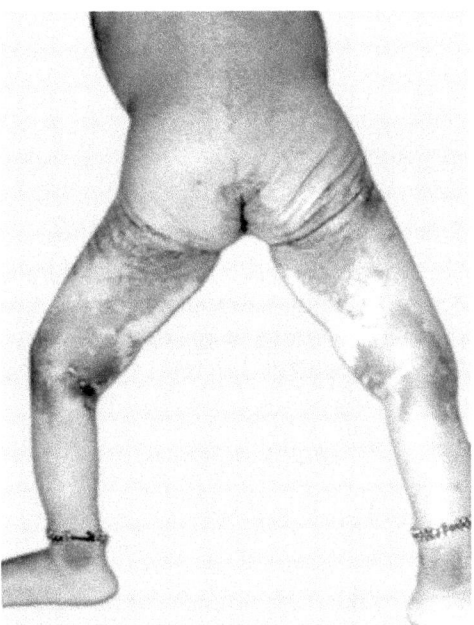

Fig. 18: Severe PEM. Note the complication of bleeding diathesis (purpura fulminans) from DIC. Superimposed sepsis is often coexisting in such a situation.

PRINCIPLES OF MANAGEMENT OF PEM

Domiciliary (Home) Management

Mild-Moderate Malnutrition

Children with mild-to-moderate malnutrition are best managed in their own homes and kept under surveillance so as to find out improvement or deterioration in their nutritional status.[15] The parents of such children are educated about the inadequacy in child's intake and guided how to correct it. The stress should be on the locally available economic foods, including **Hyderabad mix** (Table 7) rather than on expensive tinned protein preparations which should be reserved for special situations only. The parents must be apprised of the value of carbohydrates and the rationale of giving liberal amounts of semisolids and solids. They must understand why only milk will not be enough for the growing child. There is evidence that domiciliary treatment brings about gratifying results.
- It reduces the unnecessary hospital load, is much less expensive, and, in addition, gives nutritional education to the family and the community.
- Ours as well as many other workers' experience indicates that malnutrition relapses only infrequently when moderate PEM is treated at home. On the contrary, incidence of recurrences in hospital treated cases is fairly high.
- The management at home has got to be supervised and monitored by weekly visits of paramedical (say an anganwadi worker), visits to a nearby nutrition rehabilitation center or outpatient department (OPD) of a health center/hospital.

A prerequisite to domiciliary treatment is absence of severe infection(s), fulminant gastroenteritis and electrolyte imbalance. Good weight gain, as judged from the growth chart, is by and large the best yardstick of adequacy of response to nutritional rehabilitation.

Uncomplicated Severe Acute Malnutrition (SAM)

WHO had earlier categorically recommended hospitalization in case of uncomplicated SAM as well. It has now advocated home treatment for this category since it is not feasible to offer them hospital treatment and they can be managed well in domiciliary settings. This is in keeping with the IAP guidelines (Box 5).

Management in Nutrition Rehabilitation Center (NRC)

This concept, originally started in Southern America, aims at offering nutritional rehabilitation for mild-to-moderate PEM as a compromise between domiciliary

Table 7: Hyderbad protein-energy rich mixture for home treatment of PEM.

Roasted whole wheat	40 g
Roasted bengal gram	16 g
Roasted groundnut	10 g
Jaggery	20 g
Total	86 g providing 330 kcal and 11.3 g proteins

Box 5: Domiciliary (home) treatment of uncomplicated SAM as per IAP.

- **Diet:** Energy-dense therapeutic diet with low bulk in the initial phase which should be:
    - Home-based (prepared/modified from the family pot; indigenous RUTF
    - Cost-effective, easily available and acceptable
    - Fed frequently (6–8 times/24 hours)
- **Supplements:** Micronutrient and minerals
- **Oral antibiotics:** Usually cotrimoxazole or ampicillin for 7 days
- **Deworming:** Single dose
- **Warming up:** Hypothermia prevented by maintaining environmental temperature and covering the child well, especially during night
- **Immunization:** Routine
- Health education
- **Others:** Family and community participation, nutrition counseling and household food security, etc.

and hospital managements. It offers a meeting point between classical treatment and prevention, embracing the positive points of both hospital and home management.

Two types of NRCs are—(1) day care center and (2) residential center.

Day care NRC

It consists of a room for children, a kitchen, an examination room and a teaching space. At least one good meal is provided to children. Around 20–40 malnourished children along with their mothers who are expected to involve themselves in various activities are taken care of. The center remains open from 8 am to 6 pm daily.

Residential NRC

This is a larger and more organized NRC with a house-mother as the fulltime head with responsibilities that include daily work schedule of the mothers, purchase of food, issuing the correct amount of food as decided by the nutritionist, and keeping stock and maintenance of cleanliness of the center. The supervisory staff is part time and includes a doctor, a medical assistant/nurse, a home economist/nutritionist, and an agriculture teacher/extension worker. The center is attached to a health center or pediatric department of a teaching hospital, or an under five clinic. The criteria for admission to the NRC are:
- Children especially at risk.
- Children who fail to gain weight over a period of 3 months.
- Children who do not catch-up in growth after serious illness (measles, whooping cough and diarrhea).
- Failure to breastfeeding.
- Mothers and children who find it difficult to cope with their problems in spite of the health teaching they receive at the under five clinic.
- Twins and triplets.

The stress in the NRC is on nutrition and health education, household budget teaching, homecraft teaching and actual feeding, using locally available foodstuffs and local methods of cooking and preparation. The successful rehabilitation at the NRC must be followed up at home so that the knowledge acquired during stay at the center continues to be applied at home.

Hospital Management

Complicated severe acute malnutrition (SAM) needs to be managed in hospital in three phases as discussed under SAM.

Severe Acute Malnutrition(SAM)

Definition
WHO and United Nations Children Emergency Fund (UNICEF) define SAM as presence of any one of the following features in children aged 6 months to 5 years:
- Weight for height/length less than −3 SD or Z scores of the median in the 2006-2007 WHO growth charts
- MUAC less than 115 mm (11.5 cm) in children between 1 and 5 years
- Bipedal edema
- Visible severe wasting.

Infants and children suffering from SAM are at high-risk of complications which may terminate in death. SAM may further be categorized as uncomplicated or complicated.

Prevalence
Approximately 20 million children under 5 years of age have SAM. Most of them live in South Asia and sub-Saharan Africa. The mortality rate is 7.3-18.7% every year. This equates to one million child deaths every year due to SAM.

Back home in India, NFHS-3 conducted in 2005-2006 shows that 8.1 million children are suffering from SAM causing 0.6 million deaths annually. It also contributes to 24.6 million disability adjusted life year (DALY) in a year.

Etiology
A detailed description of etiology is available at the outset of this very chapter. Suffice to say here that immediate determinants include LBW, illnesses, such as diarrhea, pneumonia, measles and poor dietary intake. Three underlying household determinants that influence the immediate determinants are food, care and health. Basic determinants include low socioeconomic status, poor education status, cultural taboos, inadequacy of water and sanitation.

Diagnosis
Children with SAM can be identified by frontline community workers like anganwadi worker (AWW), accredited social health activists (ASHA) and auxiliary nurse midwife (ANM). Once the diagnosis of SAM is made, the child has to be assessed by an integrated management of childhood illness (IMCI)/integrated management of neonatal and childhood (IMNCI) trained health worker and a decision regarding the type of care (whether the child requires inpatient care or can be managed on outpatient basis) has to be made.

Management
Treatment of malnutrition is increasingly being shifted from *facility-based management* to *community-based approach*. This decentralization aims to increase access to services promoting early presentation and compliance.

Children who have coexisting human immunodeficiency virus (HIV) and tuberculosis with SAM also need simultaneous antiretroviral therapy and

Pneumocystis carinii pneumonia (PCP) prophylaxis and antituberculous therapy (ATT) for adequate response.

Uncomplicate SAM

A large chunk (85–90%) of children with SAM does not have complications. They can be managed at home or in the community. Appetite test is of value in deciding if the SAM in a particular child is complicated or uncomplicated. The test comprises of offering local therapeutic feed to the SAM child who should not have taken any feed in the preceding 2 hours. The amount consumed should be measured at the end of the test. For passing the test, the child should have consumed a minimum of 25 mL/kg. If the child fails the test, he is in need of hospital treatment. Failure of the test during the course of follow-up too is a pointer for transfer to facility-based inpatient care.

Complicated SAM

The objectives of facility-based treatment in complicated SAM are:
- To manage the complications and reduce the mortality.
- To improve the physical and psychosocial growth of children with SAM.
- To educate the mothers and caregivers about appropriate feeding of infants and young children.
- To identify any social factors that are involved in the causation of SAM.

The management of SAM is in three phases—stabilization, transition and rehabilitation.

1. **Stabilization:** In this phase, child is stabilized with treatment of acute complications and then initiated on F-75 diet. This phase lasts 1–2 days.
2. **Transition:** Child comes to this phase when he is active and alert, appetite returns; there is beginning of loss of edema, no nasogastric feeds, infusions and no severe medical problems. This phase lasts 2–3 days. There is transition from starter to catch-up diet.
3. **Rehabilitation:** Child enters this phase when he has reasonable appetite and finishes 90% of the feed, major reduction of edema and no other medical problem.
    - General principles for routine care (10 steps)
    - Emergency treatment of shock and severe anemia
    - Treatment of associated conditions.

Common Complications
- Hypothermia/sometime fever
- Hypoglycemia
- Persistent vomiting, diarrhea, severe dehydration
- Severe anemia
- Fulminant infection(s):
    - Severe lower respiratory tract infection (pneumonia)
    - Extensive superficial infection
- Lethargy, drowsiness, apathy, seizures.

Criteria for Admission
- SAM with complications
- Failed appetite test
- Child less than 6 months with SAM
- Presence of bilateral pitting edema +/++ (edema +++ always needs inpatient care).

Laboratory Investigations
- Random blood sugar
- Hemoglobin
- Serum electrolytes
- Screening for infection:
  - Total and differential count, blood culture sensitivity
  - Urine routine and culture sensitivity
  - Chest X-ray
  - Mantoux
  - HIV after counseling, if suspected
- Any other specific test based on clinical presentation.

WHO Recommended Ten Steps of Management of SAM (Fig. 19)
WHO has recommended that SAM should be treated in two major phases—namely stabilization and rehabilitation[16-19] (Box 6).

Ten steps are described in details elsewhere (Chapter 15: Severe Acute Malnutrition).

Outcome
- ***Primary failure:*** Nonresponder, i.e. no weight gain for 3 weeks or weight loss over 14 days.
- ***Secondary failure:*** Relapse—failed appetite test or 5% weight loss.

Step	Stabilization Days 1–2	Stabilization Days 3–7	Rehabilitation Weeks 2–6
1. Hypoglycemia	→		
2. Hypothermia	→		
3. Dehydration	→		
4. Electrolytes	—————————————→		
5. Infection	—————→		
6. Micronutrients	—————————————→		
7. Caution feedng	—————→		
8. Catch-up growth			————→
9. Sensory stimulation	—————————————→		
10. Prepare of follow-up			————→

Fig. 19: WHO recommended 10 steps for management of SAM. Note the time frame for stabilization and rehabilitation.

Box 6: Two major phases needing management in SAM.

1. **Stabilization phase:** Stabilization phase comprising of first 7 days of hospital treatment is a spotlight on resuscitation (restoration of homeostasis) and treating complications, such as hypothermia, hypoglycemia, dehydration and electrolyte imbalance, infections and heart failure, etc.
2. **Rehabilitation phase:** Here, spotlight is on building up the oral dietary intake over several weeks (say 2–6 weeks) in order to rebuild the wasted muscles and other tissues.

(SAM: severe acute malnutirition).

Box 7: Factors contributing to poor response to nutritional rehabilitation.

- *Feeding inadequacy*—faulty and inadequate
- Failure to adequately treat the accompanying infection(s) (pneumonia, diarrhea, UTI, AOM, intestinal parasitosis, malaria, tuberculosis, HIV)
- Failure to properly treat accompanying dehydration and dyselectrolytemia
- Failure to attend to accompanying deficiencies (say anemia)
- *Poor facilities*—untrained and poorly motivated staff, inadequate environment
- *Serious underlying diseases*—malabsorption, immunodeficiency, inborn errors of metabolism, malignancy

(UTI: urinary tract infection; AOM: acute otitis media; HIV: human immunodeficiency virus).

Box 8: Activities helpful in preventing SAM.

- Promotion of exclusive breastfeeding till 6 months of age
- Promotion of continued breastfeeding till 2 years
- Improving complementary feeding for children from 6 months to 2 years
- Improving maternal nutrition and education
- Improving availability of high quality food
- Improving access to health care
- Improving sanitation and hygiene

- **Defaulter:** Not traceable for two visits.
  Factors contributing to poor response are listed in Box 7.

Prevention
Promotion of appropriate infant and young child feeding practices and knowledge among caregivers goes a long way in preventing SAM (Box 8).

Community-Based Therapeutic Care (CTC)
Community based therapeutic care (CTC), a new concept for managing SAM is aimed at reducing the cost of treatment to the families as well as increasing the access to treatment. Its components are:
- *Community mobilization* to encourage early presentation and compliance.
- *Supplementary feeding protocols* for moderate acute malnutrition with no medical complications through outpatient therapeutic program (OTP) centers.
- *Therapeutic feeding protocols* for SAM with no medical complications through OTP centers.
- *Inpatient protocols* for SAM with medical complications. The OTP center essentially provides the following:
  - Provision of medical nutrition therapy.

- Course of oral antibiotics along with vitamin A, folic acid, antihelminthics and antimalarials, when indicated.
- Follow-up weekly/fortnightly by skilled health worker including provision of next supply of RUTF.

The principle of ***continuum of care*** from home and community to the health center and back, is critical for an effective management of SAM. A widely implemented community-based approach along with facility-based management for the complicated cases can go a long way in reducing the burden of deaths due to SAM.

Table 8 lists the type of treatment that should be given for different types of SAM as well as moderate acute malnutrition (MAM).

READY TO USE THERAPEUTIC FOOD

Background

Therapeutic diet is recommended by the WHO after stabilization in SAM, F-100, is vulnerable to bacterial contamination and has to be used within few hours of preparation. This prevents it from being used on a large scale at the community level. This paved the way for the ready to use therapeutic food (RUTF) which was developed in the mid 1990s.

RUTF as Medical Nutrition Therapy

The RUTF is a medical nutrition therapy (MNT) with a balanced composition of type I and II nutrients based on sound scientific principles. They are soft crushable ready to use foods which are energy dense and enriched with minerals and vitamins. It can be consumed without the addition of water. RUTF nutrient composition is similar to F-100, but with a greater energy and nutrient density. It also contains iron and is oil based with an extremely low water activity.

As RUTF does not contain water, it has lesser chances of getting contaminated and can be used at home without refrigeration. As it need not be cooked, there is no loss of heat labile vitamins.

Since RUTF does not contain water, plenty of safe drinking water has to be supplemented. Breastfeeding has to be continued along with RUTF.

Table 8: Recommended type of treatment for different types of SAM as well MAM.

Type of acute malnutrition	Treatment recommended
SAM with complications	Phase I treatment as inpatient at stabilization center where the treatment is on standard guidelines for complicated SAM.
SAM without complications	Home-based treatment and rehabilitation employing RUTF which is supplied on a weekly or fortnightly basis as OTP.
MAM without complications	SFP in which the family is encouraged to take home ration for the malnourished child without complications.

(SAM: severe acute malnutrition; OTP: outpatient therapeutic program; SFP: supplementary feeding program; RUTF: ready to use therapeutic food, MAM: moderate acute malnutrition).

RUTF is to be used only as a therapeutic feed for children more than 6 months and for a limited period (4-8 weeks) till the child recovers from SAM. Its use as a supplementary feed should be avoided. The amount of RUTF or any therapeutic feed to be consumed each day is given in Table 8.

RUTF has a higher success rate compared to RUTF free regimens in SAM. RUTF has also been shown to be better than F-100 in terms of weight gain, energy intake and time to recovery. The experience with of RUTF in SAM in few states of India has proved gratifying. The cost of production is about 3 USD per kg. Each child needs around 10-15 kg of RUTF over a period of 6-8 weeks during treatment.

PHENOMENA ENCOUNTERED DURING NUTRITIONAL REHABILITATION

Favorable
- Resumption of alertness as shown by a smile and interaction with mother
- Initiation of weight gain
- Disappearance of edema (by 7-10 post-therapy day)
- Disappearance of enteropathy and hepatomegaly
- Elevation of serum protein
- Attainment of normal weight for height in 1-3 months *(clinical recovery)*.

Unfavorable

Refeeding Edema

Some infants and children with marasmus may develop edema following some correction in their nutrition. The so-called **refeeding edema** results from hyperinsulinemia causing decrease in sodium excretion. It may also follow nutritional rehabilitation with a diet that is predominant in calories (energy) with relative inadequacy of proteins.

Pseudotumor Cerebri

Overenergetic nutritional correction in malnourished infants may be accompanied by a transient rise of intracranial tension. The phenomenon is benign and self-limiting.

Nutritional Recovery Syndrome (Gomez Syndrome)[19]

The term refers to interesting sequelae of events seen in children who are being treated with very high quantity of proteins during the course of rehabilitation from gross malnutrition. The syndrome is characterized by increasing hepatomegaly, abdominal distention, ascites, prominent thoracoabdominal venous network, hypertrichosis, parotid swelling, gynecomastia and eosinophilia. In some instances, splenomegaly also occurs. Though the syndrome was initially described in kwashiorkor from Africa, we have recorded its occurrence in both kwashiorkor and marasmus in India.

Etiopathogenesis

The etiopathogenesis of this syndrome remains speculative. Its development may well be related to endocrine disturbances. That in PEM the function of the pituitary and its target glands is set at a lower 'tempo' level is well known. This response of the pituitary to the state of poor dietary intake appears to be an adaptive mechanism that permits survival of the patient by reducing body activity and metabolic rate, and by retarding growth. During nutritional rehabilitation, the greater utilization of the hormone by the body stimulates the pituitary to produce its trophic hormones. This results in a response by the target glands. Thus, it appears that the nutritional recovery syndrome is caused by an increase in estrogen level and by a variety of trophic hormones produced by the recovering pituitary gland.

Encephalitis-like Syndrome

- ***Progressive deterioration in sensorium:*** About one-fifth children with kwashiorkor become drowsy within 3–4 days after initiation of dietary therapy. Most often, the condition is self-limiting. Occasionally, it may be accompanied by progressive unconsciousness with fatal outcome.
- ***Kahn syndrome:*** Even more rarely, a transient syndrome marked by coarse tremors, Parkinsonian rigidity, bradykinesia and myoclonus (Kahn syndrome) may appear 6 to several days after starting the dietary rehabilitation.
- ***Tremors during recovery (kwashi-shakes):*** Sometimes, tremors (the so-called ***kwashi-shakes***) may occur during the recovery phase and may take even months to resolve. These encephalitis-like states are considered to be the result of far too much of proteins in the diet.

Refeeding Syndrome

It denotes fluid and electrolyte disturbances, especially severe hypophosphatemia, with neurologic, pulmonary, cardiac, neuromuscular, and hematologic complications (Box 9) following rapid overloading with too much of energy (calories) during nutritional rehabilitation. Associated hypokalemia and hypomagnesemia may cause cardiac arrhythmias which may prove fatal.

Etiopathogenesis

During prolonged fasting, the body aims to conserve muscle and protein breakdown by switching to ketone bodies derived from fatty acids as the main energy source. The liver decreases its rate of gluconeogenesis thus conserving muscle and protein. Many intracellular minerals become severely depleted

---

Box 9: Clinical manifestations of severe hypophosphatemia in refeeding syndrome.

- **Neurologic:** Weakness, lethargy, paresthesia, disorientation, seizures and coma
- **Pulmonary:** Impaired contractility of diaphragm, dyspnea and respiratory failure
- **Cardiac:** Hypotension and poor stroke volume
- **Hematologic:** Leukocyte dysfunction, hemolysis and thrombocytopenia
- **Neuromuscular:** Areflexic paralysis

during this period, although serum levels remain normal. Importantly, insulin secretion is suppressed in this fasted state and glucagon secretion is increased.

During refeeding, insulin secretion resumes in response to increased blood sugar, resulting in increased glycogen, fat and protein synthesis. This process requires phosphates, magnesium and potassium which are already depleted and the stores rapidly become used up. Formation of phosphorylated carbohydrate compounds in the liver and skeletal muscle depletes intracellular adenosine triphosphate (ATP) and 2,3-diphosphoglycerate in red blood cells, leading to cellular dysfunction and inadequate oxygen delivery to the body's organs. Refeeding increases the basal metabolic rate. Intracellular movement of electrolytes occurs along with a fall in the serum electrolytes including phosphate, potassium and magnesium. Glucose, and levels of the vitamin B thiamine may also fall.

Cardiac arrhythmias are the most common cause of death from refeeding syndrome, with other significant risks including confusion, coma, convulsions and cardiac failure.

The syndrome is described in details elsewhere (Chapter 17: Refeeding Syndrome).

Prevention and Treatment

Too rapid nutritional correction with too much of carbohydrate diet should be avoided. Secondly, it is advisable to monitor phosphate levels during refeeding. Low phosphate levels (less than 1-1.5 mg/dL) are an indication for IV administration of phosphate, 0.08-0.16 mmol/kg over 6 hour.

Rickets

During nutritional recovery, as a result of rapid growth, vitamin D, calcium and phosphate consumption may fall short of the body needs, causing rickets. In some children, the pre-existing, but hidden rickets become manifest following restoration of bone growth during nutritional rehabilitation.

Anemia/Micronutrient Deficiency

In addition to the pre-existing anemia as a part of malnutrition, the child may manifest further worsening in hemoglobin status if iron and folic acid supplements are not provided during nutritional rehabilitation. Likewise, deficiencies of other micronutrients may become evident.

PROGNOSIS

With good hospital care, mortality rate in gross PEM has today considerably fallen. Against the alarmingly high figures of 20-50% in the older series, the recent reports indicate around 10% mortality.

Bad prognostic signs include severe dehydration, hypoglycemia, hypothermia, CCF, superimposed infections, xerophthalmia, bleeding diathesis, hepatic dysfunction, seizures, significant change in sensorium and cachexia (extreme weight loss).

The causes of mortality include dehydration and electrolyte imbalance (dyselectrolytemia), hypoglycemia, hypothermia, fulminant systemic infections and CCF. In our experience, dehydration and electrolyte imbalance due to diarrheal disease and fulminant systemic infections are the chief killers of malnourished children. CCF, though uncommon, carries a very bad prognosis. In some cases hypoglycemia and hypothermia may prove fatal.

LONG-TERM SEQUELAE OF PEM
Growth Retardation
Infants who suffer from significant malnutrition fairly early in life and over a prolonged period develop a permanent and irreversible stunting of growth.

Mental Impairment
Now a sort of consensus seems to have emerged concluding that IUGR and malnutrition in the first year of life, if severe enough to retard physical growth and to warrant hospitalization, may cause retardation in mental performance, eventually leading to low intelligence and impaired learning skills.

Malnutrition and Liver
It is no longer believed that PEM causes cirrhosis in the long run. The concept is based on longitudinal follow-up studies of children suffering from severe PEM and the observation that incidence of cirrhosis in Africa, the home of kwashiorkor, is fairly low.

PREVENTION OF MALNUTRITION
This is described in details elsewhere (Chapter 20: Prevention of Childhood Malnutrition).

CONCLUSION
Child malnutrition, still rampant in India, has adverse effects on the survival, health performance and progress of child population groups in particular. The survivors are likely to suffer from consequences, such as poor quality of life, low cognitive development and learning skills over and above other handicaps. Though treatment of mild-moderate malnutrition is by and large home-based, severe acute malnutrition is best treated employing WHO guidelines starting with resuscitative and stabilizing measures followed by nutritional rehabilitation and follow-up. Dietary correction that is very rapid and very rich in carbohydrate or protein foodstuffs needs to be avoided as a safeguard against adverse phenomena during nutritional correction.

> **KEY LEARNING POINTS**
>
> - Adverse effects of malnutrition are on the survival, health performance and progress of child population groups, especially in India and other resource-limited countries.
> - The undernourished survivors are likely to suffer from consequences such as poor quality of life, low cognitive development and learning skills over and above other handicaps.
> - Nutritional anemias and other micronutrient and vitamin deficiencies also contribute to significant morbidity and, at times, mortality directly or indirectly.
> - Treatment of mild-moderate malnutrition is by and large home-based.
> - Severe acute malnutrition is best treated employing the World Health Organization guidelines of 10 steps, starting with resuscitative and stabilizing measures followed by nutritional rehabilitation and follow-up.
> - Dietary correction that is very rapid and very rich in carbohydrate foodstuffs needs to be avoided as a safeguard against feeding syndrome.
> - Very high protein intake during nutritional rehabilitation should be discouraged to prevent the occurrence of adverse phenomena that become a roadblock in attaining the goal of satisfactory recovery.
> - In its prevention and treatment, early recognition, prompt stabilization and dietary correction, and good action based follow-up are crucial for favorable outcomes.

REFERENCES

1. National Family Health Survey-1, 1992-93. India Fact Sheet. Available at: rchiips.org/NFHS/nfhs1.shtml. Accessed on: 3 January 2018.
2. National Family Healthn Survey-2 1998-99. India Fact Sheet. Available at: rchiips.org/NFHS/nfhs2.shtml. Accessed on: 3 January 2018.
3. National Family Health Survey-3 2005-06. India Fact Sheet. Available at: h rchiips.org/nfhs/nfhs3.shtml rchiips.org/nfhs/nfhs3.shtml. Accessed on: 3 January 2018.
4. National Family HealthnSurvey-4, 2015-16. India Fact Sheet. Available at: http://rchiips.org/nfhs/pdf/NFHS4/India.pdf. Accessed on: 3 January 2018.
5. Earth Institute, Columbia University. India is booming—so why are nearly half its children malnourished. Available at: http://blogs.ei.columbia.edu/2011/03/24/india-is-booming-so-why-are-nearly-half-of-its-children-malnourished-part-1. Accessed on: 4 January 2018..
6. Mendelson S, Chaudhuri S. Child malnutrition in India: Why does it persist? Child in Need Institute (CINI) Available at: http://www.cini.org.uk/childmalutrition.pdf. Accessed on: 15 January 2018.
7. Jha R, Gaiha R, Kulkarni VS. Child undernutrition in India. ASARC working paper. 2010. [Last retrieved on 2010 Oct 16]. Available from: http://rspas.anu.edu.au/papers/asarc/WP2010_11.pdf
8. Svedberg P. Why malnutrition in shining India persists. 2008. Available at: http://www.isid.ac.in/~pu/conference/dec_08_conf/Papers/PeterSvedberg.pdf. Accessed on: 4 January 2018.
9. Nutritional status in infancy and early childhood. 2008. Available at: http://wcd.nic.in/research/nti1947/7.5%20iycn%203.2.2008%20prema.pdf. Accessed on: 6 January 2018.

10. Gupte S, Gomez EM. Malnutrition. In: Gupte S (Ed): *The Short Textbook of Pediatrics*, 12th edn. New Delhi: Jaypee 2016:197-224.
11. Jelliffe DB, Jelliffe EEP: Causation of kwashiorkor: Towards a multifactorial consensus. Pediatrics 1992:4:502-510.
12. Alleyne GAO, Hay RW, Picou DI, Stanfield JP, Whitehead RJ. Protein-energy Malnutrition. London: Edward Arnold 1989.
13. Gupte S. *Pediatric Nutrition*, 2nd edn. New Delhi: Peepee 2012.
14. Ramachandran P, Gopalan HS. Undernutrition and risk of infections in preschool children. *Indian J Med Res* 2009;130:579-83. [PubMed]
15. Gupta P, Shah D, Sachdev HPS, Kapil U. National workshop on development of guidelines for effective home-based care and treatment of children suffering from severe acute malnutrition. *Indian Pediatr* 2006:43:131-139.
16. Bhan MK, Bhandari N, Bahl R. Management of the severely malnourished child: Perspectives from developing countries. *BMJ* 2003:326:146-151.
17. Bhatnagar S, Lodha R, Choudhury P. IAP Guidelines 2006 on hospital-based management of severely malnourished children (adapted from the WHO guidelines). *Indian Pediatr* 2007:44:443-461.
18. Karunakara BP, Shenoy S. Severe acute malnutrition. In: Gupte S, Gupte SB, Gupte M (Eds): Recent Advances in Pediatrics-22 (Hot Topics). New Delhi: Jaypee 2014:167–182.
19. Gupte S. Nutritional recovery syndrome. *N Engl J Med* 1972:291:501.

16. Severe Acute Malnutrition

Harmesh S Bains, Manu Sharma Sareen

ABSTRACT

Severe acute malnutrition (SAM) is an important cause of child mortalty. A midarm circumference of <115 mm or a weight-for-height/length <–3 Z-scores or/and bilateral edema warrants immediate complete evaluation and hospitalization. Children having reasonable appetite and without any medical complication need to be treated as outdoor patients. Initial phase, rehabilitation phase and follow-up phase are the three major phases of management. Criteria for discharging children with SAM include: weight-for-height/length ≥–2 Z-score without edema for at least 2 weeks, or midarm circumference ≥125 mm.

Keywords: Appetite, Child mortality, Discharge criteria, Edema, Follow-up phase, Initial phase, Malnutrition, Midarm circumference, Rehabilitation phase, Severe acute malnutrtion (SAM).

INTRODUCTION

Mortality is due to severe acute malnutrition can be as high as 20%.[1-3] About 20 million children suffer from severe acute malnutrition world over and 1 million children die every year due to severe acute malnutrition, majority being from south Asia and sub-Saharan Africa.[1, 4-6]

Severe malnutrition is considered to be not only a medical but also a social disorder. Hence its treatment would be successful only if the underlying medical and social problems are identified. Such an integrated approach is also important for prevention of recurrence of relapse of this disorder.[7,8]

Measurement of midarm circumference (community level) and weight-for-height/length (hospital level) of infants and children aged 6 months to 5 years and detection of bilateral pitting edema is crucial for early identification of children with severe acute malnutrition in the community and for timely treatment or referral to reduce morbidity and mortality. A midarm circumference of <115 mm or a weight-for-height/length <–3 Z-scores (WHO growth standards) or and bilateral edema warrants immediate complete evaluation and admission of such children for the management of severe acute malnutrition. Children having appetite and without any medical complications are treated as outdoor patients. The criteria for discharging children with SAM include: Weight-for-Height/length is ≥−2 Z-score and they have had no edema for at least 2 weeks, or midupper arm circumference is ≥125 mm.[3, 7-9]

TYPES OF ACUTE MALNUTRITION

Acute malnutrition is divided into two categories which are as follows:
1. Moderate acute malnutrition
2. Severe acute malnutrition

Moderate Acute Malnutrition (Wasting)

It is defined by a weight-for-height between -3 and -2 standard deviations of the international standard or by a mid-upper arm circumference (MUAC) between 11 cm and 12.5 cm.

Severe Acute Malnutrition

In children between the ages of 6 and 59 months, severe acute malnutrition (SAM) is defined as:
- Weight/height or weight/length <-3 Z-score, using the WHO Growth Charts
  OR
- Presence of visible severe wasting
  OR
- Presence of bilateral pedal oedema of nutritional origin
  OR
- Mid-upper arm circumference <115 mm.

SEVERE ACUTE MALNUTRITION

Severe acute malnutrition is characterized by severe wasting and edema.

Severe wasting is characterized by massive loss of body fat and muscle mass. These children have old man look or monkey face.

In severe acute malnutrition, bilateral pitting edema is present on the lower limbs.

There may be skin and hair changes, hepatomegaly, etc.

Cardiovascular system: There is lower cardiac output and stroke volume, low blood pressure resulting in impaired tissue perfusion in renal, brain and skin; rapid increase in blood volume can easily produce acute heart failure.

Gastrointestinal system: There is reduction of gastric acid, pancreatic and intestinal digestive enzymes due to atrophy of pancreas and intestinal mucosa, intestinal motility and absorption of nutrients is also diminished. Metabolic functions of liver are also affected resulting in low proteins, hypoglycemia and many other disturbances.

Genitourinary system: There is decreased glomerular filtration is reduced resulting in low urinary phosphate, sodium, excretory capacity of acid.

Immune system: There is diminished cell-mediated immunity and humoral immunity. There is atrophy of lymph glands, tonsils and thymus; resulting in increased chances of infection.

Endocrine system: There are greater chances of glucose intolerance due to reduced insulin levels—insulin growth factor 1 (IGF-1) levels. Growth hormone and cortisol levels are usually increased.

History

- Appetite and feeding and dietary history. Routine diet including food and fluids being taken before the current illness and breastfeeding history.
- Duration and frequency of vomiting or diarrhea, appearance of vomit or diarrheal stools, sinking of eyes, passage of urine.
- Contact with patients having measles or tuberculosis.
- Any deaths of siblings.
- Birth weight.
- Developmental milestones reached (sitting up, standing, etc.).
- Immunizations.

Physical Examination

- Accurate recording of weight and length or height, mid-upper-arm circumference
- Checking for edema
- Appetite: Anorexia, doing an appetite test, thirst
- Enlargement or tenderness of the liver
- Abdominal distension, bowel sounds
- Pallor and its severity, cyanosis, jaundice, lymphadenopathy
- Signs of circulatory failure: Cold hands and feet, weak radial pulse, diminished consciousness, decreased urine output, prolonged capillary refill time
- Temperature: Hypothermia or fever, skin infections, purpura
- Eyes: Sunken eyes, corneal lesions indicative of vitamin A deficiency
- Respiratory rate and type of respiration: Signs of pneumonia or heart failure.

Laboratory Investigations

- Blood glucose
- Blood smear (malaria)
- Complete blood count (CBC)
- Urine culture
- Stool
- Chest X-ray (CXR)
- Purified protein derivative (PPD).

Figure 1 highlights the approach to a child with severe acute malnutrition.

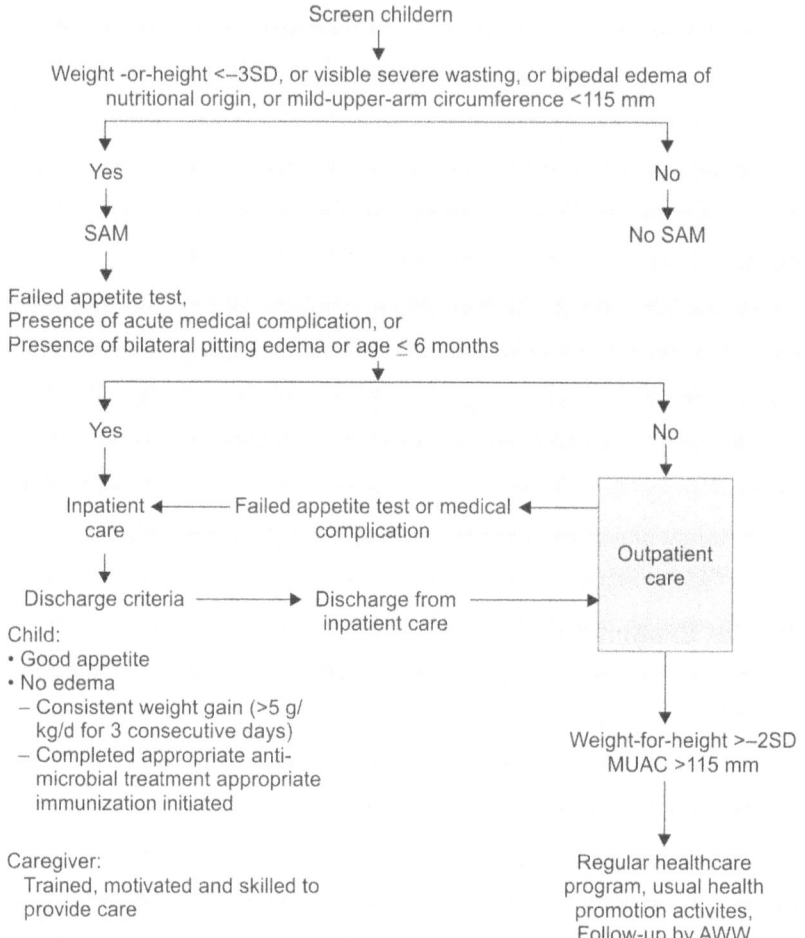

Fig. 1: Approach to a child with acute malnutrition (IAP).
(SD: standard deviation; SAM: severe acute malnutrition; MUAC: mid-upper arm circumference; AWW: anganwadi worker).

Table 1 lists the criteria for passing the appetite test.

Table 1: Criteria for passing appetite test as per IAP.

Body weight (kg)	Minimum amount of RUTF(kg) to be consumed for passing the appetite test (mL or g)
>4	15
4–6.9	25
7–9.9	35
10–14.9	50

Phases of Treatment

There are three phases of treatment of SAM:
1. Initial phase of treatment
   - Life-threatening problems identified and treated
   - Specific deficiencies/metabolic abnormalities corrected
   - Feeding begun
2. Rehabilitation phase of treatment
   - Intensive feeding
   - Emotional and physical stimulation
   - Training of mother
3. Follow-up phase of treatment
   - Prevention of relapse
   - Assure continued development.

Ten Steps for Management of Severe Acute Malnutrition

1. Treat/prevent hypoglycemia
2. Treat/prevent hypothermia
3. Treat/prevent dehydration
4. Correct electrolyte imbalance
5. Treat/prevent infection
6. Correct micronutrient deficiencies
7. Start cautious feeding
8. Achieve catch-up growth
9. Provide sensory stimulation and emotional support
10. Prepare for follow-up after recovery.

Treatment of Hypoglycemia

- Hypoglycemia = <56 mg/dL or <3 mmol/L
- Child unconscious/lethargic/hypothermic
- Immediately administer Dextrose 10% (D10), 5 mL/kg IV followed by 50 mL of 10% glucose or sucrose by nasogastric tube. If child regains consciousness start feeding
- If child regains consciousness give 50 mL of 10% glucose or sucrose or formula 75 kcal/100 mL; frequent feeding q2-3 hours with F-75 to prevent recurrence.

Treatment of Hypothermia

- Should be taken as sign of sepsis also treat for hypoglycemia
- Axillary temperature <35°C or <95°F.
- Warming efforts skin-to-skin contact (Kangaroo care) is helpful. Remove wet clothes and cover. Provide heat-by-heat lamps but need to monitor closely.

Treatment of Dehydration/Shock
- Difficult to assess in malnourished children
- Reliable signs: Watery diarrhea; increased thirst; sunken eyes; low urine output; elastic skin and dry mucous membranes are not reliable in SAM.

If dehydrated: Give rehydration solution for malnutrition (ReSoMal) orally. 5 mL/kg q30 × 2 hours followed by 5–10 mL/kg per hour for 6 hours thereafter change ton F-75.

If in shock (Weak or absent radial pulse, cold extremities/hypothermia, lethargic or unconscious, decrease urine flow): Give IV fluids under monitoring D5LR, D5 ½ NS, or D5 ½ darrows 15 mL/kg over 1 hour, also start ReSoMal.

Treatment of Infections

Children with SAM are to be considered as immunocompromised as there is atrophy of lymph glands, tonsils and thymus, severe depression of cell-mediated immunity; typical signs of infection may be absent in these children. Following guidelines are considered:

Bacterial sepsis: Cotrimoxazole 4 mg/20 mg PO BID × 5 days/ampicillin 50 mg/kg IM/IV q6 × 7 days plus gentamycin 7.5 mg/kg IM/IV qDay × 7 days.

Malaria: In severe malaria give quinine 20 mg/kg IV/IM loading dose in dextrose over 4 hours, followed by 10 mg/kg over 2 hours after 12 hours of starting the loading dose. In other cases give artemether/lumefantrine 3 day pack, other artemenisin-based combination.

Tuberculosis: Treatment should be started only after confirmed or strongly suspected TB.

Feeding

For initial re-feeding we start with F-75 feed
Composition of F-75 feed (1 L) without cereal:
- Milk: 300 mL
- Sugar: 100 g
- Vegetable oil: 20 mL
- Mineral oil and multivitamins: 20 mL
- Water: Water to make total 1000 mL

Start with 11 mL/kg/per feed (1–2 days q2 hours), 16 mL/kg/feed (3–5 days q3 hours), 22 mL/kg/feed (6 day onwards, q4 hours).

Record weight regularly and switch to F-100, when there is documented weight gain.

Composition of F-100 Feed (1 L) feed without cereal:
- Milk: 880 mL
- Sugar: 75 g

- Vegetable oil: 20 mL
- Mineral and vitamins: 1/2 spoon
- Water: 25 mL

Micronutrients

All children with SAM are to be given vitamin A, folic acid, and iron on daily basis.

Blood Transfusion

In case of Hbg <4 g/dL or <6 g/dL if child has respiratory distress, transfuse whole blood or pRBCs at 10 mL/kg slowly over 3 hours, give frusemide 1 mg/kg.

CRITERIA FOR DISCHARGE AS PER IAP GUIDELINES

- A good appetite (eating at least 120–130 Cal/kg/day) along with micronutrients
- No edema
- Consistent weight (>5 g/kg/day) on three consecutive days
- Completed antimicrobial treatment; and appropriate immunization has been initiated
- Mother or caretaker has been trained to prepare and provide appropriate feeding
- Has financial resources to feed the child
- Has been motivated to follow the advice given.

CONCLUSION

Acute severe malnutrition, if not adequately managed, is a grave challenge. Measurement of midarm circumference (community level) and weight-for-height/length (hospital level) of infants and children aged 6 months to 5 years and detection of bilateral pitting edema is crucial for early identification of children with SAM in the community and for timely treatment or referral to reduce morbidity and mortality A midarm circumference of <115 mm or a weight-for-height/length <-3 Z-scores or/and bilateral edema warrants immediate complete evaluation and admission of such children. Children having appetite and without any medical complications are treated as outdoor patients. Management consists of initial phase, rehabilitation phase and follow-up phase. Criteria for discharging children with SAM include: Weight-for-height/length ≥-2 Z-score without edema for at least 2 weeks, or mid-upper arm circumference ≥125 mm.

> **KEY LEARNING POINTS**
>
> ¤ The presence of edema is an essential feature of SAM.
> ¤ Measurement of midarm circumference and weight-for-height/length of infants and children aged 6 months to 5 years and detection of bilateral pitting edema is crucial for early identification of children with severe acute malnutrition.
> ¤ Most of the body organ systems including immune system are adversely affected in SAM.
> ¤ The management comprises initial phase, rehabilitation phase and follow-up phase.

REFERENCES

1. World Health Organization. *Guidelines for the Inpatient Treatment of Severely Malnourished Children*. Geneva: WHO 2003.
2. Collins S. Treating severe acute malnutrition seriously. *Arch Dis Child* 2007;92: 453-461.
3. UNCEF. Community-based Management of Severe Acute Malnutrition. A Joint Statement by the, the World Food Programme, the United Nations. System Standing Committee on Nutrition and the United Nations Children Fund. Geneva: UNICEF 2007.
4. Bhatnagar S, Lodha R, Choudhury P, et al. IAP Guidelines 2006 on hospital-based management of severely malnourished children. *Indian Pediatr* 2007;44:443-461.
5. World Health Organization. WHO child growth standards and the identification of severe acute malnutrition in infants and children. A joint statement by WHO and UNICEF, 2009. Available at: http://www.who.int/nutrition/publications/severemalnutrition/9789241598163_eng.pdf. Accessed on: 18 January 2018.
6. World Health Organization. *WHO Handbook for Guideline Development*. Geneva: WHO 2010. Available at: http://www.who.int/kms/guidelines_review_committee/en/) Accessed on 19 January 2018.
7. World Health Organization. *WHO Guideline: Updates on the Management of Severe Acute Malnutrition in Infants and Children*. Geneva: WHO 2013.
8. Dalwai S, Chaudhary P, Bavdekar SB, et al. Consensus Statement of the Indian Academy of Pediatrics on Integrated Management of Severe Acute Malnutrition. *Indian Pediatr* 2013,50:399-404.
9. World Health Organization. WHO protocols for treatment of severe acute malnutrition. Available at: www.who.int/nutrition/publications/malnutrition/en/ Accessed on: 19 January 2018.

17 Refeeding Syndrome

Pushwinder Kaur, Harmesh S Bains

ABSTRACT

Refeeding syndrome, a fatal complication of rapid refeeding in severely malnourished children, manifests in the form of electrolyte imbalance and/or thiamine deficiency involving various body organs. It occurs in the early stages of refeeding and can be prevented. It has a good prognosis if managed on the lines of permissive underfeeding in early stages of management.

Keywords: Electrolyte imbalance, Hypokalemia, Hypomagnesemia, Hyponatremia Hypophosphatemia, Metabolic complications, Rapid refeedng, Refeedng syndrome, Thiamine deficiency.

INTRODUCTION

Refeedng syndrome is a potential lethal complication of aggressive refeeding in children who are severely malnourished. This syndrome involves potentially fatal shifts of fluids and electrolytes in severely malnourished children exposed to enteral and parenteral nutrition. Abnormalities in fluid balance, glucose, protein and fat metabolism, vitamin deficiency like thiamine deficiency and electrolyte imbalance like hypophosphatemia, hypomagnesemia, hypokalemia and hyponatremia does occur. The hallmark biochemical feature is hypophosphatemia. Children that have the greatest risk of refeeding syndrome includes kwashiorkor or marasmus, anorexia nervosa, chronic malnutrition and prolonged fasting.[1,2] Several case reports in children range from the setting of anorexia nervosa in older children to younger children with malnutrition. The principles of management are to anticipate, prevent and treat the biochemical abnormalities and fluid imbalances returning levels to normal range. Increased awareness among healthcare professionals and identification of patients at risk lead to reduction in mortality and morbidity among children as the condition is preventable and the metabolic complications are avoidable.

PATHOPHYSIOLOGY

Carbohydrates are the main source of energy in presence of sufficient food supply. Glucose, the principal product of carbohydrate digestion, is actively cotransported along with sodium at the intestinal brush border against a concentration gradient. Glucose enters the portal circulation by facilitated diffusion and blood sugar levels rise. This stimulates the release of peptide hormone insulin from pancreatic islet cells. Insulin promotes glucose uptake and storage (glycogenesis), inhibits the breakdown of fats (lipolysis) and increases cellular uptake of potassium. When glycogen storage capacity is beyond limit, lipogenesis occurs with nonoxidized glucose being converted to fat and stored as triglycerides in adipose tissue.[3]

During starvation, glucose levels begin to fall within 24-72 hours which results in the release of the glucagon and fall in insulin secretion.[4] Glucose levels are maintained by glycogenolysis but glycogen stores rarely last more than 72 hours.[5] Glucose homeostasis is essential because certain tissues, such as brain, erythrocytes and cells of the renal medulla are obligate glucose users.[6] These demands for glucose are met by gluconeogenesis by which noncarbohydrate sources like protein alanine and fatty acid are metabolized to glucose via Cori cycle and Kreb's cycle. As a result, there is loss of body fat and protein with depletion of potassium, phosphate and magnesium. The physiological systems maintain the serum levels of these ions at the expense of intracellular stores.

The reintroduction of feeding in malnourished children causes an increase in insulin secretion which stimulates the movement of extracellular potassium, phosphate and magnesium to the intracellular compartment.[4] Rapid fall in extracellular concentration of ions drag the sodium and water into the intracellular compartment to maintain the osmotic neutrality.[7] Thiamine, a B-complex vitamin, plays an important role as a cofactor in cellular enzymatic reactions, gets depleted after reactivation of carbohydrate dependent metabolic pathways.[8] The symptoms of thiamine deficiency may be reduced with thiamine supplementation prior to refeeding.

Phosphate is a major intracellular anion that is able to shift between the intracellular and extracellular environments and acidosis can shift phosphate out of cells and into the plasma. The serum concentration of phosphate is generally kept within normal limits during starvation by adjustment of kidney excretion. Most phosphate is filtered by the glomeruli and reabsorbed in the proximal tubules, where 90% of the excretion occurs. Gastrointestinal (GI) loss of phosphate accounts for 10% of the body's phosphate excretion. Of the 500-800 g of phosphate stored in the body, 80% can be found in the bones while 20% is present in soft tissues and muscle. Depleted body stores of phosphate, in addition to increased intracellular flux caused by insulin can result in severe extracellular hypophosphatemia. Several case reports has documented the increased morbidity associated with severe hypophosphatemia in nutritional recovery syndrome.

Magnesium is an essential intracellular cationic metal that is a cofactor for many enzymes found mainly in bone and muscle. Up to 70% of dietary magnesium is eliminated and not absorbed, and the kidneys are the main route of excretion. While nutritional recovery syndrome is associated with hypomagnesemia, the mechanism by which this occurs has not been elucidated.

Potassium is a predominant intracellular cation essential for maintaining cell membrane action potentials. The kidney regulates total potassium, specifically the distal nephron secretes potassium into the urine, which is increased in the alkalosis, presence of aldosterone or high dietary intake.

Flowchart 1 summarizes the pathophysiology of refeeding syndrome.

CLINICAL FEATURES

Refeeding syndrome may have variable symptoms, manifesting in the form of simple nausea, vomiting and lethargy to respiratory insufficiency, cardiac failure, hypotension, arrhythmias, delirium, coma and death. Symptoms occur because changes in serum electrolytes affect the cell membrane potential impairing function in nerve, cardiac and skeletal muscle cells (Table 1).

Table 1: Clinical features of electrolyte abnormalities associated with refeeding syndrome.[9,10]

Electrolyte	Electrolyte abnormality	Symptoms
Phosphate	Hypophosphatemia (normal range: 0.8–1.45 mmol/L)	• *Cardiovascular:* Heart failure, arrhythmia, hypotension, cardiomyopathy, shock, death • *Renal:* Acute tubular necrosis, metabolic acidosis • *Skeleton:* Rhabdomyolysis, weakness, myalgia, diaphragm weakness • *Neurology:* Delirium, coma, seizures, tetany • *Endocrine:* Hyperglycemia, insulin resistance, osteomalacia • *Hematology:* Hemolysis, thrombocytopenia, leucocyte dysfunction
Potassium	Hypokalemia (normal range: 3.5–5.1 mmol/L)	• *CVS:* Hypotension, ventricular arrhythmias, cardiac arrest, bradycardia, tachycardia • *Respiratory:* Respiratory distress, respiratory failure. • *Skeleton:* Weakness, fatigue, muscle twitching • *GI:* Diarrhea, nausea, vomiting, anorexia, paralytic ileus, constipation • *Metabolic:* Metabolic alkalosis
Magnesium	Hypomagnesemia (normal range: 0.77–1.33 mmol/L)	• *CVS:* Paroxysmal atrial or ventricular arrhthymia • *Respiratory:* Respiratory distress, respiratory failure • *CNS:* Weakness, fatigue, ataxia, muscle cramps, hallucinations, depression • *GI:* Abdominal pain, diarrhea, nausea, vomiting, constipation • *Other:* Anemia, hypocalcemia
Sodium	Hyponatremia (normal range: 136–145 mmol/L)	• *CVS:* Heart failure, arrhythmia • *Respiratory:* Respiratory failure, pulmonary edema • *Renal:* Renal failure • *Skeleton:* Muscle cramps, fatigue, fluid retention and edema
Vitamin	Thiamine deficiency	• *CNS:* Wernicke-Korsakoff syndrome (retrograde and anterograde amnesia, confabulation), Korsakoff's psychosis (ocular abnormalities, ataxia, coma) • *CVS:* CHF, lactic acidosis, beriberi disease • *Skeleton:* Muscle weakness

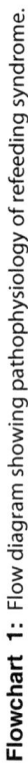

Flowchart 1: Flow diagram showing pathophysiology of refeeding syndrome.

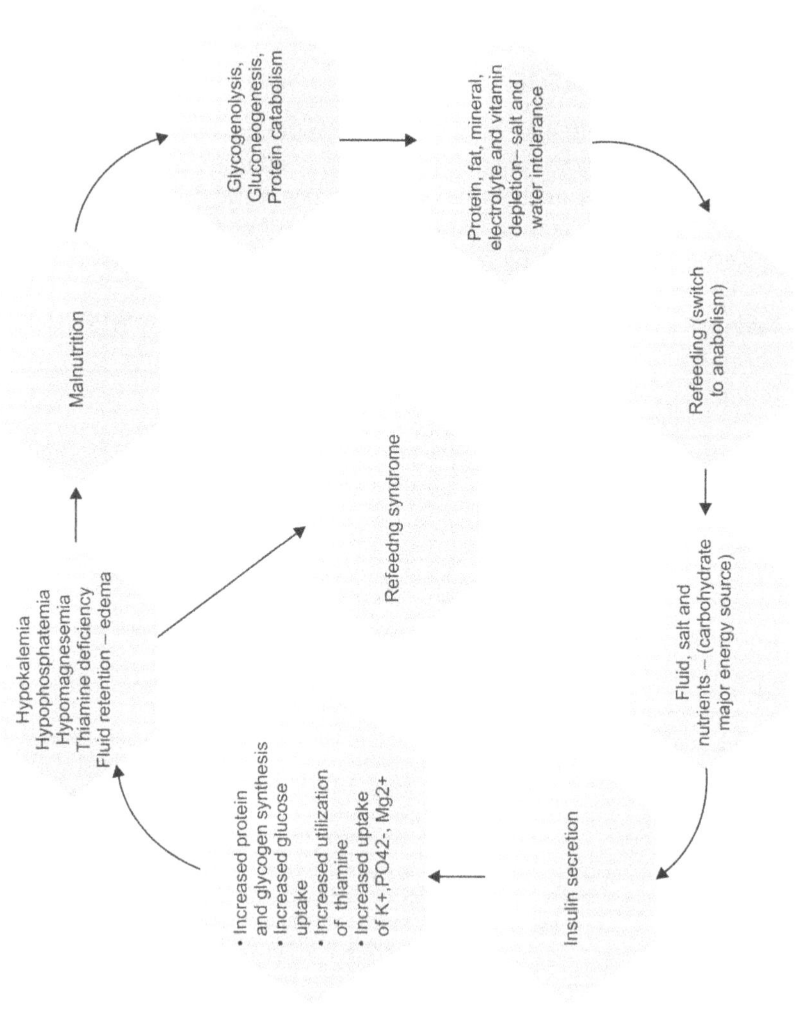

MANAGEMENT[6-10]

The objectives of management are:
- Correcton of electrolyte abnormalities.
- Correcton of fluid imbalance.

As symptoms of refeeding syndrome are uncertain and unpredictable, prevention is the best strategy for successful management so as to reduce the incidence of mortality and morbidity among children. Fundamental steps in the prevention are:[11]
- Early identification of at risk individuals
- Monitoring during refeeding (Table 2)
- Appropriate feeding regimen.

The syndrome has lethal complications which can be prevented by early identification of high-risk cases, managed by taking a detailed history and clinical examination. Various risk factors associated are:
- Severe malnutrition (marasmus/kwashiorkor)
- Anorexia nervosa
- Malabsorption diseases
- Oncology patients
- Radiation therapy
- Postoperative patients.

Meticulous monitoring during refeeding of clinical and biochemical parameters aids in prevention of syndrome. This is elaborated in Table 2.

Feeding regimen for patients at risk of developing refeeding syndrome is summarized in Flowchart 2.

CONCLUSION

Refeeding syndrome is an adverse and potentially fatal complication of far-too rapid nutritional correction, especially with high carbohydrate food-stuffs, in severe malnutrition. Manifestations result from dyselectrolytemia

Table 2: Monitoring patients at risk of developing refeeding syndrome.[9,10]

Clinical monitoring	Biochemical monitoring
Early identification of high-risk patients	Monitor basic metabolic panel, magnesium, phosphorus levels daily in the initial phase
Monitor vital signs	Monitor blood glucose levels
Monitor feeding rate (provide slow calorie repletion. At first, 20 kcal/kg/day should be provided)	ECG monitoring in severe cases
Monitor fluid intake and output chart	
Monitor change in body weight	
Monitor for neurologic signs and symptoms	
Counseling for those with eating disorders, as these have chances of recurrence	

Flowchart 2: Feeding regime for patients at risk of developing refeeding syndrome.[9]

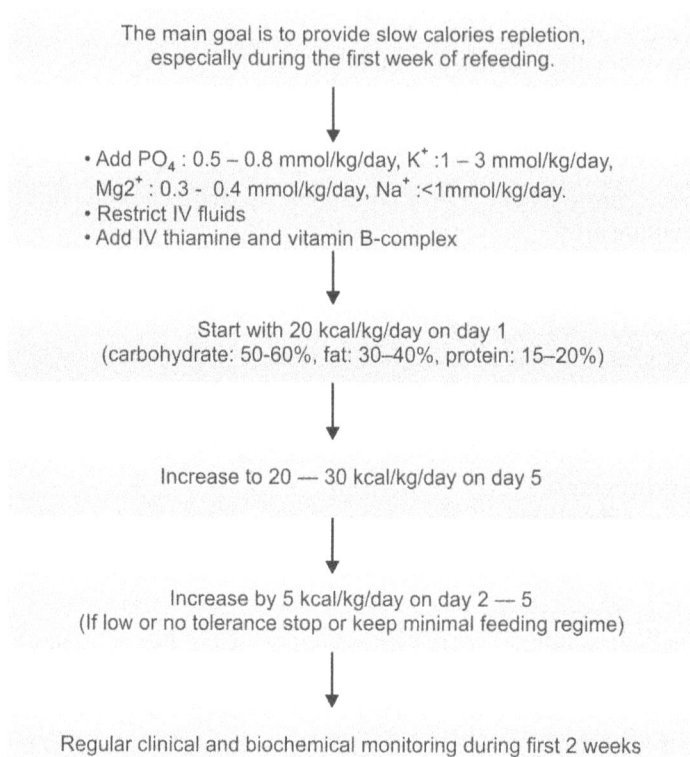

and/or thiamine deficiency involving various body organs. Permissive underfeeding in early stages of management .of severe malnutrition is critical for its prevention.

> **KEY LEARNING POINTS**
>
> ¤ Refeeding syndrome is a fatal complication of early phase of rapid refeeding in severely malnourished children.
> ¤ It results from potentially fatal shifts of fluids and electrolytes leading to electrolyte imbalance and/or thiamine deficiency involving various body organs.
> ¤ This is preventable if managed on the lines of permissive underfeeding in early stages of management.

REFERENCES

1. Gupte S. Malnutrition. In: Gupte S (Ed): *The Short Textbook of Pediatrics*, 12th edn. New Delhi: Jaypee 2011.
2. Worley G, Claerhout SJ, Combs SP. Hypophosphatemia in malnourished children during refeeding. *Clin Pediatr (Phila)* 1998;37:347-352.

3. JBerg JM, Tymoczko JL, Stryer L. *Biochemistry*. New York: Freeman 2002.
4. Allison SP. Effect of insulin on metabolic response to injury. *J Parenter Enter Nutr* 1980;4:175-179.
5. Ekberg K, Landau BR, Wajngot A, et al. Contributions by kidney and liver to glucose production in the postabsorptive state and after 60 hours of fasting "*Diabetes* 1999;48:292-298.
6. Kraft MD, Btaiche IF, Sacks GS. Review of the refeeding syndrome. *Nutr Clin Pract* 2005;20:625-633.
7. Tresley J, Sheean PM. Refeeding syndrome: recognition is the key to prevention and management. *J Am Dietet Ass* 2008;108:2105-2108. [PubMed]
8. Reuler JB, Girard DE, Cooney TG. Current concepts: Wernicke's encephalopathy. *N Engl J Med* 1985;312:1035-1039.
9. Stanga Z, Brunner A, Leuenberger M, et al. Nutrition in clinical practice—the refeeding syndrome: Ilustrative cases and guidelines for prevention and treatment. *Eur J Clin Nutr* 2008;.62:687-694.
10. Mehanna H, Nankivell PC, Moledina J, Travis J. Refeeding syndrome—awareness, prevention and management. *Head and Neck Oncol* 2009; 26;1:4. doi: 10.1186/1758-3284-1-4.

18 Immunology of Malnutrition

Ashish Simalti, Sheikh Minhaj Ahmed, Uday Bodhankar

ABSTRACT

Malnutrition, a global health problem more so in resource-constrained countries, is defined as reduced weight-for-age (underweight), weight-for-length (wasting) or length-for-age (stunting). Two forms of severe acute malnutrition (SAM) exist in children are marasmus and kwashiorkor. There may also be "marasmic kwashiorkor" with both edema and wasting. Malnutrition is associated with wider implications including increase predisposition for infections. Immunity plays the crucial role for combating these infections. Different forms of immune mechanisms exist to combat infections. These include barrier function of skin and gut, antimicrobial factors in mucosal secretions, microbial colonization, acquired, innate immunity and complement system. Many of these immune mechanisms are compromised in malnourished children. A narrative review is presented here to appraise the readers about immunology of malnutrition.

Keywords: Barrier function, Combating infection, Complement system, Edema, Immunology, Kwashiorkor, Malnutrition, Marasmus, Marasmic kwashorkor, Severe acute malnutriton, Wasting.

INTRODUCTION

Malnutrition, a public health problem globally, has wide implications. Malnourished children have higher mortality from infectious diseases. As high as 45% of deaths among children below 5 years of age can be attributed to malnutrition. Malnutrition increases susceptibility to various infections and infections further aggravate malnutrition by inducing catabolism, decreasing appetite, and altered demand for nutrients. Malnourished children are at higher risk of mortality once infected. This increase in susceptibility may be due to impairment of immune system secondary to malnutrition. It remains unclear whether these malnourished children are getting infected with opportunistic infections or same pathogens which infect well-nourished children cause infection with more severity. Although opportunistic pathogens like severe varicella and *Pneumocystis jiroveci* were reported among malnourished children, they may also represent cases of undiagnosed pediatric AIDS as recent studies have shown that pneumonia caused by *Pneumocystis jiroveci* is not so frequent in children who were malnourished but not infected with HIV.[1] Pathogens like yeast and *Cryptosporidium* are more common causes of diarrhea in malnourished group as compared to general population. These children also have increased risk of invasive bacterial infections causing pneumonia, diarrhea, and septicemia with a prominence of gram-negative bacterial infection. Current guidelines recommend empiric antibiotic administration to all children with severe acute malnutrition because of high prevalence of invasive bacterial infections although the evidence for this is not very strong.

Nonimmunological issues may also add to increased mortality in these malnourished children, for example, impairment of respiratory work due to reduced muscle mass may decrease respiratory reserve associated with lung infections, malabsorption secondary to villous atrophy, increased susceptibility to dehydration after diarrhea due to impaired concentration capacity of renal tubules; and diminished ejection fraction may precipitate cardiac failure. Thus, immune function may be an important link between malnutrition, infections and increased mortality among several other links.

DEFINITIONS OF MALNUTRITION

Malnutrition is defined by reduced weight-for-age (underweight), weight-for-length (wasting) or length-for-age (stunting).[2] Earlier weight-for-age was more frequently used but now newer studies prefer weight-for-length. Mid-upper arm circumference (MUAC) is an age independent criterion to diagnose severe acute malnutrition. It is easy to measure and predicts mortality risk better than other anthropometric indices.[3] Obesity is also considered a form of malnutrition but for purpose of this discussion it is not being considered. Specific micronutrient deficiencies like zinc or thiamine, etc. are also associated with immune system dysfunction but it does not fit in classic definition of malnutrition.

SEVERE ACUTE MALNUTRITION (SAM)

Two forms of severe acute malnutrition (SAM) exist in children:[2]
a. Marasmus is nonedematous malnutrition characterized by severe wasting and currently defined by weight-for-length Z-score <−3 SD of the WHO growth standard or MUAC 11.5 cm.
b. Kwashiorkor is a form of edematous malnutrition. It is a fulminant syndrome including mental changes, enlarged fatty liver, as well as skin and hair changes.

There may also be "marasmic kwashiorkor" with both edema and wasting. It is still not clear why some children develop kwashiorkor. It is possible that this subset of SAM is associated with different category of immune deficiency.

BARRIER FUNCTION OF SKIN

The barrier function of the epithelial surfaces is considered as the first-line of defense for the immune system. It consists of the physical integrity of skin or mucosal surface, protective commensal bacterial flora, antimicrobial factors present in secretions like secretory IgA, lysozyme, and gastric acid. Children with kwashiorkor may develop a characteristic dermatosis which is characterized by cracking and scaling of the epidermis, hyperpigmentation, resembling "peeling paint". It is a potential entry point for pathogens.[4] Small abrasions in the skin of kwashiorkor children revealed higher numbers of leukocytes predominantly granulocytes and a lower proportion of monocytes/macrophages.[5] This pattern was similar to neonatal immature immune response.

BARRIER FUNCTION OF INTESTINAL MUCOSA

The intestinal mucosa of malnourished children has been described based on autopsies from early 60s as a thin-walled intestine so called, "tissue paper intestine of kwashiorkor".[6] Biopsies from small intestine reveal mucosal thinning, villous atrophy with altered morphology and lymphocytic infiltration. These histological changes were most severe in those with kwashiorkor. Electron microscopy studies show sparse brush border with short microvilli and few endoplasmic reticulum. Intestines were found to have increased permeability to lactulose. It may predispose to bacterial translocation. High levels of lipopolysaccharide have also been documented in the blood of malnourished children most probably originating from bacteria translocating from gut. Although in malnourished children severity is much more but similar anomalies were present in otherwise well-nourished children from the same environment and they frequently persist after nutritional recovery.[7] Small intestinal biopsies from malnourished children in Gambia and Zambia reported more T-cells, more lymphocyte infiltration, and cells expressing HLA-DR in malnourished children compared to English children, remained unaltered even after nutritional recovery. The changes in colon have not been described except one article reporting increased vascularity and of the mucosal atrophy.[8] Malnourished children also have tendency for rectal prolapse.

A more recent study comparing intestinal histological findings between marasmic children with kwashiorkor has found higher numbers of T-cells and cells expressing HLA-DR in the first group, while the intestines of kwashiorkor children were deficient in sulfated glycosaminoglycan.[9]

ANTIMICROBIAL FACTORS IN MUCOSAL SECRETIONS

There are various factors secreted by epithelium and mucosa for protection against microbes. Secreted IgA (sIgA), lysozyme released in tears and saliva and acid released by gastric cells are some of the examples.[10] Levels of sIgA in saliva, urine, tears, nasal washings and duodenal fluid and small intestinal biopsies have been studied and were found to be reduced in saliva, tears and nasal washings obtained from severely malnourished children with conflicting results in mild-to-moderate SAM.

Similarly, studies of sIgA in fluid from duodenum and small intestinal biopsies showed inconsistent results. The sIgA content in urine was either increased or normal even in severely malnourished children. Lysozyme levels in malnourished children were reduced in tears but were normal in saliva. Gastric acid secretion was uniformly reduced in severe cases of SAM and it was also associated with colonization of stomach by bacteria.[11]

MICROBIAL COLONIZATION

Many microorganisms colonize skin and mucosa and protect them against infections. They do it by competing with pathogenic organisms producing specific substances with antimicrobial properties and stimulating immune function of host. Malnourished children were found to host a different flora as compared to healthy group. Their throats and mouths showed more candidiasis and upper gut mucosa considered to be almost sterile had bacterial overgrowth. While gram-positive cocci tend to predominate in the small intestine of healthy children, SAM group hosted gram-negative bacteria and candida more frequently. Sequencing of bacterial DNA from various stool samples has revealed the variable pattern of colonic flora in malnourished children with more pathogenic potential bacteria with overall flora being less diverse and less mature.

A study from Malawi suggested that microflora pattern could also play a role in developing malnutrition.[12] No difference so far has been reported in the intestinal flora in children with marasmus or kwashiorkor.

INNATE IMMUNE SYSTEM

The innate immune system delivers a nonspecific response based on granulocytes, monocytes. Most reports evaluating this have shown similar or higher numbers of total leukocyte count (TLC) in blood of children with SAM with higher proportion of granulocytes. There seems no difference in the natural killer (NK) among well-nourished or malnourished children; although few studies have reported abnormally low numbers of NK cells.

Levels of dendritic cells were also less in blood taken from malnourished children before nutritional recovery than after rehabilitation. Paradoxically, lower level of dendritic cell activation was associated with an elevated inflammation markers and high endotoxin levels suggesting a type of immune paralysis may be secondary to bacterial translocation through gut. It is not clear whether this is different from normal children having severe infections without malnutrition.

Chemotaxis, adherence to foreign material, phagocytosis and microbicidal activity of granulocytes was found to be reduced in malnourished children in five of seven studies, although few studies have reported normal microbicidal activity.[13] Production of reactive oxygen compounds which is an important requisite for bactericidal action is assessed by the Nitroblue tetrazolium (NBT) blood test. NBT test gave inconsistent results in malnourished children and production of reactive oxygen is considered factor in pathogenesis of kwashiorkor. Overall NBT test results did not show any clear pattern in children with edematous vs. nonedematous malnutrition. Levels of enzymes like acid and alkaline phosphatase were found to be increased in leukocytes among these children and markers of apoptosis (CD95) and signs of DNA damage were also more frequent in the leukocytes of malnourished children. Expression of pattern recognition molecules like toll-like receptors should also be reduced in malnourished children but so far it has not been analyzed or reported.

ACUTE PHASE RESPONSE

Crisis like infection or trauma induces a response from immune system known as acute phase response. It is mediated by cytokines like TNF-α, IL-6, etc. and involves amplification of innate and suppression of acquired immune responses. Examples of acute phase proteins are C-reactive protein (CRP), complement factors, serum-amyloid-A (SAA), α-1-acid-glycoprotein and ferritin. Certain proteins, reduce levels of which in acute phase are called 'negative acute phase proteins'; like albumin, transferrin, prealbumin, α-2-HS-glycoprotein, and α-fetoprotein. Most studies have found that acute phase proteins are elevated and negative acute phase proteins were low in malnourished children when suffering from infections.

CRP in malnourished children without apparent infections were also found to be elevated and negative acute phase proteins like transferrin, α-2-HS-glycoprotein, fibronectin and prealbumin were consistently reduced in these children, even with no infections.

COMPLEMENT

The complement system plays an important role in immunity by recruiting immune cells, opsonizing and killing the pathogens. It consists of plasma proteins which are secreted by the liver. Since these components are produced by the liver, it is probable that production of these proteins is impaired in malnutrition. Complement system is divided in three pathways: Classical pathway, alternative pathway and lectin pathway. Activated complement protein C3 plays a pivotal role in all of these three pathways. In vitro activity of complement proteins has been studied and levels of C3 were found to be depressed correlating with albumin in malnourished children. These levels were lower in children with edematous (kwashiorkor) than nonedematous (marasmus) SAM. Levels of C6, C9, and factor B were also reduced in malnourished children, more in edematous children. On the other hand, levels of C1 and C4 were almost normal in children with SAM. It appears that classical pathway activity was either unaffected or reduced only in edematous but not in marasmic SAM.[14] General opsonizing capability of serum was reduced. Both increased consumption and reduced production may be responsible for reduced levels of complement factors. High levels of C3d, which is a byproduct after activation of C3 in malnourished children was most pronounced in kwashiorkor.

ACQUIRED IMMUNITY

Specialized antibody mediated and cellular immune responses are generated by B and T-lymphocytes. This is characterized by high specificity towards antigen and long-lasting immunological memory. This system also allows tolerance to self and nonpathogenic bacteria like gut organisms. The thymus gland is the central organ in this acquired immune system and is the site for maturation followed by proliferation of T-lymphocytes. The gland is large at birth with gradual involution post-childhood, resulting in diminished release of T-lymphocytes. Thymus atrophy is a common finding in malnourished children labeled as "nutritional thymectomy". It is characterized by depleted thymocytes, replaced with connective tissue, and loss of corticomedullar differentiation. Thymic size measured by ultrasound can be correlated with nutritional status and is also reversible with nutritional rehabilitation. Thymus size correlates with nutritional status even in mild malnutrition. Breastfed children tend to have a larger thymus than top fed children. It could be due to growth factor like action of IL-7 present in breast milk. Size of thymus can be a predictor of chances of survival in infancy with bigger size being beneficial.[15] Atrophy of lymph nodes, tonsils, spleen, Peyer's patches and appendix has also been documented in SAM; although it is not as pronounced as atrophy of thymus. Histologically depletion of lymphocytes from paracortical areas, reduction in germinal centers are common findings.

CELLULAR IMMUNE FUNCTION

Cellular immune function can be assessed by dermal delayed type hypersensitivity response (DTHR), prototype of DTHR is the Mantoux test. Besides PPD in Mantoux, intradermal phytohemagglutinin (PHA), candida or local sensitizer, such as 2-4-dinitroclorobenzene (DNCB) can also be used. It is a well-known fact that malnourished children may not show positive Mantoux reaction even after tuberculosis infection. They also have diminished reactivity to candida, PHA and other common antigens. DTHR is impaired more in edematous malnutrition although this finding is not accepted universally. DTHR improves with zinc supplementation, diminished by infections and is a strong interaction was seen between infections and nutritional status.[16]

Lymphocytes in Blood

Total numbers of lymphocytes or lymphocyte subsets in blood is similar or higher in peripheral blood of malnourished children. Malnourished children with edema had atypical lymphocytes in peripheral blood resembling plasma cells. There are other functional differences noted like higher density, different pattern of genetic expression with more apoptosis in lymphocytes.

T-lymphocytes in Blood

Lower levels of T-lymphocytes were seen among malnourished children analyzed with monoclonal antibodies to CD3. However, flow cytometry based studies have not found such differences. Numbers of T-lymphocytes are also reduced in acute infections. T lymphocytes proliferate in healthy children on incubation with phytohemagglutinin (PHA); reduced proliferative response to PHA by lymphocytes in malnourished children is documented improved with zinc supplementation. In malnourished children without HIV, assessment of CD4+ cells using monoclonal antibodies and microscopy found reduced levels of CD4+ lymphocyte but flow cytometry-based studies found levels of CD4 to be similar or even higher. Bacterial infections are known to reduce the CD4-count. For HIV-infected malnourished children, nutritional rehabilitation without antiretroviral treatment resulted in CD4 counts declining further. When comparing two groups edematous vs. nonedematous malnutrition, level of CD4+ lymphocytes were higher in former.[17] Interestingly kwashiorkor is uncommon in children with HIV suggesting that CD4+ lymphocytes may play a role in development of this syndrome. Other findings related to T lymphocytes based on flow cytometry in malnourished children include fewer effector T-lymphocytes (CD62L, CD28), fewer activated T-lymphocytes (CD69, CD25) and fewer memory T-lymphocytes (CD45RO+).

B-lymphocytes: Till 1990 B lymphocytes were measured by their rosettes forming properties, when incubated with sheep erythrocytes and C3. Now monoclonal antibodies to CD20 and flow cytometry are used for the same. Rosette-based studies found B-lymphocyte counts to be unaffected or higher in children with SAM but flow cytometry-based studies using found numbers of B-lymphocytes to be reduced in this group.[18]

Antibody Levels

Levels of immunoglobulins in blood of malnourished children were similar to well nourished children. Subgroup analysis shows that IgM and IgG levels are similar but IgA was elevated in malnourished children. One study has correlated levels of IgA with severity of dermatosis in kwashiorkor. IgE was also elevated in malnourished children and IgD of which levels are low normally, was also elevated in kwashiorkor but not nonedematous malnutrition.[19]

Antibody Vaccination Responses

Studies assessing rates of seroconversion post-vaccination in children with SAM have found that these children responded with reduced titers of antibodies and it improves post-nutrition rehabilitation.[20] There seems no specific pattern in terms of responses to dead or live vaccines.

In contrast children with mild-to-moderate malnutrition tend to seroconvert normally when vaccinated.[20] Malnourished children after measles vaccine may develop pneumonia, diarrhea, and fever as against well-nourished children who usually develop mild rash.

Cytokines

Cytokines are the molecules acting as a signal among immune cells besides their own systemic effects. Levels of cytokines are measured by immunoassay in plasma, with flow cytometry in cultured leukocytes or by identifying mRNA coding for the protein. Cytokines commonly found to be reduced in malnutrition include IL-1, IL-2, IL-12 and IL-18.[21] Granulocyte macrophage colony stimulating factor (GM-CSF) and IFN-c were also found to be lower in malnutrition. In-vitro stimulation with LPS revealed blunted cytokine response in malnutrition but incubation with leptin normalized this pattern of intracellular cytokines. Few cytokines were also elevated in these children. These included tumor necrosis factor-a, IL-4, IL-6, IL-8, IL10.

Leukotrienes (LT) are derived from long chain polyunsaturated fatty acids (PUFA). These are immune modulating molecules not considered cytokines. Levels of LTC4 and LTE4 were elevated and LTB4 were lower in children with kwashiorkor as compared to nonedematous malnutrition.[22] Prostaglandin E2 were also found to be higher in children with kwashiorkor.

MECHANISMS OF ALTERATION IN IMMUNE FUNCTION: HYPOTHESES

It is not yet clear why these immunological changes take place. One possibility is inability to synthesize the basic proteins required for immune system due to lack of protein and energy but some of the immune parameters like TLC, acute-phase proteins, Th2 cytokines, plasma IgA, etc. remain intact. It is not clear as to why alteration in immunity related to malnutrition is partial to Th2-response with high immunoglobulins, thymus atrophy and reduced DTHR. Infections can contribute to these changes with interactions between malnutrition and infection impacting immune parameters. Malnutrition independently also alters immune function.

Role of hormones like prolactin, leptin, and growth hormone in growth and function of thymus is well established and fall in their levels in malnourished children could explain thymus atrophy and subsequent imbalance of Th1 and Th2 pathways.

Low leptin level corelate with a higher mortality in malnourished children. Growth hormone increases size and output of thymus in HIV patients.[23] Cortisol levels are high in children with malnutrition and cortisol is known to induce atrophy of thymus in animals, this could explain why in SAM acquired immunity is suppressed temporarily and innate immunity predominates.[24] Zinc deficiency is known to cause atrophy of thymus and acute phase reaction also cause in fall in plasma zinc contributing to the immune deficiency.

It is also possible that a state of subclinical inflammation persists in malnutrition leading to impairment of immune function. However, activated T cell and dendritic cells are reduced in malnourished children and it goes against theory of persistent inflammation. Another focus of interest is an intracellular receptor called mammalian target of Raptomycin (mTOR) which is present in most cells. It enables the cell to adapt its metabolism to available nutrition as mTOR responds to level of nutrients in the cell's surrounding and signs of stress like hypoxia. mTOR is used by immune cells to regulate activation like whether T-cells will differentiate into a proinflammatory phenotype or a tolerance-inducing one. Responsiveness of mTOR to microenvironment can explain how nutrients in this microenvironment can act as signal molecules.[25]

Depression of cellular immunity can be an adaptive response in malnutrition to avoid autoimmune reactions secondary to release of self-antigens. Unfortunately, this adaptive response can lead to increased susceptibility to infections. The pathogenesis of kwashiorkor is still not clear since many immune parameters are affected differently in these children, with higher levels of IgA, IgD, lower complement levels and predominance of Th2-response. The pattern of leukotrienes is also different in this group compared to children with nonedematous malnutrition. This immunological profile is somewhat like autoimmune disorder like lupus erythematosus representing a possible autoimmune reaction to malnutrition from a failure to induce tolerance. Elevated immunoglobulins in these children have been correlated with edema and specific manifestation like dermatosis.

IMMUNE PARAMETERS APPARENTLY NOT AFFECTED BY MALNUTRITION

As described above there are many immune parameters which remain unaffected by malnutrition. These include TLC and lymphocyte numbers, T-lymphocytes and CD4 counts when measured by flow cytometry. Elevated levels seen in many malnourished children seem to reflect ongoing infections and not the nutritional state. However, high infectious mortality is seen in these children having malnutrition and infection despite unaffected white blood cell counts.[26] Malnourished children are able to mount an acute phase reaction in response to infections with high CRP and fall in negative acute phase reactants. In fact, acute phase reaction seems rather exaggerated and not reduced. Immunoglobulin levels of IgM and IgG remain normal or elevated in malnutrition.

IMMUNE PARAMETERS AFFECTED BY MALNUTRITION

The gut mucosa as described above becomes atrophied and consequently permeable leading to enteropathy. This enteropathy affects even otherwise well-nourished children in similar communities akin to tropical sprue and has led to suggestion of labeling it as environmental enteropathy. Pathology of this mucosal atrophy seems high pathogen load and not predominantly nutrient deficiencies. It could be the cause rather than effect of malnutrition and stunting.[27] Flow of saliva and gastric acid production is reduced in SAM children. Secretory IgA is also reduced in tears, saliva, and nasal washings from these children, but it is not so in moderate malnutrition. There is overgrowth of bacteria in the small bowel of malnourished children and the pattern of commensal gut flora is different from healthy population. Phagocytosis and microbicidal properties of granulocytes are impaired. Levels of complement proteins are reduced in blood of these children especially in children with kwashiorkor. Lymphatic tissue most importantly the thymus atrophies in malnutrition as discussed above in a dose-response fashion and thymic size reduces even in milder degree of malnutrition which can be used as a predictor of survival in malnutrition. DTHR is reduced in malnourished children and lymphocytes are less responsive to PHA. Plasma IgA is usually elevated in malnourished children more so in those with edema.

Children with SAM mount a lesser specific antibody response on vaccination, although response is usually sufficient for protection.

Immune system of children with malnutrition seems to be leaning towards a Th2 response with low levels of IFN-c, IL-2 and IL-12 and high levels of IL-4 and IL-10. Induction of acute phase reaction is normal in children with malnutrition as levels of IL-6 and TNF α elevate in response to infections. Malnourished children also appear to show high levels of cytokines with anti-inflammatory action and their proinflammatory cytokines response is similar to healthy children. However, gut environment can be described as predominantly proinflammatory of these children.

CONCLUSON

Malnutrition is known to have high predisposition for infections. Immunity plays the crucial role for combating these infections. Many of the immune mechanisms that normally combat infection are compromised in malnourished children, e.g. barrier function of skin and gut, antimicrobial factors in mucosal secretions, microbial colonization, acquired, innate immunity and complement system.

KEY LEARNING POINTS

- Malnutrition in pediatrics is a global health problem particularly in resource constrained countries predisposing malnourished children for infections.
- Different forms of immune mechanisms exist to combat infections. These include barrier function of skin and gut, antimicrobial factors in mucosal secretions, microbial colonization, acquired, innate immunity and complement system.
- Barrier functions of skin and gut protects infections in these children.
- Levels of sIgA were found to be reduced in saliva, tears and nasal washings obtained from severely malnourished children with conflicting results in mild-to-moderate SAM.
- Acute phase proteins are elevated and negative acute phase proteins were low in malnourished children when suffering from infections.
- Thymus atrophy is a common finding in malnourished children labeled as "nutritional thymectomy".
- When measured by flow cytometry TLC and lymphocyte numbers, T-lymphocytes and CD4 counts are reported unaffected in malnutrition.

REFERENCES

1. Chisti MJ, Tebruegge M, La Vincente S, Graham SM, Duke T. Pneumonia in severely malnourished children in developing countries—mortality risk, aetiology and validity of WHO clinical signs: a systematic review. *Trop Med Int Health TM IH* 2009; 14:1173-1189.
2. World Health Organization, United Nations Children's Fund (2009) WHO child growth standards and the identification of severe acute malnutrition in infants and children A Joint Statement. Available at: http://www.who.int/maternal_child_adolescent/documents/9789241598163/en/. Accessed on: 5 October 2017.
3. Soler-Catalun˜a JJ, Sa´nchez-Sa´nchez L, Martı´nez-Garcı´a MA, Sa´nchez PR, Salcedo E, et al. Mid-arm muscle area is a better predictor of mortality than body mass index in COPD. *Chest* 2005;128:2108-2115.
4. Heilskov S, Rytter MJ, Vestergaard C, Briend A, Babirekere E, Deleuran MS. *J Eur Acad Dermatol Venereol* 2014;28:995-1001.
5. Thavaraj V, Sesikeran B. Histopathological changes in skin of children with clinical protein energy malnutrition before and after recovery. *J Trop Pediatr* 1989;35:105-108.
6. Burman D. The jejunal mucosa in kwashiorkor. *Arch Dis Child* 1965;40:526-531.
7. Campbell DI, Murch SH, Elia M, Sullivan PB, Sanyang MS, et al. Chronic T cell-mediated enteropathy in rural west African children: relationship with nutritional status and small bowel function. *Pediatr Res* 2003;54:306-311.
8. Redmond AO, Kaschula RO, Freeseman C, Hansen JD. The colon in kwashiorkor. *Arch Dis Child* 1971;46:470-473.
9. Amadi B, Fagbemi AO, Kelly P, Mwiya M, Torrente F, et al. Reduced production of sulfated glycosaminoglycans occurs in Zambian children with kwashiorkor but not marasmus. *Am J Clin Nutr* 2009;89:592-600.
10. Miller EM, McConnell DS. Brief communication: chronic undernutrition is associated with higher mucosal antibody levels among Ariaal infants of northern Kenya. *Am J Phys Anthropol* 2012;149:136-141.
11. Gilman RH, Partanen R, Brown KH, Spira WM, Khanam S, et al. Decreased gastric acid secretion and bacterial colonization of the stomach in severely malnourished Bangladeshi children. *Gastroenterology* 1988;94:1308-1314.
12. Smith MI, Yatsunenko T, Manary MJ, Trehan I, Mkakosya R, et al. Gut microbiomes of Malawian twin pairs discordant for kwashiorkor. *Science* 2013;339:548-554.
13. Lotfy OA, Saleh WA, el-Barbari M. A study of some changes of cell mediated immunity in protein energy malnutrition. *J Egypt Soc Parasitol* 1998;28:413-428.
14. Berczi I, Quintanar-Stephano A, Kovacs K. Neuroimmune regulation in immunocompetence, acute illness, and healing. *Ann N Y Acad Sci* 2009;1153: 220-239.
15. Garly M-L, Trautner SL, Marx C, Danebod K, Nielsen J, et al. Thymus size at 6 months of age and subsequent child mortality. *J Pediatr* 2008;153:683-688.
16. Wander K, Shell-Duncan B, Brindle E, O'Connor K. Predictors of delayed-type hypersensitivity to Candida Albicans and anti-Epstein-Barr virus antibody among children in Kilimanjaro, Tanzania. *Am J Phys Anthropol* 2013;151:183-190.
17. Bachou H, Tylleska¨r T, Downing R, Tumwine JK. Severe malnutrition with and without HIV-1 infection in hospitalized children in Kampala, Uganda: differences in clinical features, haematological findings and CD4+ cell counts. *Nutr J* 2006;5: 27-27.

18. Na´jera O, Gonza´lez C, Corte´s E, Betancourt M, Ortiz R, et al. Early Activation of T, B and NK lymphocytes in nfected malnourished and infected well-nourished children. *J Nutr Immunol* 2002;5:85-97.
19. Cripps AW, Otczyk DC, Barker J, Lehmann D, Alpers MP. The relationship between undernutrition and humoral immune status in children with pneumonia in Papua New Guinea. *P N G Med* 2008;J 51:120-130.
20. Asturias EJ, Mayorga C, Caffaro C, Ramirez P, Ram M, et al. Differences in the immune response to hepatitis B and *Haemophilus influenzae* type b vaccines in Guatemalan infants by ethnic group and nutritional status. *Vaccine* 2009;27: 3650-3654.
21. Gonza´lez-Torres C, Gonza´lez-Martı´nez H, Miliar A, Na´jera O, Graniel J, et al. Effect of malnutrition on the expression of cytokines involved in Th1 cell differentiation. *Nutrients* 2013;5:579-593.
22. Mayatepek E, Becker K, Hoffmann G, Leichsenring M, Gana L. Leukotrienes in the pathophysiology of kwashiorkor. *Lancet* 1993;342:958-960.
23. Hansen BR, Kolte L, Haugaard SB, Dirksen C, Jensen FK, et al. Improved thymic index, density and output in HIV-infected patients following low-dose growth hormone therapy: A placebo controlled study. *AIDS* 2009;23:2123-2131.
24. Barone KS, O'Brien PC, Stevenson JR. Characterization and mechanisms of thymic atrophy in protein-malnourished mice: role of corticosterone. *Cell Immunol*. 1993; 148:226-233.
25. Cobbold SP. The mTOR pathway and integrating immune regulation. *Immunology* 2013;140:391-398.
26. Hughes SM, Amadi B, Mwiya M, Nkamba H, Tomkins A, et al. Dendritic cell anergy results from endotoxemia in severe malnutrition. *J Immunol Baltim Md* 2009;1950 183:2818-2826.
27. Keusch GT, Rosenberg IH, Denno DM, Duggan C, Guerrant RL, et al. Implications of acquired environmental enteric dysfunction for growth and stunting in infants and children living in low- and middle-income countries. *Food Nutr Bull* 2013;34: 357-364.

19. Malnutrition and the Nervous System

TM Ananda Kesavan, Nithya Thuruthiyath

ABSTRACT

Malnutrition is highly prevalent in developing countries like India. A combination of poor nutrition and a lack of environment stimulation can interfere with normal cognitive development of the child. Also, malnutrition in pregnant women may adversely affect the brain growth of her offspring.

The changes in the brain depends on the duration and severity of malnutrition and the stage of brain development. The changes due to malnutrition can be prevented by proper nutritional care of the adolescent girls, pregnant women and children in younger age by proper health education and nutritional supplements.

Keywords: Brain development, Health education, Malnutrition, Nutritional deficiency, Nutritional supplements.

INTRODUCTION

Malnutrition is estimated to contribute to more than one-third of the deaths in children who are under 5 years of age worldwide. Severe acute malnutrition affects nearly 20 million preschool age children, mostly from the World Health Organization (WHO) African Region and South-East Asia Region.[1] Lack of access to highly nutritious foods, poor feeding practices, such as inadequate breastfeeding, offering the wrong foods and frequent infections—particularly frequent or persistent diarrhea, pneumonia, measles and malaria—predispose to undernutrition in children.

Malnutrition in children typically develops during the period from 6 to 24 months of age, when growth velocity and brain development are especially high. Children with severe acute malnutrition (SAM) have profoundly disturbed physiology and metabolism, such as hypoglycemia, hypothermia, electrolyte abnormalities, and severe infections which can cause high mortality and morbidity rates.

EFFECT OF NUTRITION ON BRAIN

Malnutrition directly or indirectly affects a variety of organ systems including central nervous system. The interrelations between malnutrition and the developing nervous system, and the effect of malnutrition on brain structure, function and behavior have been widely studied. Exposure to undernutrition early in life is shown to have deleterious effects on encephalic growth, myelination, neurotransmitters, behavioral and motor function, and intellectual development later in life.

MALNUTRITION OF THE MOTHER

The problem of malnutrition starts from intrauterine life. The brain weight was found to be reduced in children of mothers with malnutrition.[2] It was also noted that the brain/body weight ratio of babies of malnourished mothers are less severely impaired when compared to body weight or weight of other organs in the body which explains a certain degree of brain sparing phenomenon too.[3] Severe malnutrition is known to cause reduced head circumference.[4] The proportion of reduction in HC is proportional to the degree of maternal malnutrition. Nutritional rehabilitation can produce catch-up of the head circumference, although not complete.[5]

MORPHOLOGICAL CHANGES

The structural changes in the brain are due to malnutrition depends on the duration, severity of malnutrition and stages of brain development. Brain is severely affected during growth spurt. Animal studies have shown that early malnutrition produces growth distortion in the cerebral cortex with retarded cell division, impaired cellular differentiation and poor synaptic development.[6] Decreased cortical thickness, reduced number of dendritic spines, decreased dendritic length, and decreased synapse/neuron ratios and cellular deficit at glial level are also noted.[7]

Generally, there are two classes of CNS developmental disorders. The first occurs during the initial half of gestation and affects cytogenesis and histogenesis. The second occurs during the second half of gestation and early postnatal period and affects brain growth and differentiation. They both progressive events (neuronal maturation, connection formation, and synaptogenesis) and regressive events (cell death and selective elimination of processes). Human behavior emerges from these processes of cellular and intercellular connections which are estimated to have 100 billion cells, each with up to 10,000 connections.

The intensity of changes due to malnutrition will depend on the stage of development, during which the nutritional insults take place. According to the stages of development, the number of neurons may remain unaffected, but the number of glial cells are reduced. Cellular differentiation is also affected. There is reduction in the number of synapses per neuron in the cortex.[8]

In animals (e.g. rat model) the brain growth is mainly postnatal, whereas in humans it is perinatal. By stimulating undernourished animals it is possible to prevent severe damage, because the brain development occurs in postnatal period. However, it is not possible in humans since brain development mainly is in fetal period.[9] Greater vulnerability is observed in the cerebellum in relation to other brain regions (due to the fact that during human intrauterine life, cerebellar growth is much more than that of forebrain). Reduction in number of dendritic segments, reduction in cerebellar granule cell population and a decrease in size of the Purkinje cells are also noted.

NEUROCHEMICAL CHANGES IN MALNUTRITION

Deficits in myelin contents is noted in early malnutrition in animals.[10] It is mainly due to delay in maturation of oligodendroglial cells. Fishman et al. showed that undernutrition in animals decreases myelination though the chemical composition of the myelin remain normal.[11] However, several other studies described qualitative changes in myelin composition like decrease in proportion of phospholipids and cholesterol relative to the galactolipid fractions when compared with normal controls.[12]

Reduced brain DNA in small for dates and malnourished infants has been reported. Cerebroside-sulfatide content was significantly reduced in the small for date infants. Galactolipid sulfotransferase activity in small for date babies was also low.[13] These findings support the fact that malnutrition leads to decreased myelin content of the brain.

The normal development of neurotransmitter system is dependent partly on the availability of the plasma precursors essential for neurotransmitter synthesis as well as on appropriate activity of converting enzyme. Choline availability to the brain influences the synthesis of acetylcholine by the cholinergic neurons. Availability of tyrosine affects the function of catecholamine system and serotonin activity depends on the concentration of tryptophan. Plasma concentration of precursors of neurotransmitters depends on food intake.[14] Undernutrition in animals has shown reduction in activity of the cholinergic system in developing brain, also involving monoamine transmitter systems.

Food intake influences the plasma concentration of amino acids and can affect the synthesis of serotonin. Newborn infants receiving formula supplemented with tryptophan enter into the active sleep early than who receive a formula lacking the amino acid.[15]

CLINICAL FINDINGS IN MALNUTRITION

In acute phase of malnutrition child may have apathy, irritability, poor motivation and environmental unresponsiveness. Marasmic infants have reduced muscle tone. They may present with stereotyped head and hand movements. Dissociation of motor development described as delayed sitting and standing and hypotonia of the lower limbs with normal development of the hand and arms.[16] Poor reaction to stimulus, a monotonous wailing cry and reluctance to follow moving objects are also noted. Poor response to stimulus from the child may result in reduction in interaction between mother and the child.

Malnutrition in early life isolates the developing infant from his immediate environment. Even after nutritional rehabilitation, development depends on the intensity and duration of the previous episode of malnutrition. Early malnutrition seems to have a greater effect than malnutrition at an older age.[17]

Nerve conduction velocity is reduced to a moderate degree in malnutrition and returns to normal after recovery. Waking EEG rhythms and evoked auditory potentials show reversible alternations.[18] In infants with severe malnutrition there is increased sleep pauses during quiet sleep.[19] The cry of the malnourished child is having high pitch, lower amplitude, long duration and longer latency.

Malnutrition exerts a permanent effect on intellectual ability and motor development.[20] A difference in verbal performance and retarded psychomotor development can also be a long-term effect. In another study marked visual, motor performance and language development are also noted.[21] Recent studies have shown that stunting at a young age leads to a long-term deficit in cognitive development and school achievement up to adolescence. Such studies include a wide range of tests including IQ, reading, arithmetic, reasoning, vocabulary, verbal analogies, visual-spatial working memory, simple and complex auditory working memory, sustained attention and information processing.[22] Recent literature has also reported that malnutrition imposed at a critical development period caused an irreversible effect within the auditory primary sensory pathway in children.[23] Episodes of acute malnutrition (wasting) in young childhood also seem to lead to similar impairments.

SPECIFIC VITAMIN DEFICIENCIES AND THEIR EFFECTS

Vitamin B_1 (thiamine) deficiency is known to cause beriberi in children along with polyneuropathy. Niacin (vitamin B_3) deficiency causes pellagra including dementia and depression. Deficiency of vitamin B_6 (pyridoxine) leads to polyneuropathy and refractory seizures. Vitamin B_{12} (cobalamin) deficiency is attributable to pathology in the peripheral and optic nerves, posterior and lateral columns of the spinal cord (subacute combined degeneration), and in the brain. Folate deprivation in mothers causes neural tubal defects in fetus and cognitive dysfunction in children.

SPECIFIC MICRONUTRIENT DEFICIENCIES AND THEIR EFFECTS

Iron is essential for normal neurological function because of its role in oxidative metabolism and because it is a cofactor in the synthesis of neurotransmitters and myelin. Insufficient iron in the diet is associated with decreased brain iron and with changes in behavior and cognitive functioning.[24]

Zinc is another well studied mineral with a crucial role in memory formation and cognitive stability. Zinc plays an important role in axonal and synaptic transmission and is necessary for nucleic acid metabolism and brain tubulin growth and phosphorylation. Lack of zinc has been implicated in impaired DNA, RNA, and protein synthesis during brain development. Deficiency of zinc during pregnancy has been related to many congenital abnormalities of the nervous system in fetus. In children insufficient levels of zinc have been associated with lowered learning ability, apathy, lethargy, hyperactivity and mental retardation.[25]

Prolonged selenium and iodine deficiencies compromise thyroid hormone homeostasis in the brain due to changes in deiodinases activities and lipid peroxidation. Selenium deficiency also causes alterations in mood and behavior. Iodine deficiency can cause hypothyroidism, goiter, severe intellectual disability, behavioral changes and scholastic backwardness in children.

NEUROLOGICAL CHANGES DURING NUTRITIONAL REHABILITATION

Refeeding syndrome is caused by fluid and electrolyte abnormalities, especially severe hypophosphatemia causing neurological or neuromuscular complications, seen during nutritional rehabilitation following overloading with calories. This condition can also be associated with hypokalemia and hypermagnesemia. The predominant neurological findings include weakness, lethargy, areflexia, paresthesia, disorientation, seizures and coma. During periods of fasting, body is made to utilize ketone bodies as the main energy source, decreasing the rate of gluconeogenesis conserving muscle and protein. Insulin secretion is suppressed while glucagon levels are increased. There will be a state of intracellular depletion of electrolytes, though their serum levels may remain normal. During refeeding, insulin secretion resumes resulting in glycogen, fat and protein synthesis. This requires phosphates, magnesium and potassium and hence, their stores rapidly get depleted causing neurological manifestations. Overcorrection of nutrition in malnourished children can also result in transient rise of intracranial tension or pseudotumour cerebri which is usually a benign and self-limiting condition. Kahn syndrome is a transient syndrome marked by coarse tremors, rigidity, bradykinesia and myoclonus occurring after starting dietary rehabilitation in children. Some might experience an encephalitis like illness within 3–4 days of initiation of dietary therapy. This condition is self-limiting, but occasionally cause progressive deterioration in sensorium and fatal outcome. Tremors (Kwashi shakes) may also occur during the recovery, which might take months to resolve. Excess protein in the dietary therapy accounts for these neurological manifestations.

CONCLUSION

A combination of poor nutrition and a lack of environment stimulation can interfere with normal cognitive development of a child. Also, malnutrition in pregnant women may adversely affect the brain growth of her offspring.

The structural changes in the brain depends on the duration, severity of malnutrition and the stage of brain development. During period of fastest brain growth, there is greater vulnerability to nutritional deprivation.

Most of the malnutrition-related neurological disorders can be prevented and hence, they are of public health concern. Eradication of poverty will wipe away malnutrition in growing children. However, it is easier said than done. In such a context, provision of adequate macronutrients and micronutrients to all children at very early age is to be ensured. Prevention of micronutrient deficiencies in diet as aimed by vitamin A supplementation programs, universal iodization and fortification of food items are also important. Raising awareness in the population is the main preventive strategy.

KEY LEARNING POINTS

- Maternal malnutrition affecting the growing fetus, and poor nutrition in nfancy and early years, especially in the presence of a lack of environment stimulation are likely to interfere with normal cognitive development of a child.
- The structural changes in the brain depends on the duration, severity of malnutrition and the stage of brain development.
- Period of fastest brain growth renders the brain greatly vulnerabile to nutritional deprivation.
- Most of the malnutrition-related neurological disorders can be prevented.
- Provision of adequate macronutrients and micronutrients to all children at very early age should be ensured.
- Vitamin A supplementation, universal iodization and fortification of food items are also important programs aimed at prevention of nutritional deficiency states.
- Raising awareness in the population is the main preventive strategy.

REFERENCES

1. United Nations Children's Fund. *United Nations Interagency Group for Child Mortality Estimation. Levels and Trends in Child Mortality. Report 2012.* New York 2012.
2. Brown RE. Decreased brain weight in malnutrition and its implications. *East Afr Med J* 1965;42:584-LP.
3. Naeye RL, Blanc W, Paul C. Effects of maternal nutrition on the human fetus. *Pediatrics* 1973;52:494-503.
4. Waisman HA, Kerr GRA. Subhuman primate model for the quantitative study of malnutrition. *Proceedings of the XIII th International Congress of Pediatrics.* Vol. II: *Nutrition and Gastroenterology.* Vienna: Vorlag der Wiener Med Akademie, 1971:45.
5. Stoch MB, Smythe PM. Undernitrition during infancy and subsequent brain growth and intellectual development. In: Scrimshaw NS, Gordon JE (Eds): *Malnutrition, Learning and Behavior.* Cambridge: MIT Press 1968.

6. Bass NH, Netsky MG, Young E. Effect of neonatal malnutrition on developing cerebrum. *Arch Neurol* 1979;23:289-302.
7. Salas M, Diaz S, Nieto A. Effects of neonatal food deprivation on cortical spines and dendritic development of the rat. *Brain Res* 1974;73:139-44.
8. Thomas YM, Bedi KS, Davies CA, Dobbing JA. Stereological analysis of the neuronal and synaptic content of the frontal and cerebellar cortex of weanling rats undernourished from bitrh. *Early Hum Devel* 1979;3:109-126.
9. Frankova S. Interaction between early malnutrition and stimulation in animals. In: Cravioto Hambreaus L, Vahlquist B (Eds): *Early Malnutrition and Mental Development*. (Symposia of the Swedish Neutrition Foundation XII). Uppsala: Almqvist and Wiksell 1974;202-209.
10. Krigman MR, Hogan EI. Undernutrition in the developing rat: effect upon myelination. *Brain Res* 1976;107:239-255.
11. Fishman MA, Madyastha P, Prensky AL. The effect of undernutrition on the development of myelin in the rat central nervous system. *Lipids* 1971;6:458-465.
12. Yusuf HK M, HaqueZ, Mozaffar Z. Effect of malnutrition and subsequent rehabilitation on the development of mouse brain myelin. *J Neurochem* 1981;36: 924-930.
13. Chase HP, Welch NN, Dabiere CS, et al. Alterations in human brain biochemistry following intrauterine growth retardation. *Pediatrics* 1972;50:403-411.
14. Dyson SE, Jones DG. *Undernutrition and the developing nervous system*. *ProgNeurobiol* 1976;7:171-196.
15. Yogman MW, Zeisel SH. Diet and sleep patterns in newborn infants. *NEngl J Med* 1983;309:1147-1149.
16. Celedon JM, Andracal D. Psychomotor development during treatment of severely marasmic infants. *Early Hum Dev* 1979;3:267-275.
17. Levitsky DA, Massaro TF, Barners RH. Maternal malnutrition and the neonatal Environment. *Fed Proc* 1975;35:1583-1586.
18. Barnet AB, Weiss IP, Sotillo MV, et al. Abnormal auditory evoked potentials in early human malnutrition. *Science* 1978;201:450-455.
19. Salzarulo P, Fagiolol, Salomon F, Ricour C. Developmental trend of quiet sleep is altered by early human malnutrition and recovered by nutritional rehabilitation. *Early Hum Dev* 1982;7:257-261.
20. Hoorweg J, Stanfield J. The effects of protein energy malnutrition in early childhood on Intellectual and motor abilities in later childhood and adolescence. *Dev Child Neurol* 1976;18:330-350.
21. Chase HP, Martin HP. Undernutrition and child development. *N Engl J Med* 1970;282:933-939.
22. Grantham-McGregor S, Ani C. Cognition and undernutrition: evidence for vulnerable period. *Forum Nutr* 2003;56:272-275.
23. Penido AB, Rezende GH, Abreu RV, de Oliveira AC, Guidine PA, Pereira GS, et al. Malnutrition during central nervous system growth and development impairs permanently the subcortical auditory pathway. *Nutr Neurosci*. 2012;15:31-36
24. Domingo J. Iron in the brain: An Important contributor in normal and diseased states. *Neuroscientist* 2000;6:435-453.
25. Pfeiffer CC. Braverman ER. Zinc, the brain and behavior. *Biolog Psychiatr* 1982;17:513-532.

20 Prevention of Childhood Malnutrition

Pushwinder Kaur, Pushpendra Magon

ABSTRACT
Protein-energy malnutrition is a major cause of morbidity and mortality in the resource-limited communities. Affecting infants and children at the most crucial period of growth and development, it can lead to permanent impairments in later life. Fundamentals to its prevention are early detection of children with mild PEM, early diagnosis and treatment of common infections, promotion of exclusive breastfeeding till 6 months of age with the addition of age appropriate complementary foods after 6 months of age. Nutritional education to parents and supplementation of nutrients.

Keywords: Breastfeeding, Complementary foods, Exclusive breastfeeding, Malnutrition, Nutritional educaton, Prevention, Protein-energy malnutrition, Supplements.

INTRODUCTION

Malnutrition is a common problem faced in day to day practice and remains one of the leading cause of childhood mortality and morbidity. Protein-energy malnutrition (PEM) refers to "an imbalance between the supply of protein and energy and the body's demand for them to ensure optimal growth and function".[1] It affects particularly the preschool children (<6 years) with its dire consequences ranging from physical to cognitive growth and susceptibility to infection.[2] The human body develops differently at different steps of life. However, the so called somatic growth, has received the maximum attention in the past, as it is obvious during physical examination more than anything else. The weight of the baby could be direct consequence of maternal weight, height and nutritional status. Also the subsequent growth is more often than not related to nutrition. "Emotional or physical neglect" lead to childhood malnutrition which is initially observed as an acutely underweight child and later as stunting, if the nutritional deficiency is chronic. Hence, we need to plan our strategies to prevent acute and chronic malnutrition.

PEM is measured in terms of underweight (low weight for age), stunting (low height for age) and wasting (low weight for height). The prevalence of stunting among under five is 48% (moderate and severe) and wasting is 20% (moderate and severe) and with an underweight prevalence of 43% (moderate and severe),[3] it is the highest in the world. NFHS II reported underweight prevalence of 48.9% among girls and 45.5% among boys in India. Undernutrition makes the child susceptible to infection and complements its effect in contributing to child mortality. This accounts for 22% of the burden of disease in India and adversely affects the economic growth of the country with an estimated adult productivity loss of 1.4% of gross domestic product (GDP).[2]

In a country like India, poverty, poor education, unsupportive parenting are few of the causes which are direct stress factors on childhood growth and development. Growth is a structural event while development is more functional in nature. Lack of knowledge not only leads to poor application and practice in terms of quality and quantity of food, but also has direct bearing on later life. The poor quality of food could make a child victims of malnutrition via worm infestation, infection and nutrient deficiencies. Though poor quality of food could be a direct consequence of income and food insecurity, this gap of experienced hunger has gradually declined over the past few years due to improving socioeconomic status in our country. On the other hand poor quality of food is still an issue.

Initially, there used to be four planks to cross and prevent the child from falling in the valley of malnutrition. These were called as "**GOBI**" which stands for **G**rowth monitoring, **O**RS during diarrheal episode, prolonged and continued **B**reastfeeding up to 2 years of age and regular **I**mmunization. Later three more planks were added to make the bridge more steady which include **FFF**, i.e. **F**amily planning, **F**ood fortification and **F**emale education.

Causes of Malnutrition

- Ignorance: Lack of awareness of the nutritional qualities of food.
- Poverty
- Food fads: Highly restrictive or reservations for eating specific foods.
- Social and cultural factors: Social inequality among poor and rich families, males given more food than females.
- Traditional habits: Restriction of food intake during illnesses, continuation of breastfeeding without introduction of complementary foods at appropriate age, use of overdiluted food formulas.
- Environmental facors: Lack of sanitation and hygiene.
- Maternal malnutrition and intrauterine growth retardation.
- Congenital defects like cleft palate and cleft lip.
- Chronic illness and infections: Chronic liver disease, chronic renal failure, renal tubular acidosis, asthma, diabetes mellitus, hypothyroidism, cerebral palsy, tuberculosis, HIV, chronic diarrhea, pneumonia.
- Malabsorption.

PREVENTION OF MALNUTRITION AT NATIONAL LEVEL

Important step in prevention of malnutrition is improvement of nutritional status of each and every child independent of age, sex, religion and socioeconomic status. This has been accomplished by: (A) Nutrition supplementation and food fortification. (B) Regular Nutritional Surveillance for detecting nutritional problems at various levels. (C) Nutritional planning involving implementation of nutritional policies to upgrade the nutritional quality at national level. Various National level programs[4] started by government of India are:
- Vitamin A prophylaxis program
- National Nutritional Anemia Control Program
- National Iodine Deficiency Disorder Control Program (NIDDCP)
- Integrated Child Development Services (ICDS) Program
- Mid-Day Meal Program
- Integrated Management of Childhood Illness (IMNCI)

Vitamin a Prophylaxis Program[5]

Vitamin A prophylaxis program was started in 1970 with the objective of preventing vitamin A deficiency-associated complications like xerophthalmia, Bitot spots, night blindness and corneal xerosis. The program is to give vitamin A 100,000 unit at 9 months of age, followed by 200,000 unit every 6 months starting from 18 months to 5 years of age. However, extra dose of vitamin A is given in measles provided they have not received vitamin A in last 2 weeks.

National Nutritional Anemia Control Program[6]

This program was initiated in 1970 with the aim to prevent nutritional anemia among mothers and children. Under this program, pregnant and lactating mothers are given IFA tablet containing 100 mg elemental iron and 0.5 mg folic acid, while children in the age group of 1–5 years are given 20 mg elemental iron (60 mg ferrous sulfate) and 0.1 mg folic acid for a period of 100 days.

National Iodine Deficiency Disorder Control Program[7]

This program was launched in 1962 as National Goiter Control Program in the conventional sub. Himalayan goiter belt by replacing common salt with iodized salt with the aim to prevent goiter, mental retardation, deafmutism, cretinism, stillbirth and abortions. This program was renamed as National Iodine Deficiency Disorder Control Program in 1992. According to this program, iodine content at manufacturing level should not be less than 30 ppm on dry weight basis, while it should not be less than 15 ppm on dry weight basis at distribution level. The NIDDCP has three components:
1. Initial survey to identify endemic areas
2. Supply of iodized salt to the identified areas

3. Resurvey after 5 years of continuous supply of iodized salt to assess impact of the measures.

Integrated Child Development Service Scheme

Integrated Child Development Service scheme was started in 1975 by Government of India for early childhood development, breaking the vicious cycle of malnutrition, morbidity and mortality.[8] The beneficiaries are children under 6 years, pregnant and lactating women, women in the age group of 15-45 years. The services covered under this program are:
- Supplementary nutrition
- Immunization
- Health check-up
- Nonformal preschool education
- Nutrition and health education
- Referral services.

The administrative unit of an ICDS project is a community development block in rural areas, tribal development block in tribal areas and a group of slums in urban areas. The focal point for the delivery of ICDS is the trained local women known as "Anganwadi worker (AWW)". The impact of program on the lives of children is evident in several important areas like increased birth rate, reduced incidence of malnutrition, increased immunization coverage and a reduced infant and child mortality rate in areas covered by the ICDS (Table 1).

Mid-Day Meal Program

This program was launched in 1995 and revised in 2004 by the Government of India for Government aided schools with the aim to reduce school dropouts and improve school attendance by supplementing meals with at least 450 Kcal and 12 g protein at the primary stage and 700 kcal and protein 20 g at the upper primary stage. The meal should be a supplement, it should supply at least one-third of the total energy requirement and half of protein need, and cost of meal should be reasonably low.[9]

Integrated Management of Neonatal and Childhood Illnesses

Integrated management of neonatal and childhood illnesses (IMNCI) was started with a need to strengthen existing nutritional health policies starting from EPI in 1974 to the most recent National rural health mission. Acute malnutrition secondary to various diseases like respiratory infections, malaria, diarrhea, measles continue to haunt our country in under age 5

Table 1: Norms for supplementary nutrition in ICDS.

Beneficiaries	Calories (kcal)	Protein (g)
Children <6 years	300	8–10
Severely malnourished children	600	20
Pregnant and lactating mother	500	20–25

children, so this strategy utilizes public health approach to improve overall health of children.[10] Common interventions like immunization, exclusive breastfeeding for 6 months of age, appropriate complementary feeding, ORS and timely antibiotics may manage illnesses to great extent. However, integration of all the strategies was needed to cover overlapping signs and symptoms or more than one illness occurring simultaneously. IMNCI aims to:
- Assess the disease
- Classify and decide referral
- Identify, treatment and advice
- Treat
- Counsel mother
- Follow-up

IMNCI guidelines are targeted for two groups:
1. Newborns and young infants from birth to 2 months of age.
2. Children: 2 months–5 years.

- It is based on the principle of ask, look, listen and feel where the priority is to look for danger signs. If any of the danger signs is present, then the disease is classified into severe or very severe. Color coded standard management charts are provided to help in assessment, classification and planning further line of management.

    Color coded standard management for classification:
    - Pink classification: Child needs referral and patient care.
    - Yellow classification: Child need specific treatment, provide it at home.
    - Green classification: Child needs no medication, home care advice.

Under the gambit of IMNCI, both ARI control program and Acute Diarrheal Disease Control Program are included. ARI control program include respiratory rate taken at rest and subsequent severity of disease based presence or absence of groaning, grunting, cyanosis, difficulty in feeding from rest which classify the disease as no pneumonia, pneumonia and severe pneumonia. Prevention of ARI was specifically aimed at avoiding use of bottle, exclusive breastfeeding till 6 months of age, immunization and early diagnosis and treatment of the respiratory infections.

In the past ADD control program was separately used to assess status of dehydration, duration of loose stools and presence or absence of blood in stools, whereas the signs of lethargy, sunken eyes, lack of thirst and absence of urination were taken as signs of severity. Prevention of acute diarrheal disease and related complications mainly aimed at avoiding 5 F's, i.e. **F**ecal contamination, improper washed **F**ingers, **F**ood contamination, unhygienic conditions like **F**lies and improperly washed **F**omites in and around the child.

PREVENTION OF MALNUTRITION AT COMMUNITY LEVEL

- Health and nutritional education: Most of the people are unaware of the nutritional quality of the locally available food, contributing to

malnutrition. People should be informed of the nutritional quality of various locally available and culturally acceptable low cost foods.
- Promotion of education and literacy in the community.
- Growth monitoring: The growth of each and every child should be monitored on growth charts with regular visits to the hospital.
- Integrated health package: It includes immunization, ORS in diarrhea, periodic deworming and early diagnosis and treatment of common illnesses.
- Promotion of family planning programs.

PREVENTION OF MALNUTRITION AT FAMILY LEVEL

- Promotion of exclusive breastfeeding for first 6 months of age.
- Introduction of complementary foods at the age of 6 months.
- Timely and proper vaccination.
- Discouragement of restriction of feeding during illness.
- Proper birth spacing to ensure proper infant feeding.

Relationship Between Vitamin D and Malnutrition

Vitamin D deficiency and malnutrition are interrelated. Vitamin D deficiency a worldwide health problem especially in people with poor sun exposure has a direct impact on the intrauterine growth, bone mass, behavior and cognition. If maternal vitamin D deficiency is present, then the supply to fetus is inadequate which may have bearing on future disease in baby like allergy, asthma, rickets, language impairment, immune dysfunction and poor brain development. Several programs have been started to prevent vitamin D deficiency in the newborn and children. One can begin with sensible sun exposure of 5-10 minutes on arms, legs, face and hands, two or three times per week between 10 am-3 pm and by eating foods rich in vitamin D like mushrooms and fatty ocean fish. However, the best way to prevent vitamin D deficiency is supplementation with vitamin D. Recent study conducted by NICHD in the year 2011, concluded that 4,000 IU of vitamin D given to mother during pregnancy was ideal in achieving adequate levels of vitamin D in both mother and newborn.[11-13] The recommended vitamin D intake in newborn is 400 IU/day and in children more than 1 year of age is 600 IU/day.

Role of Zinc in Prevention of Malnutrition

Malnutrition includes both macronutrient and micronutrient or trace element deficiency. Of late, zinc has been recognized as an essential trace element required for maintaining normal body homeostasis. Zinc deficiency is associated with growth retardation, delayed sexual and bone maturation, impaired immune function, recurrent infections, dermatitis, diarrhea and mental disturbances. Meta-analysis has revealed 25% reduction in relative risk of diarrhea beyond 3 days in zinc treated children less than 5 years. Even there has been statistically significant reduction in hospital admissions for diarrhea.[14] Incorporating zinc into national programs alongwith ORS has now become policy in many developing countries including India, e.g. in NRHM, it is recommended to give zinc 10 mg/day in children less than 6 months and 20 mg/day in children >6 months for 14 days.[15,16] Various studies conducted till date have shown low serum zinc levels in children with malnutrition.[14]

Role of Breastfeeding in Prevention of Childhood Malnutrition

All of us know that survival instinct of the baby makes him crawl and latch on breast soon after birth. To that effect breastfeeding promotion network of India has formulated several policies to support breastfeeding, thereby reducing the neonatal mortality rate, infant mortality rate and under 5 mortality rate. The Baby-Friendly Hospital Initiative (BFHI) was also launched in the year 1991 by WHO and UNICEF to implement practices that protect, promote and support breastfeeding to reduce morbidity and mortality among children.

Quenching thirst using watery foremilk is a nature's way to provide micronutrients to the baby, while hindmilk fat provide satiety. Breast milk contributes to the child health, growth and development due to its unique composition of macro- and micronutrients; digestive enzymes; hormones; anti-inflammatory substances; growth modulators and prebiotics, such as bifidus factors which enhance the maturation of the gastrointestinal tract and stimulate the growth of bifido bacteria. Breast milk has high bioavailability of iron, calcium and zinc.

Breast milk has antimicrobial activity due to the presence of immunoglobulins, macrophages, lymphocytes which lead to lower risk of infections like sepsis, diarrhea and respiratory tract infections in exclusively breastfed infants as compared to the partially breastfed or non-breastfed infants.[17,18]

Various measures like initiating breastfeeding immediately after birth, continuing exclusive breastfeeding up to 6 months of age with the addition of complimentary food 6 months onwards, ensuring appropriate use of breast milk substitutes in situation of need (i.e. death of mother), controlling the aggressive advertising practices of the formula industry can protect the breastfeeding and breastfeeding related malnutrition in the children.

Other recommendations for the prevention of childhood malnutrition are:
- Continue night feeds.
- Proper feeding techniques by offering small, frequent feeds through a motivated gentle loving parent/caregiver.
- Free supply of family foods stored in hygienic conditions.
- Check for any untreated infection like urinary tract infection (UTI), tuberculosis and giardiasis which are often occult.
- In case of abnormal behavior like stereotype, rumination and attention seekers proper environment and emotional attachment would help apart from diet itself.

- The caregivers are advised to ensure the child is regularly followed up especially for immunization, vitamin A and given energy dense foods whenever required. They are also advised play therapy for better emotional bonding.

CONCLUSION

The aim of any intervention should be to break the cycle of malnutrition, so that children should grow healthier and lead a good life. For this, one need to establish priorities, so as to trigger decision making of the mother towards utilization of 5 A's: **A**vailability of food, **A**ffordability, **A**ccesibility, **A**ttractiveness and time **A**ppropriateness of food.

KEY LEARNING POINTS

- Protein-energy malnutrition affects children at the most crucial period of growth and development which can lead to permanent impairments in later life.
- Early detection of children with mild PEM, early diagnosis and treatment of common infections, promotion of exclusive breastfeeding till 6 months of age with the addition of age appropriate complementary foods 6 months onwards, nutritional education to parents and supplementation of nutrients are the basic steps in preventing the childhood malnutrition.
- PEM is a serious health issue responsible for high childhood mortality and morbidity in children.

REFERENCES

1. Onis MD, Blossner M. WHO Global database on child growth and malnutrition. WHO.1997. Available at: http:/whqlibdoc. Who.int/hq/1997/WHO_NUT_97.9pdf. Accessed on: 15 January 2018.
2. Gragnolati M, Shekar M, Gupta MD, Bredenkamp C, Lee YK. *India's Undernourished Children: A Call for Reform and Action*. Washington: World Bank 2005.
3. UNICEF. *The State of the World's Children*. Adolescence: Children with disabilities. 2013. Available at: http://www.Unicef.org/sowc2011. Accessed on: 16 January 2018.
4. Kundra S, Singh T, Gupte S. Community pediatrics. In: Gupte S (Ed): *The Short Textbook of Pediatrics,* 12th edn. NewDelhi:Jaypee 2016:135-152.
5. Government of India1970. *Maternal and Child Health scheme for prophylaxis against nutritional blindness in children caused by Vitamin A deficiency. Family planning Program, Fourth Five year Plan Technical information:* MCH No2;PP1-22. 1970.
6. Kapil U, Chaturvedi S, Nayar D. National Nutrition Supplementation Programs. *Indian Pediatr* 1992;29:1601-1613.
7. Government of India. New Delhi. *National Rural Health Mission Iodine Deficiency Disorder and Nutrition Cell.Revised Policy Guidelines on National Iodine Deficiency Disorder Control Program*. New Delhi: Ministry of Health and Family Welfare 2006.
8. Government of India. Revised *Nutritional and Feeding Norms for Supplementary Nutrition in ICDS Scheme*, New Delhi : Ministry of Women and Child Development 2009.

9. Nutritional Foundation of India. *A Report of the Workshop on "Midday meal programs in school in India-The Way Forward",* July 31- August 01 2003, New Delhi 2003.
10. Government of India. *Integrated Management of Neonatal and Childhood Illnesses. Training Modules for Physicians.* New Delhi: Ministry of Health and Family welfare 2003.
11. Hollis BW, Jhonson D, Hulsey T, Vitamin D supplementation during pregnancy: NICHD, RCT. Available at: htttps://www.google.co.in/search?safe=off&q=Hollis+BW,+Johnson+D,+Hulsey+T+:+Vitamin+D+supplementation+during+pregnancy+:+NICHD+,+RCT.&sa=X&ved=0ahUKEwiD77ao1-HYAhUBY48KHXVrAXwQ7xYIJSgA&biw=1280&bih=694 Accessed on: 14 January 2018.
12. Specker BL, Valanis B, Hertberg V, Edwards N, Tsang. Sunshine exposure and serum 25-hydroxy vitamin D concentrations in exclusively-breastfed infants. *J Pediatr* 1985;107:372-376.
13. Balasubramanian S, Dhanalakshmi K. Vitamin D deficiency in childhood—A review of current guidelines on diagnosis of vitamin D deficiency. *Indian Pediatr* 2013l;50:669-675.
14. Bahl R, Bhandari N, Hambidge KM, Bhan MK. Plasma zinc as a predictor of diarrheal and respiratory morbidity in children in an urban slum setting. *Am J ClinNutr* 1998;68:414S-417S.
15. World Health Organization. *Clinical Management of Acute Diarrhea.* Geneva/NY. WHO/UNICEF 2004.
16. World Health Organization. *implementing the New Recommendations of the clinical Management of Diarrhea.* Geneva: WHO 2006.
17. Khan J, Vesel J, Bahl R, Martines JC. Timing of breastfeeding initiation and exclusivity of breastfeeding during the first month of life: effects on neonatal mortality and morbidity–A systematic review and meta-analysis. *Matern Child Health J* 2014;19: 468-479.
18. Debes AK, Kohli A, walker N, Edmond K, Mullany LC. Time to initiation of breastfeeding and neonatal mortality and morbidity: A systematic review. *BMC Public Health* 2013;13:S19-23.

21 Feeding of Low Birth Weight Babies

Anita Singh, Anup Thakur

ABSTRACT

Low birth weight babies are a heterogeneous population of preterm and growth restricted babies who are at increased risk of morbidities, growth failure, poor neurodevelopmental outcomes and death. Early aggressive enteral nutrition is a recommended feeding strategy in these infants. Mother's own milk should be the first choice of feeding. Human milk fortification and supplementation should be a standard of care to meet nutritional recommendation and achieve target growth. Monitoring of nutrition and growth should be done during hospital stay and post-discharge.

Keywords: Enteral nutrition, Feeding, Fortification, Human milk, Growth, Low birth weight, Nutrition.

INTRODUCTION

Low birth weight (LBW) babies have been defined as those weighing less than 2,500 g at birth. They account for 15.5% of total birth globally and 96.5% of them are born in developing countries.[1] Low birth weight babies are either preterm (born before 37 completed weeks of gestation) or small for gestational age (SGA, defined as weight for gestational age less than 10th percentile on appropriate growth chart) or both. A small proportion of LBW babies are born at term and are not SGA. LBW babies are at increased risk of early and late morbidities, such as growth failure, infections, neurodevelopmental delay and under-five mortality.[2,3] They contribute to 60–80% of all neonatal deaths.[4] Interventions like temperature maintenance, optimum feeding, identification and treatment of complication can improve the overall outcome.

Nutritional interventions have a positive impact on survival and long-term neurodevelopmental outcomes of these infants. Significant proportions of LBW babies are born preterm and are often sick at birth. Many nutrients being transferred in last trimester, these babies require supplementation with them. In addition, preterm and growth restricted babies are at increased risk of feed intolerance due to immaturity of gastrointestinal tract.[5]

FEEDING OF LBW BABIES

Low birth weight babies comprise of heterogeneous groups of preterm, growth restricted and appropriate for gestational age babies. Some cardinal issues related to feeding of LBW babies are discussed as follows:

Nutritional Requirements of LBW

In order to achieve postnatal growth similar to fetal growth and satisfactory functional development, European Society of Paediatrics Gastroenterology and Nutrition (ESPGHAN) guidelines of 2010 provide important recommendations on quantity and quality of nutrients needed for preterm infants. The recommendations relate to ranges of enteral intakes for stable growing preterm infants up to a weight of approximately 1,800 g. There is no specific recommendation for infants weighing less than 1,000 g because data are lacking for this group for most nutrients, except for protein needs. The recommended intake of macro- and micronutrients in infants <1,800 g is shown in Table 1.[6]

Initiation of Feeds in LBW

Initial feeding method in a LBW baby depends on birth weight and gestational maturity. Even all infants born at a particular gestation may not have same feeding skills. Gestational age, birth weight, presence or absence of sickness and feeding effort in a baby determines how an infant should be started on feeds or fluids to provide nutrition.

Babies who are able to breastfeed should be put to the breast as soon as possible after birth. Sick babies including those with shock requiring inotropic support, seizures, necrotizing enterocolitis, symptomatic hypoglycemia and surgical condition of the gastrointestinal tract are initially started on intravenous fluids or parenteral nutrition. Enteral feeding is initiated once they are hemodynamically stable unless contraindicated otherwise. Breastfeeding requires coordination of sucking, swallowing and breathing. These skills mature with increasing gestation. Fetal sucking and swallowing has been observed as early as 12 weeks of gestation. Esophageal contraction is poorly coordinated until 32 weeks of gestation and coordinated contractions are usually absent for several days after birth.[7] Effective sucking and swallowing occurs only at 34 weeks of gestation.[8,9] Immature sucking pattern termed as non-nutritive sucking (NNS) in these babies may not meet the fluid and nutritional requirements but helps in rapid maturation of their feeding skills and improves the milk secretion in mothers. A Cochrane meta-analysis demonstrated a significant effect of NNS on the transition from gavage to full oral feeding, transition from start of oral feeding to full oral feeding, and length of hospital stay.[10] NNS helps in initiation and maintenance of successful breastfeeding during hospital stay and after discharge. The coordination between suck/swallow and breathing is not fully achieved until 37 weeks of gestation.

Initial choice of feeding method has been described in Table 2.

Table 1: Recommended intake of macro and micronutrients expressed per mg/kg/day and per 100 kcal unless otherwise denoted

Max-Min	Per/kg/day	Per/100 kcal
Fluid, mL	135-200	
Energy, kcal	110-135	
Protein, g < 1 kg body weight	4.0-4.5	3.6-4.1
Protein, g 1-1.8 kg body weight	3.5-4.0	3.2-3.6
Lipids, g (of which MCT<80%)	4.8-6.6	4.4-6.0
Linoleic acid, mg*	385-1540	350-1400
A Linoleic acid, mg	>55(0.9% of fatty acid)	>50
DHA, mg	12-30	11-27
AA, mg†	18-42	16-39
Carbohydrate, g	11.6-13.2	10.5-12
Sodium, mg	69-115	63-105
Potassium, mg	66-132	60-120
Chloride, mg	105-177	95-161
Calcium salt, mg	120-140	110-130
Phosphate, mg	60-90	55-80
Magnesium, mg	8-15	7.5-13.6
Iron, mg	2-3	1.8-2.7
Zinc, mg‡	1.1-2.0	1.0-1.8
Copper, µg	100-132	90-120
Selenium, µg	5-10	4.5-9
Manganese, µg	≤27.5	6.3-35
Fluoride, µg	1.5-60	1.4-55
Iodine, µg	11-55	10-50
Chromium, ng	30-1230	27-1120
Molybdenum, µg	0.3-5	0.27-4.5
Thiamin, µg	140-300	125-275
Riboflavin, µg	200-400	180-365
Niacin, µg	380-5500	345-5000
Pantothenic acid, µg	0.33-2.1	0.3-1.9
Pyridoxine, µg	45-300	41-273
Cobalamin, µg	0.1-0.77	0.08-0.7
Folic acid, µg	35-100	32-90
L-ascorbic acid, mg	11-46	10-42
Biotin, µg	1.7-16.5	1.5-15
Vitamin A, µg RE, 1 µg ~3.33 IU	400-1000	360-740
Vitamin D, IU/day	800-1000	
Vitamin E, mg (α-tocopherol equivalents)	2.2-11	2-10
Vitamin K1, µg	4.4-28	4-25
Nucleotides, mg		≤5
Choline, mg	8-55	7-50
Inositol, mg	4.4-53	4-48

AA=arachidonic acid; DHA=docosahexaenoic acid; IU=international unit; MCT=medium-chain triacylglycerols. Calculation of the range of nutrients expressed per 100 kcal is based on a minimum energy intake of 110 kcal/kg.

*The linoleic acid to a-linolenic acid ratio is in the range of 5 to 15:1 (wt/wt).

† The ratio of AA to DHA should be in the range of 1.0–2.0 to 1 (wt/wt), and eicosapentaenoic acid (20:5n-3) supply should not exceed 30% of DHA supply.

‡The zinc to copper molar ratio in infant formulae should not exceed 20.

Table 2: Feeding skills and initial method of feeding.

Gestational age	Maturation of feeding skills	Initial feeding method
<28 weeks	No proper sucking efforts No propulsive motility in gut	Intravenous fluids
28-31 weeks	Sucking bursts develop No co-ordination between suck, swallow and breathing	Oro-gastric/ nasogastric tube feeding with occasional spoon/ paladai feeding
32-34 weeks	Slightly mature sucking pattern Co-ordination between breathing and swallowing begins	Feeding by spoon/paladai/cup
>34 weeks	Mature sucking pattern More co-ordination between breathing and swallowing	Breastfeeding

The approach to feeding in low birth weight babies should be as under:
- **Less than 28 weeks:** These babies should be started on parenteral nutrition or intravenous fluids as soon as the baby is admitted in neonatal intensive care unit (ICU). Once the baby is hemodynamically stable, baby should be started on minimal enteral nutrition (MEN). MEN is a practice of giving trophic feeds in the form of expressed breast milk (EBM) at 10-15 mL/kg/day through orogastric tube in 3-6 hourly schedule. MEN shortens time to regain birth weight, improves feeding tolerance, enhances enzyme maturation, improves gastrointestinal motility, improves mineral reabsorption and lowers incidence of cholestasis.[11] Orogastric feeds are gradually increased to full enteral volume feeds and as maturity improves, baby can be tried on spoon and *paladai* feeds along with non-nutritive sucking on the mother's breast. Gradually, the baby can be switched to breastfeeding.
- **28-31 weeks:** These neonates can be started on MEN by orogastric feeding along with parenteral nutrition. Orogastric feeds are gradually increased to full feeds and further the infants may be transitioned to spoon feeds and then direct breastfeeding.
- **32-34 weeks:** These babies can be started on spoon feedings and transitioned to breastfeeding.
- **More than 34 weeks**: These babies can be started directly on breastfeeding and if required, supplementation with spoon feeding can be done.

Progression of Feeds

Total fluid requirement on first day of life is approximately 60 mL/kg/day and 80 mL/kg/day in infants with birth weight ≥1,500 g and <1,500 g, respectively. The optimal feed volume and speed of increment of feeds in very low birth weight- and preterm babies are not clear. A Cochrane systemic review of 9 randomized controlled trials have assessed the effect of slow vs. fast (15-24 mL/kg vs. 30-40 mL/kg) of feed increments on necrotizing enterocolitis (NEC), mortality and other morbidities in very, preterm very or low birth weight infants. This meta-analysis did not show any significant effect of rate of feed increment on NEC [risk ratio (RR): 1.02, 95% CI: 0.64-1.62] or all-cause mortality (RR: 1.18, 95% CI: 0.90-1.53). Slow feeding delayed the time to full feeds by 1 to 5 days and increased the risk of invasive infection (RR: 1.46, 95% CI:1.03-2.06).[12] For preterm very low birth weight babies (<32 weeks, birth weight <1500 g), volume of starting and upgrading feeds can be 20-25 mL/kg/day. For extremely preterm babies (<28 weeks, birth weight <1,000 g), corresponding volumes can be as small as 10-15 mL/kg/day. Such smaller feeds increments are also safe in babies who are small for gestational age due to intrauterine growth restriction.

It is reasonable to start and advance feeds cautiously in preterm and low birth weight babies. However, it has been observed in some studies that full feeds can be started soon after birth in very preterm and very low birth weight babies (birth weight: 1,000-1,500 g)[13,14] This provides optimal nutrition and avoids need of intravenous fluids. Feasibility of such practice has been studied in hemodynamically stable in very low birth weight (VLBW) infants and gestational age of 30-34 weeks in a randomized controlled trial (RCT) from India. Study group was started on 80 mL/kg/day of feed on first day of life and increased by 20 mL/kg/day to a maximum volume of 180 mL/kg/day. Control group was started on feeds by 20 mL/kg/day along with parenteral nutrition and subsequently increased by 20 mL/kg/day up to 180 mL/kg/day. Mean time to full feeds was shorter (6.94 ± 2.86 vs.10.33 ± 3.53 days, p < 0.0001) and mean number of days on intravenous fluid were lesser (1.5.8 ± 3.61 vs. 5.82 ± 3.98 days, p <0.0001) in study as compared to control group.[13] In a similar study by Sanghvi et al. on hemodynamically stable babies weighing between 1,200-1,500 g, it was observed that median time to regain birth weight was shorter and duration of hospital stay was lower in study vs. control group.[14] More robust studies are required with NEC as their primary outcome before such feeding strategy can become a recommended practice.

The maximum volume at full feeds is usually 150-170 mL/kg/day in preterm very low birth weight babies.[15] In a RCT by Kuschel et al. 54 preterm infants (<30 weeks) were randomised after reaching full feeds to remain on either 150 mL/kg/day (150 group) or increase to 200 mL/kg/day (200 group). The primary outcome was growth at 35 weeks corrected gestational age. There was significant crossover between the groups. Increased feed was required in 43% of infants in 150 group, whereas volume has to be reduced in 54% of infants in 200 group. Infant in 200 group had greater daily weight gain (16.7 vs. 15.2 g/kg/day, p = 0.047) and weighed more (2020 vs. 1885 g, p = 0.014) at 35 weeks corrected gestational age with a greater arm fat area (282 vs. 218 mm^2, p = 0.009). It was thought that increased weight gain may be due to increased fat deposition.[16] There was no effect on length and head circumference. There was no difference in growth parameter in 1 year. Pending results of further research, more important is to provide optimum protein calorie ratio than excess calorie alone.

Feeding Intervals and Modes

Two Hourly vs. Three Hourly Feeding Intervals

Two small randomized controlled trials have studied outcomes of 2 hourly vs. 3 hourly feeds in VLBW infants. Ibrahim et al. randomly allocated 150 VLBW infants to either 2 or 3 hourly feeds. Mean time to full feeds was 11.3 vs. 10.2 days in 2 hourly vs. 3 hourly feeding. The mean time to regain birth weight was shorter in 3 hourly group (12.9 vs. 14.8 days, p = 0.04). The 3 hourly feeds were comparable to 2 hourly feeds in achieving full feeds without increased adverse events.[17] Dhingra et al. compared the incidence of feed intolerance, apnea and hypoglycaemia in healthy infants weighing <1,750 g. The 3 hourly feeds did not decrease the incidence of feed intolerance, or increase the risk of apnea and hypoglycemia. However, it provided a practical convenience.[18]

Nasogastric vs. Orogastric Feeds

According to a recent Cochrane review, there is insufficient evidence to support the use of naso-versus orogastric feeding tubes as their effects on feeding, growth, development, and the incidence of adverse events in preterm or low birth weight infants is not very clear.[19] However, orogastric tubes should be preferred to nasogastric tubes because nasogastric tubes increase airway resistance. Moreover the displacement and vagal stimulation which are considered disadvantages with orogastric tubes are not significant practical issues.[20]

Push vs. Gravity for Administering Feeds

Investigators comparing push vs. gravity for administering gavage feeding has reported no significant difference in time required to administer the feeds regardless of methods used.[21] Some reports a trend towards higher respiratory rate following push feeds.[22] Further studies are needed to confirm these results.

Intermittent vs. Continuous Feeds

Intermittent feeding is preferred over continuous feeding since it is more physiological.[23] A systematic review of randomized controlled trials (7 trials, N = 511) reported no significant difference in time to reach full feeds in preterm very low birth weight infants randomized to continuous vs. intermittent feeds.[24]

Methods of Assisted Feeding

Babies who are not able to feed directly on breast are given feeding by alternative methods in (Figs. 1A and B). In gavage feeding method, feeds are delivered through a tube placed in the stomach either by orogastric or nasogastric route. This feeding method is generally used in neonatal intensive care unit but it can be used at home by educated parents after

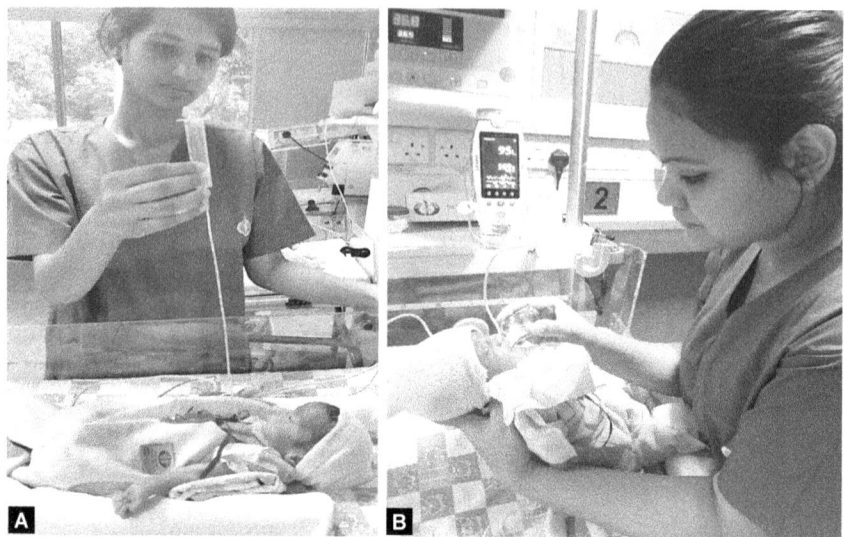

Figs. 1A and B: Methods of assisted feeding: A. Gavage Feeding; B. Paladai feeding.

appropriate training. Cup feeding or *katori* spoon feeding or *paladai* feeding methods are used in asymptomatic low birth weight- and preterm babies above 32–34 weeks of gestation till adequate weight gain or good sucking reflex is established. Bottle feeding is better avoided because of obvious hazards of increased risk of infections and later difficulty in establishment of breastfeeding. A Cochrane review has analyzed the effect of avoidance of bottle during establishment of breastfeeding on the likelihood of successful breastfeeding to find safe alternatives to bottle feeds. Seven trials with 1,152 preterm infants were involved in analysis. The results suggested that use of cup instead of bottle may increase the extent and duration of breastfeeding in preterm infants. However, there was insufficient evidence to recommend tube alone approach.[25] Recently, a RCT was conducted with aim of testing bottles with novel teat designed to simulate sucking mechanism comparable to breastfeeding. The teat is designed in a way to release milk when vacuum is applied and also encourages tongue motion similar to the term breastfed infants. One hundred infants <34 weeks who were establishing breastfeeding were randomized to bottle with a conventional teat or bottle with a novel teat if suck feed was scheduled and mother was not available. The study results showed that length of hospital stay was shorter, breastfeeding rates were higher and lesser formula was fed at discharge in the group receiving novel teat.[26]

FEEDING IN INTRAUTERINE GROWTH RESTRICTED BABIES

Initiation of feeds is often delayed in low birth weight intrauterine growth restricted infants (birth weight <10th percentile), considering a higher risk of necrotizing enterocolitis. Shah et al. studied the nutritional outcome of extremely preterm intrauterine growth restriction (IUGR) babies and observed that the IUGR neonates reached full feeds at significantly late median postnatal age and took longer time to reach this outcome. Postnatal growth restriction was significantly higher in IUGR vs. non IUGR neonates.[27]

Preterm growth restriction with absent end diastolic flows (AEDF) increases the odds of all stages of NEC by a factor of 2 and for confirmed NEC by a factor of 6 to 7. The multicentric abnormal doppler enteral prescription trial (ADEPT) studied the effect of delay in starting feeds in this population. Preterm (<35 weeks, median 31 weeks) growth restricted neonates with abnormal antenatal umbilical artery waveforms were randomly (202 per group) allocated to commence enteral feeds early "day 2" or late "day 6". Feeds increment were guided by a protocol common for both the groups. Primary outcomes were time to full feeds sustained for 72 hours and necrotizing enterocolitis. The median age at full feeds was 18 vs. 21 days in early vs. late group [hazard ratio (HR) 1.36; 95% CI: 1.11–1.67], respectively with no difference in incidence of NEC [early: 18% vs. late: 15%; RR: 1.2 (95% CI: 0.77-1.87)]. Early feeding reduced the duration of parenteral nutrition and high dependency care lowered the incidence of cholestatic jaundice and improved SD score for weight at discharge. Overall early feeding was judged safe.[28] However, a subsequent post hoc analysis of data from this trial showed that neonates born <29 weeks of gestation failed to tolerate feeds as per the conservative feeding protocol of the trial. The median [interquartile range (IQR)] age at full feeds [28(22-40) vs. 19(17-23) days (HR 0.35: 95% CI: 0.3-0.5)] and the incidence of NEC was higher [(39% vs. 10%, RR: 3.7(95% CI: 2.4-5.7)] in <29 vs. ≥29 weeks. Neonates tolerated very little milk and reached full feeds 9 days later than predicted.[29] It was concluded from the study that early introduction of feeds in preterm IUGR resulted in earlier achievement of full feeds without increase in risk of NEC. But as infants below 29 weeks with IUGR and AEDF failed to tolerate even careful graded feeding regimen used in ADEPT trial, they may require an increased duration of MEN and slower increments to decrease intolerance and establish full-feeds.

Type of Milk

Mother's own milk is the first choice for feeding low birth weight infants as it contains bioactive protective components, such as immunoglobulins, antibodies, interleukins, lactoferrins, lysozymes and stem cells.[30-33] It is a source of beneficial microbes and oligosaccharides which helps in host defence.[34,35] Breast milk provides ideal whey casein ratio (60:40) and contains long chain polyunsaturated fatty acid (LCPUFA) which is important for brain and retinal growth. From the clinical perspective human milk is tolerated better and is associated with benefits, such as lower risk of late onset sepsis, death, NEC and better long-term neurodevelopment.[36-38] The economic benefits of human milk in preterm very low birth weight relates to better growth and reduced risk of morbidities.[39] Breastfeeding also reduces under five child mortality by 13–15%.

If mother's own milk is not available then pasteurized donor human milk is second best choice followed by preterm formula for babies weighing less than 1,800 g and term formula for babies weighing ≥1,800 g. A few human milk banks have started recently in our country.

Fortification of Human Milk

Human milk has several benefits for preterm and LBW babies. However, feeding unfortified human milk to a preterm baby <32 weeks may have certain disadvantages. Though preterm milk initially contains higher protein but the protein content gradually declines over next 3-4 postnatal weeks. It also contains inadequate amounts of calcium and phosphate. A growing preterm needs higher protein, calorie, calcium, phosphate that can be provided by breast milk alone. Exclusive feeding of unfortified human milk has been associated with poor growth and nutritional deficits during and beyond the period of hospitalization.[40] Mother's own milk can be supplemented by combining with a commercially prepared multicomponent fortifier to provide increased protein, energy and minerals. Indications of fortification of human milk include all preterm infants with a birth weight <1,800 g to meet recommendations suggested by ESPGHAN. Infants weighing >1,800 g also benefit from the addition of human milk fortifier (HMF) particularly if they are SGA or demonstrate poor postnatal calorie intake and/or growth.

In one study from India by Mukhopadhyay et al. observed that fortification resulted in better growth till discharge or 2 kg weight in preterm VLBW babies as compared to unfortified group. The data was insufficient to evaluate long-term neurodevelopmental and growth outcomes, although there appears to be no effect on growth beyond 1 year of life.[41] A systematic review of 14 trials concluded that feeding preterm infants with multinutrient fortified breast milk compared with unfortified breast milk leads to slightly increased in-hospital growth rates, i.e. weight, length and occipitofrontal circumference but that did not translate into important outcomes of long-term growth and development.[42] In a randomized controlled trial by Dogra and Thakur et al. fortification of expressed human milk with fortifier containing higher protein resulted in better head growth and weight gain at 40 weeks postmenstrual age in preterm infants less than 32 weeks or 1,500 g without any benefits on long-term growth and neurodevelopment at 12-18 months corrected age.[43] HMF is started once baby has reached 100 mL/kg/day of feeds. Fortification should be continued till the infant reaches 2-2.5 kg or 40 weeks postmenstrual age whichever comes later, however it may be continued till 9-12 months.[44] There are concerns about high osmolality, feed intolerance, NEC, risk of Contamination and added cost associated with use of HMF. However, the cochrane review of available studies comparing infants fed unfortified and fortified human milk did not indicate other potential benefits or harms and provided low-quality evidence that fortification does not increase the risk of necrotizing enterocolitis in preterm infants (typical RR 1.57, 95% CI 0.76 to 3.23).[42] Currently, there are 3 HMF brands available in India: Lactodex HMF (Raptakos, Brett & Co. Ltd), HIJAM (Endocura Pharma Pvt Ltd) and Prenan (Nestle). Composition of these fortifiers is given in Table 3.

Table 3: Composition of HMFs available in India.

Components	Lactodex HMF* 4 Sachets	HIJAM HMF** 4 Sachets	Prenan HMF*** 5 Sachets
Energy	13.48	14	15
Protein (gm)	1.08	1	0.9
Fat (gm)	0.16	1	0
Carbohydrate (g)	1.96	0.2	3.4
Vitamin A (IU)	800	620	946
Vitamin D (IU)	531.2	400	120
Vitamin E (IU)	3.72	2.48	3.5
Vitamin K (mcg)	4.4	2.2	6.4
Vitamin B1 (mcg)	74	40	100
Vitamin B2 (mcg)	80	24	150
Nicotinamide (mcg)	920	460	1200
Vitamin B6 (mcg)	100	50	100
Folic acid (mcg)	50	80	32
Vitamin B12 (mcg)	0.2	0.1	0.1
Pantothenic acid (mcg)	400	200	550
Biotin (mcg)	2	1	2.8
Vitamin C (mg)	20	10	14
Copper (mcg)	57.2	50	50
Manganese (mcg)	6.8	3.4	5
Magnesium (mg)	7	8	3.2
Zinc (mg)	0.160	0.16	0.7
Calcium (mg)	63.2	100	60
Phosphorus (mg)	31.6	50	36
Sodium (mg)	7.6	16	20.8
Potassium (mg)	36	7.8	52.8
Chloride (mg)	38	8.8	19.4
Iron (mg)	1.2	1.44	1.45
Choline (mg)	–	–	1.36
Taurine (mg)	–	–	0.28
L-carnitine (mg)	–	–	0.56

HM-Human milk
*4 sachets to be dissolved in 100 ml of expressed breast milk
**4 sachets to be dissolved in 100 ml of expressed breast milk
***5 sachets to be dissolved in 100 ml of expressed breast milk

Supplementation

Micronutrient stores are lower in low birth weight babies as majority of them are preterm and significant accretions of these nutrients occur predominantly in later trimester. Calcium, phosphorus and vitamin D are important for bone health. Supplementation of these nutrients is critical for very low birth weight infants considering their low levels in human milk. For babies weighing less than 1,800 g recommended daily vitamin D intake should be 800–1,000 IU/day. Babies who are on EBM with HMF do not require additional multivitamin supplements except vitamin D and iron.

Iron is essential for neurodevelopment and deficiency can have adverse effects, such as irreversible long-term neurodevelopment, growth failure and altered immunity. ESPGHAN recommendation emphasize on starting 2-3 mg/kg/day of iron as early as 2 weeks and continuing till 6-12 months of age depending upon diet. Iron supplementation should be delayed in infants who have received multiple blood transfusions and have higher ferritin concentration. For babies weighing between 1,800-2,500 g do not require multinutrient supplementation but vitamin D still needs to be supplemented in dose of 400 IU/day. This group is also at risk of iron deficiency and World Health Organization recommends iron supplementation to all LBW infants as 2-3 mg/kg/day from 2 to 8 weeks of age until 12 months of age.[45]

Low birth weight babies less than 1,800 g who are on exclusive breast-feed should be supplemented with calcium and phosphorus to meet the recommended daily intake of 120-140 mg/kg/day and 60-90 g/kg/day, respectively. Those infants who are on fortified EBM or formula feeds do not need additional calcium or phosphorus supplementation.

Feed Intolerance

Low birth weight babies are often preterm and are at increased risk of feed intolerance due to gastrointestinal immaturity. There are no standard criteria to define feed intolerance and it is often difficult to differentiate feed intolerance with NEC stage I. Signs and symptoms of feed intolerance include abdominal distension, increased gastric residuals, vomiting, lethargy, apnea, abdominal tenderness and reduced or absent bowel sounds. Bile stained and large gastric residuals are common in first few weeks of life and have been used to predict feed intolerance. Interpretation of gastric residuals in LBW baby continues to be controversial. In a recently published study from India, it was observed that babies in whom feed intolerance was measured by abdominal circumference monitoring had fewer feed interruption days [0 (0-2) vs. 2.0 (1,5), P<0.001] and shorter duration of parenteral nutrition (P<0.001) in comparison to those in whom it was monitored by gastric residual volume.[46] Feeding intolerance can be defined as increase in abdominal girth by >2 cm between feeds or presence of bile stained or hemorrhagic gastric residuals or presence of abdominal signs like abdominal wall discoloration, erythema/tenderness. In the event of feed intolerance, feeds should be stopped for 12-24 hours and infants should be reassessed. In the event of suspected NEC, standard guidelines for its management should be followed.

Postdischarge Nutrition

Most follow-up studies of VLBW and extremely low birth weight (ELBW) infants show that at discharge these infants fall below 10th percentile and this growth failure continues for next few years.[47] Although, there is no clear evidence on the added benefit of administering a nutrient-enriched diet to preterm infants after discharge, a few reviews suggest an improvement in growth parameters with no effect on neurodevelopmental outcomes.[48,49]

Studies indicate that variations in dietary nutrient intake can contribute significantly to growth deficits in preterm infants, thus highlighting the choice of appropriate nutrition in this cohort.[50,51] Policy of aggressive nutrition for preterm VLBW and ELBW infants should continue beyond discharge to improve growth during early infancy and childhood.

Practical guidelines at discharge are as under:
1. For babies <1,800 g at birth discharged on direct breastfeeding, continue calcium/phosphorus, iron and multivitamin drops and follow-up on the growth chart. If baby continue to follow the target percentile; continue the same.
2. For babies <1,800 g on human milk but not direct feeds: Add human milk fortifier to EBM, supplement with multivitamin, vitamin D drops and iron. Calcium/phosphorus supplementation is not required. Alternative is preterm special formulae.

Monitoring of Growth and Nutrition

Assessment of growth and nutrition in LBW babies can be done by a simple ABCDE approach which is as follows:

Anthropometry

Weight in the neonatal intensive care unit is measured daily and length and head circumference are measured weekly. These should be plotted on Fenton's gender specific growth charts till 50 weeks postmenstrual age and subsequently on WHO growth standards.[52] Growth velocity should be measured weekly and it helps in assessment of adequacy as per recommended standards for LBW babies, i.e. weight = 18-20 g/kg/day, length = 1.1-1.4 cm/week and head circumference = 0.9-1.1 cm/week.[53] Serial growth monitoring also helps in early identification of growth faltering.

Biochemical

Biochemical assessment is needed occasionally in an otherwise healthy LBW baby receiving recommended nutrient intake. Periodic measurements of phosphorus, calcium and alkaline phosphatase may reveal bone health status. If iron intake meets recommendations then, biochemical assessment of iron status (serum ferritin, iron status, etc.) is not needed in most infants.

Clinical

Clinical signs of undernutrition, i.e. macronutrient and micronutrient deficiency are largely invisible in NICUs. Zinc deficiency may manifest with perioral and perineal rash. Calcium, phosphorus and vitamin D deficiency may result in signs of rickets. Inadequate iron intake will result in anemia and in pale infant but it would be late sign. Low iron intake is also likely to compromise brain development before anemia is clinically apparent.

Diet

Calculation of macro- and micronutrient intake is easy when parenteral and enteral nutrition is prescribed in appropriate format. Intake from parenteral and enteral feeds should be combined to calculate energy (kcal/kg/day) and protein (g/kg/day) intakes. Absolute intakes should be compared with recommended guidelines.

Evaluation of Nutritional Status

Growth, biochemical, clinical and dietary factors should be collectively used to decide nutritional status. It can help in determining how current illness may have affected a growth lag or how a low protein intake can be optimized with adding fortifier?

CONCLUSION

Optimal feeding of LBW babies is important for their survival and overall growth. This is a heterogeneous group with different feeding abilities and nutritional requirements. They are often preterm and are at higher risk for feed intolerance and micronutrient deficiency. Increased risk of critical sickness during NICU stay further accentuates the risk of inadequate nutrition and growth faltering. Hence, one should adopt early aggressive nutrition with vigilant monitoring for feed intolerance.

KEY LEARNING POINTS

- Low birth weight babies have increased risk of early neonatal complications and long-term adverse neurodevelopmental outcome.
- Optimal nutrition is essential for growth, metabolism and immunity in preterm LBW infants.
- Early and rapid initiation of enteral feeding has several advantages compared to late and slow feeding.
- EBM should be the first choice for feeding preterm infants due to its numerous inherent advantages; donor pasteurized human milk is the second choice.
- Considering the high nutrient requirements of preterm infants especially the requirements of proteins, EBM or donor milk should be fortified with HMF.
- Comprehensive monitoring of growth and nutrition is important for identification of growth faltering.

REFERENCES

1. WHO, UNICEF. Low birthweight: country, regional and global estimates. Geneva, UNICEF and WHO, 2004. Available at: https://www.unicef.org/publications/files/low_birthweight_from_EY.pdf. Accessed on: 20th July 2017.
2. Edmond KM, Kirkwood BR, TawiahCA, Agyei SO. Impact of early infant feeding practices on mortality in low birth weight infants from rural Ghana. *J Perinatol* 2008;28:438-444.

3. Chen A, Rogan WJ. Breastfeeding and the risk of postneonatal death in the United States. *Pediatrics* 2004;113:e435-439.
4. Lawn JE, Cousens S, Zupan J. Lancet Neonatal Survival Steering Team. 4 million neonatal deaths: When? Where? Why? *Lancet* 2005;365(9462):891-900.
5. Dorling J, Kempley S, Leaf A. Feeding growth restricted preterm infants with abnormal antenatal Doppler results. *Arch Dis Child Fetal Neonatal Ed* 2005;90: F359-F363.
6. Agostoni C, Buonocore G, Carnielli VP. Enteral nutrient supply for preterm infants: commentary from the European Society for Paediatric Gastroenterology, Hepatology and Nutrition Committee on Nutrition. *J Pediatr Gastroenterol Nutr* 2010;50:85-91.
7. Gryboski JD. Suck and swallow in the premature infant. *Pediatrics* 1969;43:96-102.
8. deVries JI, Visser GH, Prechtl HF. The emergence of fetal behaviour. I. Qualitative aspects. *Early Hum Dev* 1982; 7:301-22.
9. Bisset WM. Intestinal motor activity in the preterm infants. In: Milla PJ(Ed) *Disorders of Gastrointestinal Motility in Childhood*. Chichester: John Wiley 1998:17-27.
10. Foster JP, Psaila K, Patterson T. Non-nutritive sucking for increasing physiologic stability and nutrition in preterm infants. *Cochrane Database Syst Rev* 2016;(10): CD001071.
11. Schanler RJ. Enteral Nutrition for the High-Risk Neonate. In: Taeusch HW, Ballard RA, Gleason CA (Eds): *Avery's Diseases of the Newborn*, 8th edn. Philadelphia, Saunders 2005:1043-1060.
12. Morgan J, Young L, McGuire W. Slow advancement of enteral feed volumes to prevent necrotising enterocolitis in very low birth weight infants. *Cochrane Database Syst Rev* 2015;(10):CD001241.
13. Chetry S, Kler N, Saluja S, Soni A, Garg P. A randomized controlled trial comparing initiation of total enteral feeds on first day of life with standard feeding regimen in stable VLBW infants between 30-34 weeks gestation and 1000-1500 gms. Poster presented at: Pediatric Academic Societies and Asian Society for Pediatric Research Joint Meeting, Vancouver, 3-6th May 2014.
14. Sanghvi KP, Joshi P, Nabi F, Kabra N. Feasibility of exclusive enteral feeds from birth in VLBW infants >1200 g--an RCT. *ActaPaediatr* 2013;102:e299-304.
15. Klingenberg C, Embleton ND, Jacobs SE, O'Connell LA, Kuschel CA. Enteral feeding practices in very preterm infants: An international survey. *Arch Dis Child Fetal Neonatal Ed* 2012;97:F56-61.
16. Kuschel C, Evans N, Askie L, Bredermeyer S, Nash J. A randomized controlled trial of enteral feeding volumes in infants born before 30 weeks. *J Pediatr Child Health* 2000;36:581-586.
17. Ibrahim NR, Kheng TH, Nasir A, Ramli N, Foo JLK. Two-hourly versus 3-hourly feeding for very low birthweight nfants: A randomised controlled trial. *Arch Dis Child Fetal Neonatal Ed* 2016;102, F225-F229.
18. DhingraA, Agrawal SK, Kumar P, NarangA. A randomized controlled trial of two feeding schedules in neonates weighing ≤1750 g. *J Matern Fetal Neonatal Med* 2009;22:198-203.
19. Watson J, McGuire W. Nasal versus oral route for placing feeding tubes in preterm or low birth weight infants. *Cochrane Datab Syst Rev* 2013;2:CD003952.
20. Zeigler EE, Carlson SJ. Early nutrition of very low birth weight infants. *J Mat Fet Neonat Med.* 2009;22:191-197.
21. Symon A, Cunningham S. Nasogastric feeding methods in neonates. *Nurs Times* 1994;90:56-60.

22. Dawson JA, Summan R, Badawi N, Foster JP. Push versus gravity for intermittent bolus gavage tube feeding of premature and low birth weight infants. *Cochrane Database Syst Rev* 2012;(11): CD005249.
23. Maggio L, Costa S, Zecca C, Giordano L. Methods of enteral feeding in preterm infants. *Early Hum Dev* 2012;88(Suppl 2):S31-3.
24. Premji SS, Chessel L. Continuous nasogastric milk feeding versus intermittent bolus milk feeding for premature infants less than 1500 grams. *Cochrane Database Syst Rev* 2011;9(11):CD001819.
25. Collins CT, Gillis J, McPhee AJ, Suganuma H, Makrides M. Avoidance of bottles during the establishment of breast feeds in preterm infants. *Cochrane Database Syst Rev* 2016;(10):CD005252.
26. K Simmer, Kok C, Nancarrow K, Hepworth AR, Geddes DT. Novel feeding system to promote establishment of breastfeeds after preterm birth: a randomized controlled trial. *J Perinatol* 2016;36:210-215.
27. Shah P, Nathan E, Doherty D, Patole S. Optimising enteral nutrition in growth restricted extremely preterm neonates—a difficult proposition. *J Matern Fetal Neonatal Med* 2015;28:1981-1984.
28. Leaf A, Dorling J, Kempley S, McCormick K, Mannix P. Abnormal Doppler Enteral Prescription Trial Collaborative Group. Early or delayed enteral feeding for preterm growth-restricted infants: a randomized trial. *Pediatrics* 2012;129:e1260-e1268.
29. Kempley S, Gupta N, Linsell L, Dorling J, McCormick K. ADEPT trial collaborative group. "Feeding infants below 29 weeks' gestation with abnormal antenatal Doppler: analysis from a randomised trial". *Arch. Dis. Child. Fetal Neonatal Ed* 2014;99:F6-F11.
30. Hsieh CC, Hernández-Ledesma B, Fernández-Tomé S, et al. Milk proteins, peptides, and oligosaccharides: Effects against the 21st century disorders. *BioMed Res Int* 2015; doi.org/10.1155/2015/146840.
31. Lönnerdal B. Human Milk: Bioactive Proteins/Peptides and Functional Properties. *Nestle Nutrtr Inst Workshop Ser.* 2016;23;86:97-107. [Epub ahead of print]
32. Albenzio M, Santillo A, Stolfi I, et al. Lactoferrin levels in human milk after preterm and term delivery. *Am J Perinatol* 2016;33:1085-1089.
33. Briere CE, McGrath JM, Jensen T, Matson A, Finck C. Breast Milk Stem Cells: Current Science and Implications for Preterm Infants. *Adv Neonat Care* 2016;16:410-419.
34. Fitzstevens JL, Smith KC, Hagadorn JI, Caimano MJ, Matson AP, Brownell EA. Systematic Review of the Human Milk Microbiota. *Nutr Clin Pract* 2017;32:354-364.
35. Kulinich A, Liu L. Human milk oligosaccharides: The role in the fine-tuning of innate immune responses. *Carbohydr Res* 2016;432:62-70.
36. Slomski A. Human Milk protein prevents infections in preterm infants. *JAMA* 2016;316:2078.
37. Sisk PM, Lovelady CA, Dillard RG, Gruber KJ, O'Shea TM. Early human milk feeding is associated with a lower risk of necrotizing enterocolitis in very low birth weight infants. *J Perinatol* 2007;27:428-433.
38. Belfort MB, Anderson PJ, Nowak VA, et al. Breast milk feeding, brain development, and neurocognitive outcomes: A 7-year longitudinal study in infants born at less than 30 weeks' gestation. *J Pediatr* 2016;177:133-139.
39. Mahon J, Claxton L, Wood H. Modelling the cost-effectiveness of human milk and breastfeeding in preterm infants in the United Kingdom. *Health Econ Rev* 2016;6:54.
40. Cooper PA, Rothberg AD, Pettifor JM, Bolton KD, Devenhuis S. Growth and biochemical response of premature infants fed pooled preterm milk or special formula, *J Pediatr Gastroenterol Nutr* 1984;3:749-754.

41. Mukhopadhyay K, Narang A, Mahajan R. Effect of Human Milk Fortification in Appropriate for Gestation and Small for Gestation Preterm Babies: a randomized controlled trial. *Indian Pediatr* 2007;44:286-290.
42. Brown JV, Embleton ND, Harding JE, McGuire W. Multi-nutrient fortification of human milk for preterm infants. *Cochrane Database Syst Rev* 2016;(5):CD000343.
43. Dogra S, Thakur A, Garg P, Kler N. Effect of differential enteral protein on growth and neurodevelopment in infants <1500 g: a randomized controlled trial. *J Pediatr Gastroenterol Nutr* 2017;64:e126-e132.
44. Nzegwu NI, Ehrenkranz RA. Post-discharge nutrition and the VLBW infant: to supplement or not supplement?: a review of the current evidence. *Clin Perinatol* 2014;41:463-474.
45. Edmond K, Bahl R. Optimal Feeding of Low-Birth-Weight Infants. Geneva, Switzerland:World Health Organization; 2006. Available at: http://whqlibdoc.who.int/publications/2006/9789241595094_eng.pdf. Accessed on: 13th July 2017.
46. Kaur A, Kler N, Saluja S, Modi M, Soni A. Abdominal circumference or gastric residual volume as measure of feed intolerance in VLBW infants. *J Pediatr Gastroenterol Nutr* 2015; 60:259-63.
47. Lemons JA, Bauer CR, Oh W, Korones SB, Papile LA. Very low birth weight outcomes of the National Institute of Child Health and Human Development Neonatal Research Network, January 1995 through December 1996. *Pediatrics* 2001;107:e1-8.
48. Henderson G, Fahey T, McGuire W. Nutrient-enriched formula milk versus human breast milk for preterm infants following hospital discharge. *Cochrane Database Syst Rev* 2007;(4):CD004862.
49. Teller IC, Embleton ND, Griffin IJ, van Elburg RM. Post-discharge formula feeding in preterm infants: a systematic review mapping evidence about the role of macronutrient enrichment. *Clin Nutr* 2016;35:791-801.
50. Embleton NE, Pang N, Cooke RJ. Postnatal malnutrition and growthretardation: an inevitable consequence of current recommendations inpreterm infants? *Pediatrics* 2001;107:270-273.
51. Olsen IE, Richardson DK, Schmid CH, Ausman LM, Dwyer JT. Intersite differences in weight growth velocity of extremely premature infants. *Pediatrics* 2002; 110:1125-1132.
52. Bhatia J. Growth curves: How to best measure growth of the preterm infant. *J Pediatr* 2013;162(Suppl 3):S2-6.
53. Ehrenkranz RA, Dusick AM, Vohr BR, et al. Growth in the neonatal intensive care unit influences neurodevelopmental and growth outcomes of extremely low birth weight infants. *Pediatrics* 2006;117:1253-1261.

22   Pediatric Obesity

Noopur Singhal Sud, Harmesh S Bains

ABSTRACT

Obesity in children and adolescents has assumed epidemic proportions due to modern energy dense diets, sedentary lifestyles and numerous other environmental and genetic factors. Its treatment is critical to prevent complications and improve quality of life. Body mass index (BMI) for age is used to define obesity in pediatric population. A thorough clinical and laboratory evaluation should screen for associated comorbidities in obese children. Treatment includes nutritional and behavioral modifications, increased physical activity with family and societal support. Severe and poorly responding cases may require pharmacotherapy and weight loss (bariatric) surgery despite the associated risks. Continuous efforts targeted at prevention and behavioral modification on the part of both patients with their families and healthcare providers will be instrumental in providing much needed education and support to decrease this burgeoning problem.
Keywords: Adolescence, Behavioral modification, Body mass index, Clinical evaluation, Diet, Laboratory evaluation, Obesity, Physical activity.

INTRODUCTION

Pediatric obesity has emerged as the most grave epidemics of the 21st century. It is the forerunner of metabolic syndrome, type 2 diabetes mellitus, pediatric sleep apnea, nonalcoholic fatty liver disease, dyslipidemia, hypertension and polycystic ovarian syndrome (PCOS). Even more significant are the psychosocial morbities due to obesity in adolescence including social marginalization, poor self-esteem, depression and poor quality of life which can extend into adulthood.

An alarming 3- to 4-fold increase has been observed in obesity prevalence in the last 4 decades. The calculated global prevalence of overweight (including obesity) in children aged 5–17 years is 10%, and the prevalence varies from over 30% in America to <2% in sub-Saharan Africa. National health and nutrition examination survey (NHANES) data from 2011–2014 reports prevalence of obesity among 2–19 years old as 17% with prevalence being higher in older children, males, and certain racial and ethnic minorities.

However, nationally representative data from India is scarce with only few sporadic reports on prevalence in specific age groups. Obesity in developing countries coexists with undernutrition and its rising prevalence is largely attributable to rapid nutrition and lifestyle transition.[1-3]

ETIOPATHOGENESIS

Obesity occurs due to a complex interplay between genetic predisposition and environmental influences. The combination of our genetic propensity to store fat, the ready availability of calorie dense foods, and sedentary lifestyle promotes overweight thus making it multifactorial.

Prenatal Growth

Prenatal growth is a critical growth period that influences the future weight. Prenatal growth deprivation, gestational diabetes, and high birth weights correlate positively with rates of obesity later in life.

Childhood Growth

Certain growth periods in childhood strongly influence adolescent weights.

Some studies have found that breastfeeding may have a protective influence against childhood obesity. Early onset of "adiposity rebound" (defined as the age at which adiposity reaches a postinfancy low point and then increases) is inversely associated with BMI and positively correlated with impaired glucose tolerance later in life. Pubertal changes and early menarche also increase the risk of developing obesity and metabolic syndrome later.

Diet

Calorie intake disproportionate to energy expenditure is a major contributor to weight gain. A child's food environment and patterns of family eating play a pivotal role in the development of obesity. Aggressive advertising practices by the food industry and relatively lower cost of energy dense foods promote poor dietary habits in young people.

Convenience foods and fast foods which are inexpensive, high calorie and have high levels of fats, simple carbohydrates, and sodium and low levels of fibers and micronutrients are being consumed in increasing amounts by the youth.

Unhealthy snacking in between meals is also a contributory factor to the development of overweight.

Diets containing foods with a high glycemic index, or propensity to cause a rise in blood glucose level after a meal have been shown to be associated with higher insulin and glucose levels in obese adolescents.

Sweetened beverages including soda, juices and energy drinks have been linked to increased calorie intake and higher weight gain.

Dairy foods have been shown to have a protective influence on body weight as the intake of calcium from dairy foods is associated with reduced insulin resistance.

Having the television on during mealtimes is associated with poor quality food intake in children.

Sedentary Behaviors

Unhealthy and inactive lifestyles are often established in adolescence. It has been seen that children who have greater daily activity from ages 4–11 years have consistently smaller weight gain, BMI and triceps skinfold throughout childhood.

Television and newer forms of media viewing is largely responsible for sedentary behavior by substituting more active modes of entertainment in children. Almost one-fourth of children's waking hours are spent watching television or playing video games. This has been correlated with increased BMI and the development of type 2 diabetes. In addition, television constitutes a predominant source of media influence on food choices and obesity. Even brief exposures to televised food commercials have been found to influence food preferences and demands in children.

Suboptimal Physical Activity

Decreased physical activity has been shown to be predictive of a higher BMI in adolescents. Activity patterns in children have shifted from outdoor play to indoor entertainment like television, internet, and computer games due to changed familial, home and environmental patterns. There is also a dearth of safe open spaces and playgrounds in schools and communities. An increasing pressure on academics and reduced emphasis on physical activity in schools is another contributory factor.

Psychosocial

Disordered eating behaviors especially erratic dieting and subsequent binge-eating episodes have been shown to be associated with greater weight gain.

Depressed adolescents and children in troubled or broken families are also more likely to have a higher BMI in adult life.

Genetic

Genetic syndromes associated with obesity includes Prader-Willi, Turner, and Lawrence-Moon syndromes. These disorders are generally accompanied by poor linear growth relative to an excessive body weight and mental deficiency and hypogonadism are frequent features.

Alterations in the gene that encodes for the melanocortin 4 receptor have been shown to lead to binge-eating and obesity phenotypes.

Endocrine

Obesity due to endocrine disorders (hypothyroidism, Cushing's syndrome, growth hormone deficiency (GHD), pseudohypoparathyroidism) are very rare. Hormones contributing significantly to weight and energy balance

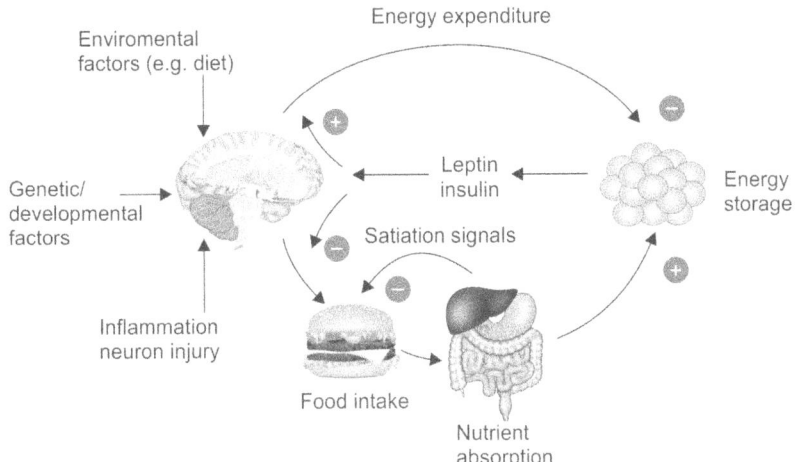

Fig 1: Hormonal control of obesity.

include insulin and leptin. Insulin resistance has been shown to increase weight gain, and fasting plasma insulin levels are significantly greater in obese adolescents than in lean controls.

Leptin is secreted from adipocytes and helps to moderate food intake and energy expenditure, and circulating levels correlate with body fat and BMI (Fig. 1).

Another gastric hormone, ghrelin has adipogenic properties, and increased levels are thought to contribute to hyperphagia.

Hormones, such as corticotropin-releasing hormone (CRH), arginine vasopressin, melanocyte-stimulating hormone, glucocorticoids, neuropeptide Y (NPY), and catecholamines, norepinephrine and epinephrine helps to promote weight gain, and may increase visceral abdominal fat stores.

COMORBITIES

Box 1 shows the comorbities of obesity.

DIAGNOSIS

According to the Wold Health Organization (WHO), obesity is defined as a condition of abnormal or excessive fat accumulation in adipose tissue, to the extent that health may be impaired.

Measuring total body fat directly is complex and expensive. Therefore, other inexpensive clinical criteria are used as markers of obesity.

Body Mass Index

Body mass index (BMI), a measure of body weight adjusted for height, is a useful tool to assess body fat.

Box 1: Comorbidities of obesity.

Cardiac
- Hyperlipidemia
- Hypertension
- Metabolic syndrome

Endocrine
- Diabetes type 2
- Polycystic ovarian syndrome

Pulmonary
- Obstructive sleep apnea
- Asthma
- Restrictive lung disease and obesity hyperventilation syndrome

Gastrointestinal
- Nonalcoholic fatty liver disease
- Gastroesophageal reflux disease
- Gallstones

Orthopedic
- Blount disease
- Slipped capital femoral epiphysis

Neurologic
- Idiopathic intracranial hypertension

Others
- Stress incontinence
- Varicose veins
- Deep venous thrombosis

It is defined as weight (in kilograms) divided by the square of height (in meters).

Experts recommend BMI because it can be obtained easily, it is correlated strongly with body fat percentage (especially at extreme BMI levels), it is associated only weakly with height, and it identifies the fattest individuals correctly, with acceptable accuracy at the upper end of the distribution (e.g. 85th or 95th percentile for age and gender).

Reference charts widely used are the Center for Disease Control (CDC) 2006-07 growth charts with percentiles based on gender and age.

As per recommendations of American Academy of Pediatrics:
- Children with BMI >95 percentile are labeled as "obese"
- Children with BMI >85 percentile but <95 percentile are labeled as "overweight".

Exceptions to the use of 85th and 95th percentile BMI values as cutoff points occur for older and younger children:
- For older adolescents, BMI of 95th percentile is higher than BMI of 30 kg/m^2, the adult obesity cutoff point. The committee therefore recommends that obesity in youths be defined as BMI of 95th percentile or BMI of >30 kg/m^2 whichever is lower.
- For children <2 years of age, BMI normative values are not available. Weight-for-height values above the 95th percentile in this age group can be categorized as overweight.

Weight for Height
Weight for height >120% is diagnosed as obesity.

Skin Fold thickness
Skin fold thickness measured over the subscapular, triceps or biceps region is a sensitive indicator of subcutaneous fat.

However, lack of normative age specific reference values and inter-observer variations in measurement prevents recommendation of its routine use.

Waist-to-Hip ratio
It is a measure of fat distribution rather than total body fat. However, it has not shown any added advantage over BMI and skin fold thickness.

Direct Estimation of Body Fat
Bioelectric impedance analysis can be used to estimate total body fat content and fat free mass. It is a noninvasive and reliable measure and uses a portable instrument. However, it is not recommended for routine use as it requires experienced personnel and adequate hydration status.

Dual-energy X-ray absorptiometry (DEXA) provides accurate measurement of body fat, but it is expensive and involves radiation exposure limiting its use.

CT scan and MRI are emerging as useful tools for the estimation of body fat stores.

EVALUATION[4]
The first step in evaluating an overweight child is proper anthropometric measurements and plotting of BMI for age and gender.

History
A focused history taking in the obese child has three major aims:
1. To rule out an underlying organic disorder,
2. To identify the presence of comorbidities, and
3. To assess the risk of developing comorbidities.

Specific Points
1. Pregnancy history—maternal gestational diabetes or hypertension, birth weight (to identify those born small or large for gestational age).
2. Grandparental, parental, and sibling anthropometrics to rule out familial cases.
3. Family history of cardiovascular disease, diabetes, dyslipidemia, hypertension.
4. History of medication use (Box 2).
5. Review of systems for complications (Table 1).

Box 2: Drugs causing weight gain.

Drugs
- Antipsychotic agents
- Selective serotonin reuptake inhibitors
- Tricyclic antidepressants
- Anticonvulsants
- Conventional mood stabilizers
- Prednisone
- Oral contraceptives

Table 1: Review of systems for weight related problems.

Symptoms	Explanation
• Sleep problems – Loud snoring – Daytime sleepiness, later onset	 Obstructive sleep apnea Disordered sleep
• Respiratory problems – Shortness of breath, exercise intolerance	 Asthma
• Gastrointestinal problems – Dysphagia, chest pain – Right upper quadrant pain – Recurrent abdominal pain	 Gastroesophageal reflux Gallbladder disease Nonalcoholic fatty liver disease
• Endocrine problems – Polyuria, polydypsia	 Type 2 diabetes mellitus
• Menstrual problems – Oligomenorrhea or dysfunctional bleeding	 Polycystic ovary syndrome
• Orthopedic problems – Hip pain, painful gait – Foot pain	 Slipped capital femoral epiphysis Increased weight bearing
• Mental health – Loss of interest, body dissatisfaction – Poor self-esteem, binge eating	 Depression

Nutrition Assessment

Nutritional assessment should include an evaluation of current intake in detail to enable a calorie count and an overview of meal and snack patterns. Specific points to be assessed include:

- Identify timing and locations of meals—snacking patterns in between meals during evening and night. Ask about where the meals are eaten, such as in the kitchen/dining room, living room, or bedroom, and if they are eaten in front of the television or computer.
- Quantify sweetened beverage consumption including fruit juices and flavored milk.

- Assess positive components of the diet, such as fruit and vegetables, fish, and grains which can be reinforced.
- Assess portion sizes in comparison with parents and other family members.
- Ask what the child eats during school time.
- Assess risky eating behaviors, such as purging or diet pill usage, binge eating and night eating.

Physical Activity Assessment

Energy expenditure through physical activity is an important part of the energy balance equation that determines body weight. Modern lifestyles have significantly reduced children's regular daily physical activity levels. It is essential to assess the child's activity level to allow for identification of areas in which small changes, individually or together with the family or friends, can provide a significant benefit. Specific points to be assessed include:
- Assess hours per day of sedentary activities (TV and computer viewing)
- Any additional activity or participation in organized sports outside of the school system.
- Mode of transport to school—walking, cycling, car, public transport.
- Assess family activities—do the parents and siblings engage in any physical activity?

Physical Examination

An obese child should undergo a standard physical examination in detail. In particular, it should aim at ruling out the presence of established obesity-related complications and searching for specific signs of an organic cause of the obesity or its comorbidities.

Anthropometry: The most important step in evaluating an overweight child is proper anthropometric measurements (weight and height) and plotting of BMI for age and gender on standard BMI centile charts. Short stature and decreasing growth velocity suggest an endocrine cause for obesity.

Waist circumference can also be measured as an indicator of visceral adiposity and marker for cardiovascular and metabolic risk. The child should stand erect with the abdomen relaxed, arms at the sides, and the feet together. Measurement should be done at the end of normal expiration at the narrowest part of the torso between the ribs and iliac crest.

Vital signs: Radial pulse is measured and compared with age-specific standards. Increased pulse rates in the resting state could be consistent with low fitness levels, whereas decreased pulse rates could be consistent with hypothyroidism.

Blood pressure should be recorded with an appropriate sized cuff in a relaxed environment after 10 minutes of rest to avoid 'white coat hypertension'.

Head and neck: Optic disks should be examined for papilloedema or decreased venous pulsations of pseudotumor cerebri, particularly if there is a significant history of headache. The neck should be examined for goiter to rule out acquired autoimmune hypothyroidism. The pharynx should be examined for enlarged tonsils or soft tissues causing obstructed breathing.

Skin: Look for acanthosis nigricans (hyperpigmented, hyperkeratotic, velvety plaques on the dorsal surface of the neck, in the axillae, body folds, and over joints). It is noted to be an indicator of insulin resistance and decreased plasma HDL cholesterol levels. Keratosis pilaris, or skin tags are even more stronger signs of insulin resistance. Intertrigo and furunculosis may develop independently in skin folds and increase pigmentation. The deep purple striae and buffalo hump of Cushing syndrome and xanthelasmas of dyslipidemias should be noted.

Cardiopulmonary: The heart should be auscultated for irregular rhythms or sounds and the lungs for evidence of pulmonary edema if heart failure is considered.

Abdomen: The abdomen may be difficult to palpate because of abdominal girth and excess adiposity. Look for hepatomegaly of nonalcoholic fatty liver.

Secondary sexual characters: Obesity is associated with premature pubarche (≤7 years for girls or, ≤9 years for boys) which may be an early marker for later polycystic ovary syndrome in girls. Examine for early onset of comedones, acne, or axillary odor and hair. Early enlargement of the penis in boys (9 years), microphallus and gynecomastia should be looked for. Early appearance of breast tissue in girls may occur due to an estrogen effect. Hirsutism involving the body or face in girls or excessive acne should be noted as an indication of polycystic ovary disease.

Limbs: The lower extremities should be evaluated for limitations of motion or pain, including hips (slipped capital femoral epiphyses), knees (Blount disease) and ankles. Slipped capital femoral epiphyses are indicated by a waddling gait or limited hip motion. Examination for neurologic signs is important in suspected cases of hypothalamic obesity (previous history of head trauma or surgery).

Syndromic signs: Signs of syndromes should be evaluated. Prader-Willi syndrome manifests as short stature, small hands and feet, almond-shaped eyes, round face, hypogonadism, and developmental delay. *POMC* mutation manifests as red hair and pale skin and is associated with adrenal insufficiency attributable to corticotropin deficiency.

Pseudohypoparathyroidism, when manifesting as Albright hereditary osteodystrophy, is associated with round face, short fourth and fifth metacarpals, and developmental delay, and it may present with hypocalcemia. Individuals with Laurence-Moon or Bardet-Biedl syndromes have retinitis pigmentosa, polydactyly with short stature, elevated BMI, and developmental delay.

MC4R4 mutation is associated with tall stature and rapid growth with rapid bone age advancement.

Mentation may be decreased in other syndromes associated with obesity, such as Down syndrome, Prader-Willi syndrome, and fragile X syndrome.

Laboratory Investigations

Table 2 lists the primary care investigations and Table 3 lists the investigations for comorbidities.

Table 2: Primary care investigations dictated by the level of BMI.

Body mass index	Tests
>85th–94th percentile with no risk factors	Fasting lipid levels
>85th–94th percentile with risk factors (e.g. family history of obesity-related diseases, elevated blood pressure, elevated lipid levels, or tobacco use)	Fasting lipid levels, AST and ALT levels, fasting glucose levels
≥95th percentile	Fasting lipid levels, AST and ALT levels, fasting glucose levels

(AST: aspartate aminotransferase; ALT: alanine aminotransferease)

Table 3: Investigations for comorbidities.

Comorbidities suspected	Tests
Cardiac disease	Electrocardiography, assessing length of QTc interval and cardiac rhythm, and echocardiography; consider measurement of lipoprotein(a)
Hypertension	24-hour ambulatory blood pressure monitoring
Nonalcoholic fatty liver disease	Ultrasonography of liver and α1- antitrypsin, ceruloplasm, antinuclear antibody, and hepatitis antibody measurements; liver biopsy if recommended by pediatric gastroenterologist
Goiter or hypothyroidism	Serum free/total thyroxine, serum TSH and antithyroid peroxidase and antithyroglobulin antibody measurements
Diabetes	Glucose tolerance test and urinary microalbumin (first morning void) or microalbumin/creatinine ratio measurement
Sleep apnea	Polysomnography, oxygen saturation and carbon dioxide measurement for carbon dioxide retention
Orthopedic disease	Radiographs of hip, knee, and foot
Cushing syndrome	24-hour urinary free cortisol or salivary cortisol measurement at bedtime
If hirsutism and oligomenorrhea is present	Plasma 17-hydroxyprogesterone, plasma DHEAS, testosterone and free testosterone, LH and FSH measurements
Precocious puberty	Sensitive LH and FSH, testosterone (for boys) or estradiol (for girls), and DHEAS
Specific syndromes	*MCR4* evaluation, fluorescent in situ hybridization for Prader-Willi syndrome, or fragile X evaluation (high-resolution chromosomal analysis)

(TSH: thyroid stimulating hormone; DHEAS: dehydroepiandrosterone; LH: luteinizing hormone; FSH: follicle stimulating hormone)

TREATMENT[5,6]

Goals of Therapy

Behavior goals: Behavior modification strategies are needed to develop and sustain healthy eating and activity habits. The family should be involved in awareness of current eating habits, activity, and identification of problem behaviors, such as specific high-calorie foods or eating patterns and obstacles to activity.

Families should be given the goal to make a few small, permanent changes at a time and make additional changes only after the previous changes are firmly in place.

Medical goals: Resolution of any secondary complication of obesity is an important medical goal much before the child reaches the ideal body weight.

If needed changes in eating and activity should be done to achieve weight loss of about 1 pound per month.

An appropriate weight goal for all obese children is a BMI below the 85th percentile but it is secondary to the primary goal of healthy eating and activity (Table 4).

Principles of Therapy

- Intervention should begin early
- The family must be ready for change
- Education of family about medical complications of obesity
- Involvement of the family and all caregivers in the treatment program
- Treatment programs should institute permanent changes, not short-term diets or exercise programs aimed at rapid weight loss
- A family should learn to monitor eating and activity and make small, gradual changes
- Encourage and empathize and not criticize.

Table 4: Weight goals.

Age	Weight goals
• <2 years	Weight maintenance

• 2–7 years
– BMI 85th –94th percentile
– BMI ≥ 95th percentile
  - No complications
  - With secondary complications
	Weight maintenance (gradual decline in BMI as child grows in height)
	
	Weight maintenance
	Weight loss

• >7 years
– BMI 85th –94th percentile
  - No complications
  - With secondary complications
– BMI ≥ 95th percentile
	
	Weight maintenance
	Weight loss
	Weight loss

Staged Treatment

According to the American Academy of Pediatrics recommendations, treatment of overweight children be approached with a staged method based on the child's age, BMI, related comorbidities, parents' weight status, and progress in treatment.

Stage 1: Prevention Plus

Recommendations include:
- Consume 5 servings of fruits and vegetables per day
- Minimize or eliminate sugar-sweetened beverages
- Limit screen time to <2 hours per day with no television in the room where the child sleeps
- Engage in >1hour of daily physical activity.

The following eating behaviors should be facilitated:
- Eating a daily breakfast
- Limiting meals purchased from outside
- Eating family meals at least 5 or 6 times per week
- Allowing the child to self-regulate his/her meals and avoiding overly restrictive behaviors.

The goal should be weight maintenance with growth resulting in decreasing BMI as age increases.

Monthly follow-up assessment should be performed. After 3–6 months, if no improvement in BMI or weight status has been noted, then advancement to stage 2 is indicated.

Stage 2: Structured Weight Management

Recommendations in addition to those in stage 1 include:
- A planned diet balanced in macronutrients, emphasizing small amounts of energy dense foods
- Provision of structured daily meals and snacks (breakfast, lunch, dinner, and 1 or 2 snacks per day)
- Supervised active play of >60 minutes per day
- Screen time of <1 hour per day
- Increased monitoring (e.g. screen time, physical activity, dietary intake, and restaurant logs) by provider, patient, and/or family
- Reinforcement for achieving targeted behavior goals (not weight goals).

The goal should be weight maintenance that results in decreasing BMI as age and height increase. Weight loss should not exceed 1 lb/month for children 2–11 years of age or an average of 2 lb/week for older overweight/obese children and adolescents.

If there is no improvement in BMI or weight status after 3 to 6 months, then the patient should advance to stage 3.

Stage 3: Comprehensive Multidisciplinary Intervention

Eating and activity goals are the same as in stage 2. Activities within this category should also include the following:
- Planned negative energy balance achieved through structured diet and physical activity (ME)
- Structured behavioral modification program including food and activity monitoring and development of short-term diet and physical activity goals (CE)
- Provision of training for all families to improve the home environment
- Weekly office visits for a minimum of 8-12 weeks, and subsequent monthly visits help to maintain new behaviors
- Systematic evaluation of body measurements, dietary intake, and physical activity should be conducted at baseline and at specific intervals throughout the program.

Stage 4: Tertiary care

Recommended for children >11 years of age with BMI of >95th percentile who have significant comorbidities and who have not been successful in stages 1 to 3 or children with BMI of >99th percentile who have shown no improvement in stage 3 (comprehensive multidisciplinary intervention).

Stage 4 is a tertiary care protocol which include continued diet and activity counseling and the consideration of such additions as meal replacement, very low-calorie diet, medication, and surgery.

Reduce Calorie Intake

The dietary goals for patients and their families should be well-balanced, healthy meals and a healthy approach to eating. These changes should be considered permanent rather than a temporary eating plan for rapid weight loss. The most helpful guide to healthy eating is the food guide pyramid (Fig. 2).

Counting calories is tedious, difficult, and inaccurate. Reduction or elimination of specific foods may reduce calories without making patients feel hungry or deprived.

Another approach, the "stoplight diet," stresses an appropriate balance of high-, medium-, and low-calorie foods. In this diet, "green light" foods contain 20 fewer calories per average serving than standard food in that group, "yellow light" foods contain less than 20 calories above the standard for food in that group, and "red light" foods contain more than 20 calories above the standard for food in that group and should be eaten infrequently. (Fig. 3).

Medications

Pharmacotherapy for obesity is indicated in children with BMI >95th percentile with severe comorbidities and poor response for stage 1 to 3 intervention. Only two drugs have been approved for clinical use.

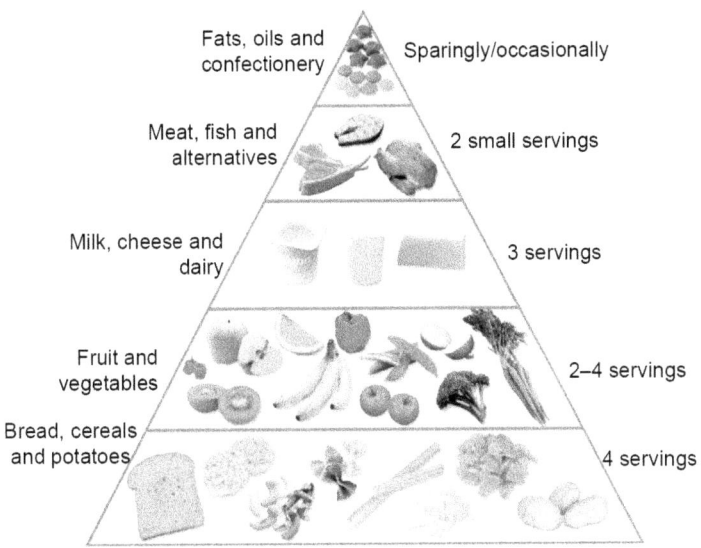

Fig. 2: Food guide pyramid. The triangular diagram represents the optimal number of servings to be eaten each day from each of the basic food groups.

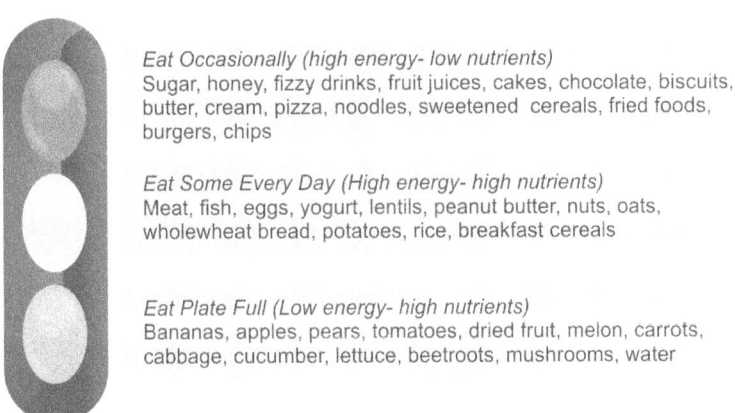

Fig. 3: Traffic light eating.

Sibutramine, a serotonin reuptake inhibitor was approved for use by the food and drug administration (FDA) in 1997 but was removed after a few years due to increased frequency of cardiovascular side effects including hypertension, tachycardia, premature ventricular contractions, prolonged interval QTc.

Orlistat, an inhibitor of gastrointestinal lipases, prevents the breakdown of triglycerides into absorbable fatty acids and monoglycerols. When orlistat 120 mg capsules are taken three times a day with meals approximately one-third of dietary triglycerides are excreted intact rather than absorbed. Side effects of this medication include oily stools, flatulence, and uncontrolled leakage of oil from the rectum. Diminished fat absorption also limits absorption of the fat soluble vitamins A, D, E, and K; therefore, a multivitamin should be part of the diet regimen with consumption of the vitamin more than 2 hours apart from administration of orlistat.

Drugs undergoing clinical trials include metformin which decreases insulin resistance, octreotide for hypothalamic obesity and leptin hormone injections.

Weight Loss Surgery

The most common weight-loss procedure performed in adolescents is Roux-en-Y gastric bypass (RYGB). It is restrictive malabsorptive, by creating a small (1/3 to 1-oz) gastric pouch by either separating or stepling the stomach. This pouch drains via a narrow passage way to the middle part of the small intestine, jejunum, and thereby bypasses the duodenum. The two other forms of bariatric surgery involve decreasing the size of the stomach to impact satiety and food intake without producing malabsorption because no bypass is involved. These are vertical banded gastroplasty and laparoscopic adjustable silicone gastric banding (LAGB) (Box 3).

Contraindications to surgery include a medically correctable cause of obesity, recent history of substance abuse, any condition that would impair adherence to postoperative dietary or medication regimens, current lactation or pregnancy, or planned pregnancy within 2 years after the surgery.

Potential postoperative complications can include intestinal leakage, strictures, small-bowel obstruction, infection, cholelithiasis, nutritional deficiencies or thromboembolism.

Box 3: Criteria for bariatric surgery.

- BMI ≥ 40 and at least 1 of the following:
  - Diabetes mellitus type 2
  - Sleep apnea
  - Pseudotumor cerebri
- BMI ≥50 with less-serious comorbidities:
  - Hypertension
  - Dyslipidemia
  - Nonalcoholic steatohepatitis (NASH)
  - Venous stasis
  - Impaired activities of daily living
  - Gastroesophageal reflux disease
  - Weight related arthropathies
- Additional criteria:
  - Skeletal maturation
  - Girls >13-year-old
  - Boys >15-year-old
  - Psychiatric evaluation that shows no contraindication and cognitive maturity to make decisions and comply with recommendations
  - Good social support system
  - Participation in at least 6 months of organized attempts at weight management or other good demonstration of an ability to comply with medical recommendations overtime

PREVENTION

At Family Level
- Limiting consumption of sugar-sweetened beverages
- Encouraging diets with recommended quantities of fruits and vegetables
- Limiting television and other screen time by allowing no more than 2 hours per day and removing television and computer screens from children's primary sleeping areas
- Eating breakfast daily
- Limiting consumption of energy dense foods and eating at restaurants
- Encouraging family meals in which parents and children eat together
- Limiting portion sizes
- Eating a diet with balanced macronutrients and rich in calcium and fiber
- Total 60 minutes of accumulated moderate to vigorous physical activity per day for children of healthy weight.

At Community Level
- Increase physical activity and sports at schools
- Efforts to preserve and to enhance parks as areas for physical activity, inclusion of walking and bicycle paths
- Actively engaging families with parental obesity or maternal diabetes because these children are at increased risk for developing obesity even if they currently have normal BMI
- Encouraging parents to model healthy diets and portions sizes, physical activity, and limited television time.

CONCLUSION

Therapy of obesity requires a multidisciplinary approach with nutritional, physical and behavioral modifications. The family needs to adopt changes as a unit. Community level interventions are needed with involvement of schools, daycare centers and media as these areas have a strong influence on the diet and lifestyles of children.

KEY LEARNING POINTS

- Obesity has a multifactorial etiology and causes numerous systemic complications.
- Body mass index for age and sex as per CDC charts is the standard diagnostic tool.
- A detailed history including nutritional and physical activity assessment and a meticulous physical examination should be performed before treatment.
- Staged treatment includes reduction in calorie intake, increasing physical activity, medications and bariatric surgery if needed.

REFERENCES

1. Barlow SE, Expert Committee. Expert committee recommendations regarding the prevention, assessment, and treatment of child and adolescent overweight and obesity: summary report. *Pediatrics* 2007;120 (Suppl) 4:164-192.
2. Peebles R. Adolescent obesity: Etiology, office evaluation, and treatment. *Adolesc Med State Art Rev* 2008;19:380-405.
3. Raychaudhuri M, Sanyal D. Childhood obesity: determinants, evaluation, and prevention. *Indian J Endocrinol Metabol* 2012;16:192-194.
4. Krebs NF, Himes JH, Jacobson D, Nicklas TA, Guilday P. Assessment of child and adolescent overweight and obesity. *Pediatrics* 2007;120(Suppl 4):S193-228.
5. Crocker MK, Yanovski JA. Pediatric obesity: etiology and treatment. *Pediatr Clin North Am* 2011;58:1217-1240.
6. Harish R, Pande D, Sharma S, Dang K. Management of Childhood obesity. In: Gupte S, Gupte SB, Gupte M (Eds): *Recent Advances in Pediatrics-26 Hot Topics*. New Delhi: Jaypee 2018:63-73.

PART 6: PEDIATRIC PRACTITIONER AND NUTRITION

23 Handling Nutritional Problems in Office Practice

Anuradha Bansal, Harmesh S Bains

ABSTRACT

Nutrition and immunization are two major issues faced by a pediatrician in office practice. Moreover, there are subtle symptoms and signs of micronutrient deficiency which might be missed by parents and even doctors if not specifically looked for. Hence, pediatricians need to include nutrition in routine care of infants and children in office practice.

Assessment and management of pediatric nutritional problems in routine day-to-day practice, right from undernutrition to obesity to behavioral eating problems like picky eaters are important. A quick nutrition history and anthropometric assessment may be done in the office, cases of borderline undernutrition, and normally growing children with micronutrient deficiencies especially iron and vitamin D should be carefully identified and managed. Overweight and obese children need to be assessed and parents counseled appropriately. Picky eaters tend to avoid certain food items, but they are growing normally and usually outgrow their symptoms by 5 years of age. Parents should be reassured regarding benign nature of problem and child to be kept under follow-up for any deviation from normal growth.

Keywords: Behavioral eating disorders, Growth, Growth charts, Nutrition, Office practice, Obesity, Overweight, Picky eaters, Undernutrition.

INTRODUCTION

Pediatric office practice has come a long way from the management of fever, upper respiratory infections, diarrhea, etc. only to immunization and dietary counseling in addition.[1,2] Rather, every visit to the pediatrician is an opportunity for the parents to get answers to their questions regarding their child's nutrition and also a window for the pediatrician to assess and manage borderline malnutrition. Even the parents of children who are not sick seek pediatrician's appointment regarding what to feed, what not to feed their kids and solutions to their trivial nutritional concerns.

Moreover, adequate nutrition is the key to good immunity.[1-3] Hence, good nutrition largely ensures freedom from infections. Also, urbanization and improvement of living standards have given rise to the problem of overnutrition and obesity leading to "dual nutrition burden". Obviously, we need to devote increased time for early recognition of nutritional problems and early intervention by increasing parental awareness of both inadequate and excess weight gain. Also, from examination point of view, pediatric postgraduates/residents should be able to recognize and manage borderline malnutrition and mild-to-moderate malnutrition. Disorders of severe malnutrition like kwashiorkar and marasmus that are easy to recognize have become less frequent, thereby largely taking a backseat.

This chapter focuses on these issues and covers approach to malnutrition (both undernutrition and obesity), outpatient management and preventive counseling.

Key topics are:
- Nutrition history
- Quick anthropometric assessment
- Micronutrient deficiencies in normally growing children
- Outpatient management of undernutrition
- Feeding guidelines for normally growing children
- Picky eaters
- Childhood obesity—risk factors, prevention and management.

NUTRITION HISTORY

Nutrition history is important in any child presenting with problems of growth and nutrition.[2] When asked an open ended question, parents may just say that the child eats normally. However, at the same time, it might not be possible to ask for "3 to 5 days" diet diary in a busy OPD. Hence, the age old 24 hour diet recall is the solution. Table 1 shows leading questions to be asked while eliciting dietary history in different age groups and Table 2 shows sample diet chart for 24 hours diet recall.

DOCUMENTATION OF GROWTH

At every outpatient visit, growth data of the child should be generated.[2] Weight, length and head circumference are measured and plotted on WHO growth chart for children under 3 years. For children younger than 2 years weight for length can be calculated and plotted on the growth chart (Table 1). It is possible to attach a copy of growth chart to the outpatient slip at first visit and use it on every visit. Current internationally accepted index is weight-for-height z-score based on WHO growth charts.

Children with severe acute malnutrition definitely need hospital admission, however, mild to moderate undernutrition can be managed on outpatient basis with dietary counseling and micronutrient supplementation (vide infra).

In addition, for children 2 years and older, body mass index (BMI) can be determined and plotted annually. BMI is a weight for height index determined by dividing weight in kg by height in m^2, and interpreted as follows:

BMI <5th percentile — Undernutrition
5th–85th percentile — Normal
85th–95th percentile — Overweight
>95th percentile — Obesity

Moreover, a yearly increase or decrease of 3 units should be a matter of concern.

Age independent criteria: Many uneducated mothers may not remember age of the chid and hence, standard anthropometric measures cannot be applied. In these cases, mid-arm circumference (MAC) can be measured as it remains constant between 1–5 years of age. MAC is classified according to Arnold's classification is as follows:

MAC >16 cm — Normal
13.5–16 cm — Mild undernutrition
12.5–13.5 cm — Moderate undernutrition
<12.4 cm — Severe undernutrition

Table 1: Leading questions for eliciting dietary history.

Age group	Questions
Neonate	When was the breastfeeding started after birth? Clostrum given or not? Any prelacteal feeds? Exclusive breastfeeding? If not, ask about additional feed
Infant	When was complementary feeding started? What does it consist of? Is the breastfeeding being continued?
Older children	Is the diet predominantly vegetarian or nonvegetarian? What is the kind of food usually being taken? 24 hour diet recall (Table 2) Is the child beneficiary of a noon meal scheme? What are the food habits of the child? Does he/she have any strong likes and dislikes for any particular food item? Is there any custom related to nutrition that the family follows, e.g. fasting, strict vegetarianism, excess fried food, etc.
Miscellaneous	Is the mother pregnant again? (breastfeeding compromised) Do both the parents stay with and care for the child?

Table 2: Sample diet chart for 24 hour diet recall.

Time	Food item	Quantity	Caloric value	Protein content
7 am				
9 am				
11 am				
1 pm				
4 pm				
8 pm				
Total				

WHO classification (Table 3) is quite helpful in busy practice.

Table 3: WHO classification of undernutrition.

Parameter	Moderate undernutrition	Severe undernutrition
Symmetrical edema	Absent	Present
Weight for height[a] (measure of wasting)	z score[b] or SD score between −2 and −3	z score or SD score <−3
Height for age[c] (measure of stunting)	z score or SD score between −2 and −3	z score or SD score <−3

a. Weight (wt) for height (ht) = (wt of the child/ wt of a normal child with same height) × 100
b. z score = (observed value−median reference value)/standard deviation of reference population
c. height for age = (length or ht of child/length or ht of normal child of same age) × 100

Only problem lies withe dematous children, where MAC will overestimate the nutritional status.

It is not possible to measure all anthropometric parameters in OPD. However, weight, height and MAC can be taken by a trained personnel in the waiting lounge and this usually suffices to assess nutritional status of the child. There are many other indices for assessment but all of them cannot be applied in a busy office practice and hence are not being discussed here.

Also, in adolescents, it will be prudent to document Tanner staging of pubertal status.

MICRONUTRIENT DEFICIENCIES IN APPARENTLY HEALTHY CHILDREN[2,6,7]

In general, it is easy to identify the classic signs of micronutrient deficiency as they are grossly evident but in apparently healthy children with normal anthropometry usually seen in office practice, subtle signs are often overlooked. Iron and vitamin D are the two most common nutrient deficiencies encountered in normally growing children accounting for frequent illnesses and sickness absenteeism. Quick assessment and office management of these micronutrient deficiencies is being discussed here:

Iron Deficiency [5,6]

Since years, iron deficiency has been the most common nutritional deficiency in children especially in developing countries.

Moderate to severe anemia can be easily recognized by palmar and conjunctival pallor, lethargy, irritability and poor feeding but mild anemia is usually missed. Typical presentation is mild to moderate microcytic hypochromic anemia in an otherwise asymptomatic, well-nourished infant.

Pica (craving for non-nutritive substances) and pagophagia (craving for ice) are associated with iron deficiency even with normal hemoglobin (Hb). Iron supplementation leads to improvement in symptoms before any increase in Hb. In addition, iron deficiency has been linked to impaired psychomotor and cognitive development in infants, poor school performance in children, and cognitive impairment and poor exercise performance in adolescents even in the absence of anemia.

Risk factors for iron deficiency include:
- Low socioeconomic status
- Infants born prematurely and low birth weight
- Non-breastfed babies especially those who are fed nonfortified formula or cow's milk
- Infants born to iron deficient mothers or breastfed by iron deficient mothers
- Early introduction of whole cow's milk (before 6 months of age) due to increased intestinal blood loss.

Hence, children with above risk factors should be carefully assessed for anemia at every outpatient visit.[7] However, anemia (Hb <11g/dL) is neither a sensitive nor specific indicator of iron status because only one-third of iron deficient children will have low Hb. Hence, an appropriate screening tool may be dietary history. Some of the pointers include:
- <5 servings each of grains, meat, fruits and vegetables per week
- >480 mL of milk per day
- > 480 mL of soft drinks per day
- Daily intake of fatty snacks or sweets.

For suspected cases, hemoglobin and peripheral blood film should be done and those with microcytic hypochromic anemia started on iron. Earliest sign of iron deficiency is increase in red cell distribution width (RDW) and diagnosis is confirmed by serum ferritin levels less than 12 ng/mL. However, ferritin is an acute phase reactant, hence, rate of false positives will be high. Most cost effective method is to give a therapeutic trial of iron in all cases of microcytic hypochromic anemia with a presumptive diagnosis of iron deficiency anemia (IDA). Flowchart 1 shows outline of management of IDA.

Vitamin D and Calcium Deficiency

Vitamin D is essential for absorption of calcium from gastrointestinal tract and deficiency of vitamin D causes hypocalcemia and hypophosphatemia leading to nutritional rickets in children. In some children, nutritional rickets may occur despite normal serum vitamin D levels due to low dietary intake of calcium. It has been seen that calcium and vitamin D content of complementary foods is <50% of required which is a major contributor towards nutritional rickets, incidence being highest between 3 months to 3 years of age. Most of the patients with vitamin D deficiency are asymptomatic, only few develop secondary hyperparathyroidism and characteristic bony abnormalities of rickets. Vitamin D deficiency has three stages:

Stage 1: Hypocalcemia due to decreased calcium absorption, serum phosphate is normal.
Stage 2: Hypophosphatemia with normal serum calcium.
Stage 3: Florid rickets with hypocalcemia and hypophosphatemia. This stage presents with delayed closure of anterior fontanelle, frontal bossing,

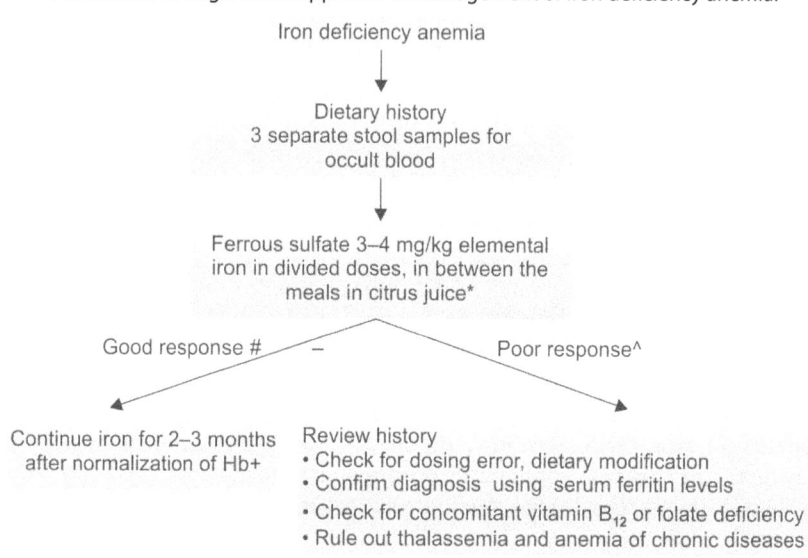

Flowchart 1: Algorthmic approach to management of iron deficiency anemia.

*Citrus fruits increase the absorption of iron.

rachitic rosary (enlargement of costochondral junction visible as beading along anterolateral aspect of chest), Harrison's groove (due to muscular pull of diaphragm on softened ribs), wrist widening, double malleoli and genu valgum (due to bowing of tibia) or coxa vara (bending of femur due to increased head-neck distance). Diagnosis is clinical and may be established by X-ray wrist (widening of epiphysis and metaphysis, cupping and fraying of margins at the end of bones and rarefaction of diaphysis).

Secondary hyperparathyroidism is present in all stages. If stage 1 and 2 are recognized and managed in office practice, skeletal abnormalities may be avoided thus reducing the burden of disease. As child is usually asymptomatic in early stages, look for subtle signs like irritability, bone pains, increased dental caries, delayed walking and poor growth. Moreover, similar to ID, a careful dietary history may provide a clue, for example, whether milk is fortified with vitamin D and is the child taking animal foods in diet. Also, vitamin D deficiency has been linked to increased susceptibility to respiratory infections and reactive airway disease and hence, children with these issues should receive vitamin D supplementation. Normal infants and young children should receive 200–400 IU/day of vitamin D to prevent deficiency. Flowchart 2 outlines the management of vitamin D deficiency in children.

OUTPATIENT MANAGEMENT OF ACUTE UNDERNUTRITION

Severely malnourished children who have no complications, have a good appetite and are clinically well can be managed on outpatient basis with regular follow-up every 2 weeks. At each visit, parents should be provided

Flowchart 2: Outline of management of nutritional rickets.

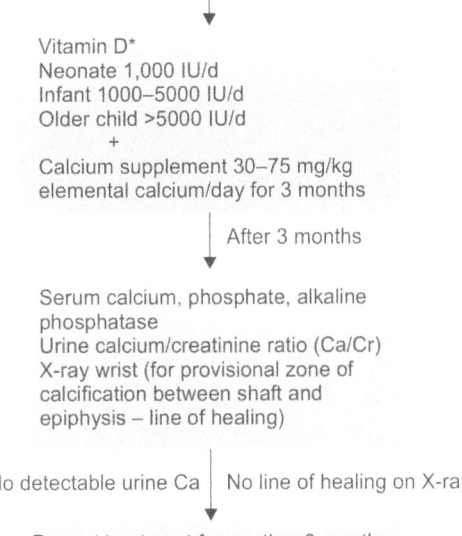

*Another option is stoss therapy which refers to single mega dose of vitamin D. 6 lakhs units in a day which is equivalent to 5000 IU/d for 3 months especially in patients where compliance or follow-up is a problem. However, this dose carries the risk of hypocalcemia.

health and nutrition education regarding how to prepare cheap, balanced and nutritious meals for the child.[8,9] Anthropometry should be done and ready to use therapeutic food (RUTF) should be advised for catch-up growth. This includes multimix foods and Hyderabad mixture which can be easily prepared at home.

Multimix food: This mixture provides around 500 calories and 15 g of protein and can be advised in addition to home-made nutritious food. Its components include:

Staple food (40 g)	Rice/wheat
Protein (15 g)	Beans/groundnuts/fish/egg
Vitamins/minerals	Green leafy vegetables/fruit
Energy supplement	Vegetable oil/ghee/sugar

Hyderabad mix: Developed by National Institute of Nutrition, Hyderabad, this mixture is rich in calories and proteins. Each 86 g of mixture provides 330 calories and 11.5 g of protein. It consists of:

Whole wheat (40 g)
Bengal gram (16 g)
Groundnut (10 g)
Jaggery (20 g)

Parents should be informed that RUTF should be used as a medicine for the child and should not be shared within the family. In addition, the child should be dewormed with single dose of albendazole (400 mg), given vitamin A (2 lakh units if weight >8 kg and 1 lakh unit if weight <8 kg) and iron folate supplementation.

Child can be discharged from follow-up after a minimum of three visits if:
- Weight-for-height is >-2SD
- Midarm circumference > 13.5 cm
- There is no edema
- Clinically well
- No clinical evidence of micronutrient deficiency.

In these cases, parents are provided with one week supply of RUTF, counseled regarding home-made nutritious food and micronutrient supplements as prescribed and can be followed after 1 month or at next visit for immunization.

FEEDING GUIDELINES FOR APPARENTLY HEALTHY[11]

In day-to-day practice, we see many well looking children whose parents want to know what and how they should feed their child? It is important to advise them regarding balanced diet and healthy eating habits to form a strong foundation for adolescence and adulthood.

The following points are from the comprehensive review of Infant and Young Child Feeding (IYCF)[11] and American Academy of Pediatrics (AAP) guidelines:

- Exclusive breastfeeding should be recommended as the gold standard for the first 6 months of life. All breastfed babies should receive vitamin D supplementation 400 IU/day since birth through first year of life.
- Appropriately thick, homogenous complementary home-made foods made from locally available ingredients should be initiated at 6 months along with continued breastfeeding. Because of small stomach size, infants tend to eat less hence, foods may be made energy dense by adding jaggery/sugar/ghee/butter/oil. To enrich the food, fermented porridge, germinated or sprouted flour may be used. Iron supplementation should be started at 6 months at a dose of 1-2 mg/kg per day and continued till 1 year of age to protect against iron deficiency anemia.

Baby should receive three meals and one or two nutritious snacks in between. Snacks are in addition and should not replace meals. They should not be confused with foods, such as sweets, chips or other processed foods.

The food should be a balanced diet consisting of various (as diverse as possible) food groups/components in different combinations. Easily available, cost-effective seasonal uncooked fruits, green and other dark colored vegetables, milk and milk products, pulses/legumes, animal foods should be given. Oil/butter, sugar/jaggery may be added in the staples gradually.

Food items that supply micronutrients should be encouraged like green, yellow, orange and red (GYOR) vegetables and fruits.

A balanced diet should consist of carbohydrates 55-60%, proteins 10-15% and fats 30-35%. Energy derived from cereals should not be >75%. And maximum protein intake should be 15-20% of total calories required. Minimum amount of green leafy and other vegetables should not be less than 50 g/day.[10] A quick guide is mentioned here:

Calories: 1,000 kcal for 1st year

Add 100 kcal per year up to 12 years, for example, energy requirement of a 5-year-old child is 1,000 + (100 × 4) = 1,400 kcal

Proteins: 1.5-2 g/kg/day

Encourage handwashing and hygienic practices during food preparation, storage and feeding. Practice responsive feeding. Self-feeding should be encouraged despite spillage. Each child should be fed under supervision in a separate plate to develop an individual identity. Forced feeding, threatening and punishment interfere with the development of good/proper feeding habits. As a general rule, parents should decide when and what to eat and children should decide how much and whether to eat.

Babies usually have 'neophobia'. Hence, any new food needs to be tried several times before it is accepted by them. Granular or lumpy food should be introduced by 9-10 months. By 1 year, baby should be eating from the family pot.

Avoid junk and commercial food which are high in sugar, salt, fat, additives/preservatives and pesticides (SSFAP). Avoid giving ready-made, processed commercial food from the market.

- Eat meals as a family. Parents should try to be a good role model.
- For children 1-3 years of age, ensure >30 minutes of structured play and >60 minutes of free, structured play daily. For older children, seek 1 or more hour of vigorous play daily. Reduce television and other screen time to less than 2 hours a day.

PICKY EATERS[12]

Although, classified as eating disorder, this problem is being discussed here as it is frequently encountered in office practice. Picky eaters are children who reject certain types of food, are unwilling to try unfamiliar foods and have discerning preferences in the taste, texture and smell of food, different from their parents or other individuals.

Child usually consumes adequate calories in a day but tends to refuse certain food items, pushes away the plate or hides the food when that specific food item is offered.

Usually seen in toddlers and preschool children, it disappears by 5 years of age. If it persists beyond 9 years, it may develop into more serious eating disorder like anorexia or bulimia nervosa.

This is a benign disorder more common in girls and is related to the problem of "plenty" or "easy availability" of food. Hence, it is more commonly seen in children of upper middle class and higher class families.

Predisposing factors

- Child-related
  - There is a higher incidence of this problem at around 2-3 years of when the rate of rapid growth and metabolism slows down leading to physiological anorexia
  - Child recognizes himself as an individual and likes to exert authority
  - Early age at joining school
  - Working mother
  - Failure to introduce diverse different textured foods during later half of the first year of life.
- Family-related
  - Undue parental concern regarding child's weight and feeding
  - Authoritative feeding behavior adapted by caregiver.
- Environment related
  - Exposure to various advertisements in media related to fast food predisposes to picky eating.

Clinical Features

There are no characteristic clinical features but these children are usually thin built with normal weight and height for age. Some of them may be picky eaters at home but may eat well in school, parties, restaurants, friends' place or with television.

Picky eating in toddlers usually does not lead to any nutritional or psychological consequences but if it persists beyond 9 years of age, it may lead to malnutrition, impaired growth and cognition and increased susceptibility to infections.

Assessment

Main aim of assessment of these children is to rule out any underlying pathology. It includes:
- Detailed dietary history
- Anthropometry (weight, height, mid-upper arm circumference)
- Complete blood count, Mantoux test, urine and stool examination, chest X-ray and blood sugar are done only if the nutrition or growth is below the normal centiles.
- In select situations, renal and liver function tests, contrast studies of the gastrointestinal (GI) tract and upper GI endoscopy may be required to rule out malabsorption syndromes.

Management

- Toddlers with picky eating usually outgrow their symptoms and only reassurance is required.

- If the problem persists beyond 5 years of age, after ruling out an organic cause, following interventions should be done:

Meal Time Suggestions
- Parents should take care of the taste of food by using gentle spices to mask unpleasant flavors.
- The texture of the food should be generally a little dry. Slimy, chunky, mushy food should be avoided including over-ripe fruits.
- They should be fed only when they are hungry.
- The meal times should be a pleasant family time and children should join the family meals at the earliest age.
- Television, storybooks, arguments should be discouraged during meal times.
- Child should not be forced to finish the food.
- The child should get involved in preparing and serving meals.
- The nonpreferred food should not be sneaked into the regular meal.
- Realistic portions of food should be served and the child encouraged to taste new food.
- Beriberi, threats should not be practiced.
- Drinking fluids and snacking in between meals should be restricted.

Behavioral Modifications
- Time out and reinforcement
- Positive and negative reinforcement.

CHILDHOOD OBESITY[13,14]

Obesity may be defined as a maladaptive increase in the mass of somatic fat stores. Unlike adults, where obesity simply correlates with increased incidence of chronic diseases, childhood obesity is related to other issues also like association with congenital and genetic disorders, predisposition to eating disorders like anorexia and bulimia nervosa and psychosocial issues. This chapter deals with nutritional aspects of childhood obesity in office practice. Further details of this disorder have been discussed elsewhere.

As mentioned earlier, BMI is a surrogate measure of body fatness and children with BMI between 85th and 95th percentile for age are overweight and BMI >95th percentile are obese. However, during risk assessment for obesity following points should be kept in mind:
- Risk of persistence of pediatric obesity into adulthood increases with age irrespective of length of time the child has been obese.
- The risk of obesity related complications like diabetes, hypertension, hyperlipidemia, asthma, etc. is strongly influenced by positive family history of these disorders regardless of family history of obesity.
- A mildly overweight child with a family history of adulthood obesity may be at higher risk of subsequent obesity than an obese child with negative family history.

Hence, any child with a history of first degree relatives with obesity, type 2 diabetes, hypertension, hyperlipidemia or premature myocardial infarction and any child with BMI >85th percentile for age is "at risk" of adiposity-related morbidity.

Management

Evaluation: Initial evaluation consists of detailed dietary history, family eating habits and physical activity history. A baseline record of blood pressure, fasting and postprandial blood sugar and lipid profile should be obtained.

Targets for obesity management: Major issue in all age groups is weight maintenance through dietary and lifestyle modification. For children between 2-11 years of age, a weight loss of 0.5 g/kg per month should be attempted. However, if the BMI is >99th percentile, a target loss of 1g/kg per month may be attempted if the age is more than 5 years. For adolescents, a weight loss of 1 g/kg should be the target.

Most important aspect of obesity management is the motivation of child and parents as family-based therapy is the best approach to successful treatment.

Dietary management: Dietary management should aim at weight maintenance or weight loss without compromising appropriate calorie intake and normal nutrition. Due emphasis should be given to initiate and maintain healthy eating patterns (vide supra). A standard protocol is to recommend a fat intake of 30-40% kcal in children 1-3 years old with a reduction of 25-35% in children 4-18 years old; a carbohydrate intake of 45-65% kcal in all children and protein intakes of 5-20% kcal in children 1-3 years old with gradual increase to 10-30% kcal in children 4-18 years old. Cholesterol intake should be less than 75 mg/1,000 kcal, not to exceed 150 mg per day. Age-appropriate serving sizes including 5 or more servings of fruit and vegetables, 3 or more servings of low fat milk or dairy products, and 6 or more servings of whole-grain and grain products per day as well as adequate amounts of dietary fiber (age in year + 5 g/d) should also be encouraged.

Both parents and child should be counseled to reduce eating outs, avoid sugary beverages, eat healthy snacks and increase the intake of fresh fruits, vegetables and dietary fiber.

Enhancement of physical activity: In general, children and adolescents should engage in not less than 60 minutes of moderate to vigorous physical activity per day to achieve optimum cardiovascular health. However, overweight and obese children should target higher levels. Longer periods of moderate intensity exercises like brisk walking are excellent for reducing body fat as they burn more fat and calories. Children should be prescribed physical activity that is safe, developmentally appropriate, interesting, practical and has a social element. Involving other members of the family in the exercise program and supervising the activity on a regular basis will improve compliance.

Restriction of sedentary behavior: Every hour of sedentary activity increases the chance of obesity and contributes to failure of weight management strategies, hence, screen time should be restricted as mentioned above.

In addition, parents should be advised to encourage their child and provide positive reinforcement for healthy lifestyle changes. Food should not be used as a reward or punishment. There should be a regular schedule of meals, snacks and exercise. Parents should adopt similar lifestyle changes as the child is being asked to make. Calorie dense harmful foods should be removed from the home for everyone.

CONCLUSION

A focused attention to nutrition with reference to undernutrition, obesity and behavioral eating problems, such as picky eaters, in routine care of infants and children in office practice are mandatory. Following a quick nutrition history and anthropometric assessment, cases of borderline undernutrition and normally growing children with micronutrient deficiencies especially iron and vitamin D should be carefully identified and managed. Overweight and obese children need to be assessed and parents counseled appropriately. In case of picky eaters, parents should be reassured regarding benign nature of problem which is usually over by 5 years of age.

KEY LEARNING POINTS

- Nutritional history and assessment of nutritional status should be an important part of pediatric office practice.
- Baseline anthropometry should be regularly charted for all the pediatric patients.
- Iron and vitamin D deficiency are the most common micronutrient deficiencies in children and should be carefully looked for in routine practice.
- Exclusive breastfeeding is the gold standard in first 6 months of life followed by complementary feeding starting at 6 months with transition to balanced diet by 1 year of age.
- Parents should be role models for children to establish healthy and hygienic eating habits.
- Physical activity should be encouraged and screen time restricted.
- Healthy lifestyle changes should be encouraged to control both persistent undernutrition and growing overnutrition.
- Picky eaters should be handled carefully with simple dietary and behavioral modifications and parents reassured regarding benign nature of the problem.

REFERENCES

1. Kleinman RE. Nutrition, physical activity and health: an office-based approach. In: *Pediatric Nutrition Handbook*, 6th edn. New Delhi: Jaypee 2010:29-42.
2. Gupte S, Gomez EM. Malnutriton. In: Gupte S (Ed): The *Short Textbook of Pediatrics*, 12th edn. New Delhi: Jaypee 2016:197-224.

3. Suskind DL. Nutritional deficiencies during normal growth. *Pediatr Clin North Am* 2009;56:1035-1053.
4. Ziegler EE, Formon SJ, Nelson SE, et al. Cow milk feeding in infancy: further observations on blood loss from the gastrointestinal tract. *J Pediatr* 1990;116: p11-18.
5. Sherriff A, Emond A, Bell JC, et al. Should infants be screened for anemia? A prospective study investigating the relation between haemoglobin at 8, 12 and 18 months and development at 18months. *Arch Dis Child* 2001;84:480-485.
6. Halterman JS, Kaczorowski JM, Aligne CA, et al. Iron deficiency and cognitive achievement among school-aged children and adolescents in the United States. *Pediatrics* 2001;107:1381-1386.
7. Boutry M, Needlman R. Use of dietary history in screening for iron deficiency. *Pediatrics* 1996;98(6 Pt 1):1138-1142.
8. Khan Y, Bhutta ZA. Nutritional deficiencies in the developing world: current status and opportunities for intervention. *Pediatr Clin North Am* 2010;57:1409-1441.
9. Lutter CK, Rivera JA. Nutritional status of infants and young children and characteristics of their diets. *J Nutr* 2003;294:1s-9s.
10. Kim SA, Grimm KA, May AL, et al. Strategies for pediatric practitioners to increase fruit and vegetable consumption in children. *Pediatr Clin North Am* 2011;58: 1439-1453.
11. Tiwari S, Bharadva K, Yadav B, et al. Infant and young child feeding guidelines, 2016. *Indian Pediatr* 2016;53:703-713.
12. Sathiyasekaran M, Ganesh R. Picky eaters. *Indian J Pract Pediatr* 2007; 9: 254-258.
13. Kleinman RE. Pediatric obesity. In: *Pediatric Nutrition Handbook*. 6th edn. New Delhi: Jaypee; 2010:733-782.
14. Raj M, Kumar KR. Obesity in children and adolescents. *Indian J Med Res* 2010;132: 598-607.

PART 7: NUTRITION IN SYSTEMIC DISEASES

24   Nutrition in Diabetes

Shaveta Kundra

ABSTRACT

Effective dietary management of children with type 1 diabetes helps to optimize glycemic control and leads to improvements in clinical and metabolic outcomes. Current recommendations are based on healthy eating principles for children and families with the aim to promote healthy lifelong eating habits while maintaining social and psychological well-being. The intake of energy and essential nutrients should aim to maintain ideal body weight, promote health and growth, optimize glycemic control, whilst minimizing the risk of chronic complications.

Recent advances include the use of intensive insulin regimes together with accurate and consistent carbohydrate counting, as well as low glycemic index food choices which have been shown improve glycemic control. The use of continuous glucose monitoring has provided us with an insight into the effect of the composition of meals on glucose levels and the opportunity to tailor insulin therapy and dietary advice on an individual basis.

Keywords: Diet, Dietary allowances, Dietary intake, Glycemic index, Insulin regimens, Nutrition, Type 1 diabetes.

INTRODUCTION

Nutrition is of critical importance in the management of children with diabetes. Consumption of adequate calories is essential to meet the normal body requirements for energy expenditure, growth, and pubertal development during infancy, childhood and adolescence. Although the nutritional requirements of a diabetic child are not different from healthy children; effective dietary interventions can significantly improve the clinical and metabolic outcomes in children with type 1 diabetes.[1-3] There is no ideal diet which can be prescribed to all diabetic patients. It requires individualization as per the nutritional goals, cultural, family traditions as well as the psychosocial needs of the individual child.[4,5]

The dietary recommendations in diabetes have evolved over the years. Earlier the dietary management was based primarily on severe restriction of calorie intake leading to starvation diets.[6] After the invention of insulin, the concept shifted to high fat and low carbohydrate diet followed by low fat and high carbohydrate.[7] The recommendations of 60–70% calories from a combination of carbohydrates and monounsaturated fats is supported by the fact that high-carbohydrate diet leads to more hyperglycemia than a high monounsaturated fat diet with no differences in the lipid profile.[8,9] In general, the food intake of a diabetic child as well as that of any healthy child should be balanced, i.e. it should contain adequate amounts of carbohydrates, protein, fat, minerals, vitamins, fiber, and water. A pediatric dietitian should be part of the multidisciplinary pediatric diabetes team. Their role is to provide education, monitoring and support to patients, parents, caregivers and families both at diagnosis and during ongoing management.[10-12]

GOALS OF DIETARY MANAGEMENT

The nutritional strategies must be planned to achieve the desired goals of healthy eating, optimal glycemic control and reduction of cardiovascular risk factors.[6] This involves:
- Encouraging healthy eating behaviors
- Three balanced meals a day with healthy snacks if appropriate
- Providing sufficient energy intake for optimal growth and development
- Maintaining an appropriate body mass index (BMI)
- Maintaining a balance between food intake, energy expenditure and insulin action profiles to attain optimal glycemic control without excessive hypoglycemia
- Prevention and treatment of hypoglycemia, hyperglycemia and exercise-related problems
- Reducing the risk of microvascular complications by optimizing glycemic control
- Modifying nutritional intake to prevent and treat dyslipidemia, hypertension and obesity
- Maintaining a good quality of life.

ENERGY BALANCE, ENERGY INTAKE AND FOOD COMPONENTS

As already stated, nutritional requirements of children with type 1 diabetes are the same as their healthy counterparts. They require a regular intake of recommended starchy carbohydrates, unsaturated fats and lean protein to meet their requirements for energy and protein, for optimal growth and development (Table 1). Regular healthy diet of three meals a day provides the required nutrients, calories and also prevents nutritional deficiencies (Fig. 1). Young children should be given additional snacks in between the meals to meet their higher calorie requirements. At the time of diagnosis children with diabetes often have increased appetite; hence energy intake should be increased to restore preceding catabolic weight loss. However, this increased

Table 1: Distribution of different food components.

Distribution of total energy intake amongst different food components

Total energy intake should be distributed as follows:
Carbohydrate 50–55%
- sucrose <10%

Fat 30–35%
- <10% saturated fat þ trans fatty acids
- <10% polyunsaturated fat
- >10% monounsaturated fat (up to 20%)

Protein 10–15%

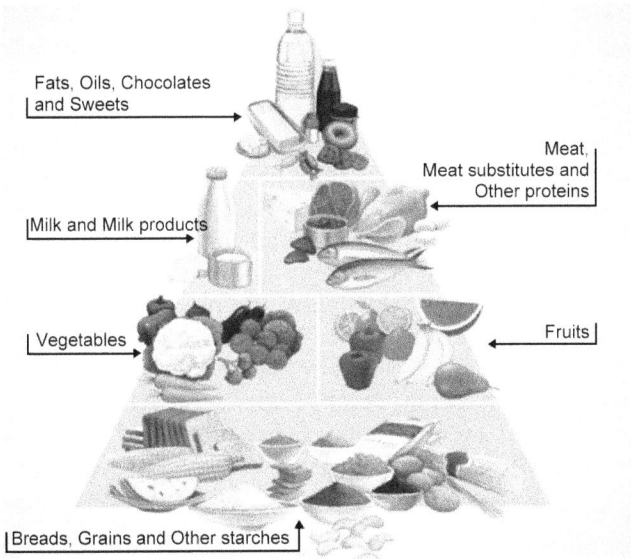

Fig. 1: Diabetes food pyramid.

energy intake must be reduced once pre-illness weight is restored.[13] Failure to reduce energy intake after the cessation of rapid growth periods can lead to excessive weight gain. In addition, insufficient physical activity, over insulinization, snacking and treatment of hypoglycemia may also contribute further to obesity in these children.[14] Hence, strict monitoring of growth and BMI, promoting regular physical activity, prevention and appropriate treatment of hypoglycemia are crucial in achieving a healthy BMI.[14,15]

In general, few important points to be remembered while planning diet for children with diabetes.
- The amount of food in diabetic diet should be flexible and revised regularly to meet the changes in appetite and insulin regimens, and to ensure optimal growth.[16]
- The amount and type of insulin should also be adapted as per child's appetite and eating pattern.
- The increased energy and nutritional requirement during puberty warrants significant increase in insulin dose.

- The practice of making a child eat without an appetite or withholding food in an effort to control blood sugar should be discouraged. This adversely affects the growth and development of children.

FOOD COMPONENTS

Carbohydrates

Carbohydrates are the main dietary source of glucose and body's principal supply of readily available energy. It should form 50–55% of total energy in children with and without diabetes.[4,5,17,18] Digestible carbohydrates are classified as starches and sugars. Starches are complex carbohydrates; these are slowly digested and absorbed and hence do not produce a rapid or sharp rise in blood glucose. It also contains other nutritional components and fiber. These are consumed in natural or in refined forms—the former should be preferred. Simple sugars produce sharper swings in blood glucose. Sugars (glucose, fructose, lactose and sucrose) occur naturally in foods (fruits, milk, and vegetables) or may be added during manufacturing or before consumption. Up to 10% of the total calories may be consumed as "added sugar" provided it is part of a fiber rich meal, and adequately spaced throughout the day.[17,19] However, sucrose provides only "empty" calories, has an adverse effect on dental health.[20] Snacks with sucrose (e.g. sweets, ice creams and chocolates) are also usually high in saturated fat content. Such snacks should not be given for reversal of acute hypoglycemia, as the fat content slows down sugar absorption. Hence, in general adding sucrose to beverages or eating sucrose containing snacks should be avoided.[20]

Carbohydrate counting: Since carbohydrates are the chief proximate principal in food that influences blood glucose. Insulin needs to be matched to the carbohydrate intake (rather than calorie content) at each meal. It aims to improve glycemic control and allow flexibility of food choices.[21] For this the carbohydrate content of common foods and snacks should be taught to patients and insulin to carbohydrate ratio for different times of the day for each patient should be established. Those on a basal-bolus regimen can calculate the pre-meal insulin to match the anticipated carbohydrate intake at each meal. If patient is on split-mixed insulin regimen taking a fixed insulin dose from day-to-day, the carbohydrate content should also be fixed for a given meal from day-to-day.

Glycemic index (GI): The GI compares postprandial blood glucose (PPBG) response to constant amounts of different carbohydrate containing foods. It measures the rise above fasting in BG area in first 2 hours after ingestion of 50 g of the carbohydrate under study compared with the response to a reference food (glucose or white bread).[22] Foods that produce lower (PPBG) excursions are to be preferred, these foods are said to have a low GI. Glycemic Index depends on multiple factors other than the type of carbohydrate—these include method of cooking, state of ripeness, degree of processing and

macronutrient distribution of the meal. A recent meta-analysis showed a 0.4% decline in HbA1c with low GI foods as against high GI foods.[17,23]
- Examples of low GI foods include oats, barley, beans, lentils, legumes, soybeans, kidney beans, cashew nuts, pasta, noodles, strawberries, apple, orange, fructose, full cream milk and yogurt.[23]
- Foods with high GI include white bread, white rice, puffed rice, bajra, jowar, ragi, maize, semolina, tapioca, cornflakes, baked potato, and honey.
- Foods with moderate GI include sugar, basmati rice, honey, popcorn, ice cream, dried rice noodles, black gram, green gram and croissants[24].

Fat

Fats should provide 30% of total calories (higher in infants below 2 years of age).[25] All fats provide the same number of calories (9 calories per g), but attention needs to be paid to the amount and the quality of fat in diet. Less than 10% of calories should be derived from saturated fats and up to 10% from polyunsaturated fats; the remaining fat-derived calories should be derived from monounsaturated fats (10–15%).[26,27] Polyunsaturated-to-saturated fat intake ratio is adjusted to approximately 1.2:1.0. Higher intakes of saturated fat are associated with increased risk of cardiovascular disease.[4,26,28] In patients with raised LDL cholesterol, the saturated fat intake needs to be further reduced to below 7% of total calories, while cholesterol intake should be less than 200 mg per day. Dietary fats derived from animal sources should be, therefore, reduced and replaced by polyunsaturated fats from vegetable sources.[26] Substituting butter by margarine, animal oils by vegetable oil in cooking, lean cuts of meat, poultry and fish for fatty meats; and less consumption of egg yolks is advisable.[29] These simple measures reduce cholesterol intake and serum LDL cholesterol, a predisposing factor to atherosclerotic disease.

Polyunsaturated fatty acids (PUFA) are essential fatty acids (not synthesized in the body). These are classified as omega-6 and omega-3 fatty acids.

Omega-6 PUFA: It is found in various cooking oils (safflower, sunflower, soya, cottonseed, corn, peanut and sesame) and in pulses, vegetables, cereals, nuts, seeds, eggs and poultry.

Omega-3 PUFA: It on may have a beneficial influence on coronary heart disease, serum triglycerides and immune system and they are found particularly in cold water fatty fish. For the vegetarian, flaxseeds, walnuts, soybean, canola oil, kidney beans, tofu, broccoli, spinach, cauliflower, and chinese cabbage are good sources of omega-3 fatty acids.

Monounsaturated fatty acids (MUFA): It should make up about 10–15% of your total daily calories.[26] It is found in olive, canola, groundnut, peanut, sesame, rice bran, mustard oils in almonds and avocados. A diet using monounsaturated fat rather than carbohydrate to lower saturated fat in diet gives better postprandial blood glucose levels with equivalent lowering of

LDL cholesterol; however, it may cause undesirable weight gain and does not significantly improve HbA1c levels.[19,30]

Protein

Protein intake should make 10-15% of the caloric requirement. It promotes growth only when sufficient amount of calories are available. Higher protein intakes >25% are not recommended as it may impact on growth vitamin and mineral intake. The protein requirement is 2 g/kg at 1 year, 1 g/kg at 10 years and 0.8-0.9 g/kg in adolescence.[31] Proteins from animal sources (fish, milk, egg white, poultry and meats) are of better quality than those from vegetarian sources (soya, beans, and lentils) as these provide all essential amino acids. However, proteins from vegetarian sources are accompanied with fiber and complex carbohydrates and contain less of saturated fat in contrast to those from animal sources which are more likely to be associated with higher salt and saturated fat content. Protein intake should be restricted to 10% of the total calories if patient develops microalbuminuria, as increased glomerular perfusion or filtration is a key factor in progression to nephropathy. However, there is insufficient evidence to restrict protein intake for prevention of microalbuminuria.[32]

Fiber

Indigestible carbohydrates present in food are designated as "dietary fiber" or "unavailable carbohydrates". A fiber intake equal to the child's age in years plus 5 g is known to be beneficial. The traditional Indian diet is naturally high in fiber content. To increase fiber intake, patients should be advised to consume whole fruits with skin and edible seeds, vegetables, legumes, oats, beans and whole grain cereals. Soluble fiber (found in dried beans, peas, oat bran, barley, apples, prunes, citrus fruits, watermelon, carrots and potatoes) improves total and LDL cholesterol levels by binding to bile salts, slows carbohydrate absorption by delaying gastric emptying thus giving a flatter blood glucose curve and may reduce insulin requirement.[33,34] Insoluble fiber (present in whole wheat products, fruit skin, green beans, dark green leafy vegetables, seeds and nuts) helps bowel movement and prevents constipation.

A high fiber diet is not recommended in children below 2-3 years of age as they need a calorie dense diet. Certain precautions need to be taken when using high fiber diet—introduce gradually; step up water intake; anticipate flatulence, abdominal cramps and bloating; and provide supplements of calcium and trace elements particularly iron and zinc.

Salt

Children with T1DM are more likely than nondiabetic children to develop hypertension. They also are more likely to consume higher amounts of salt as the stress is on a "nonsweet" diet. It would be prudent to restrict salt to 2 g per 1,000 calories.[35] Further restriction may be indicated if the child develops hypertension. Canned or packaged foods, baked products, pickles, pappad, sauces, and chinese foods should be restricted. However, flavor enhancers, such as herbs, lemon juice, vinegar, spices, onions, tamarind, and green pepper can be used.

Vitamin and Mineral Supplementation

Vitamin and mineral requirements are same as healthy children. Routine provision of vitamins and minerals are not indicated except in patients who are on a restrictive diet, or have celiac disease, pernicious anemia or achlorhydria. Potassium supplementation is important for patients recovering from DKA till they reach pre-DKA weight. Many fresh fruits and vegetables are naturally rich in antioxidants (tocopherols, carotenoids, vitamin C, and flavonoids) and are recommended for young people with diabetes for cardiovascular protection. Vitamin D supplementation should be as per recommendations if vitamin D levels are low.[36]

Sweeteners

Sweeteners are classified as nutritive and non-nutritive. Of the nutritive sweeteners, fructose contains calories similar to sucrose but with a lower GI: Fructose has a GI of 29 as against 69 of sucrose. However, added fructose may have an adverse effect on serum lipids and hence its use as a replacement for sucrose in the diet is not recommended.[37]

Sugar alcohols, such as xylitol, sorbitol and mannitol contain half the calories of sucrose and have a better GI. They are considered safe, though in excess, they may cause diarrhea.

Nutritive sweeteners are included in diabetic snacks.

Non-nutritive (artificial) sweeteners are virtually calorie free. These include aspartame, sucralose, saccharin, and acesulfame potassium. All are fairly safe in amounts recommended by the American Diabetes Association, but most children can do without it.

GUIDELINES FOR DIET, EDUCATION, AND MEAL PLANNING

A pediatric dietician should be a part of multidisciplinary diabetes management team. Initial dietary advice should be sought as soon as possible after the diagnosis is made.[11] A detailed dietary history should be obtained with special attention to:
- Pre-existing dietary habits, family traditions, and beliefs.
- The child's usual food intake including energy, carbohydrate distribution and fat intake, quality of food choices, fast foods and mealtimes, or patterns of food intake.
- Details of child's daily activities, physical activity, and exercise schedules.

Based on the dietary assessment individualized diet plan should be provided. Regular follow-up care should be maintained with the dietician initially at monthly interval followed by every 3 months for the first year and then annually. Review assessment should include identification of any body image or weight concerns. Dietary education should be individualized and appropriate for the age and maturity of the child help to engage the child in active learning.[38]

Regular dietician visits are necessary to monitor child's growth, diabetes management, psychosocial adaptation, lifestyle changes, and the identification of specific dietary problems, such as dysfunctional eating habits, family issues, obesity, and eating disorders. Certain circumstances, such as changing insulin regimen, dyslipidemia, poor dietary knowledge, excessive weight gain, and comorbidities, such as celiac disease require extra education and dietary intervention with more frequent review.

DIETARY RECOMMENDATIONS FOR DIFFERENT INSULIN REGIMES

Flexibility is the key to optimizing nutritional outcomes. Insulin regimes should be adapted where possible to the child's appetite and eating pattern. Most patients are now using intensive insulin regimes, such as multiple daily injections and pumps. This enables a more flexible approach to eating patterns and food intake allowing the insulin dose to be matched to carbohydrate intake.[4, 39-41] Rapid acting analogue insulin is given with carbohydrate intake immediately before meals and snacks according to insulin to carbohydrate ratios (ICRs) set for different meals in each individual. Many blood glucose monitors have bolus advisors which calculate insulin doses based on blood glucose levels (BGLs), carbohydrate amount to be eaten and ICR.[42] The use of bolus calculators have been shown to assist insulin dose calculations and improve postprandial glycemia. Preprandial and 2 to 3 hours postprandial BGLs are used to monitor the accuracy of the ICR. Studies have shown improvements in glycemic control and improved quality of life outcomes on these regimes. Giving the insulin dose after a meal and frequent snacking have been shown to worsen glycemic control.[43,44]

Advantage of insulin pump therapy is the ability to tailor mealtime insulin delivery according to the composition of the meal by using different types of boluses. A dual wave bolus prior to a low GI meal, especially those meals high in fat and protein can significantly reduce the postprandial excursion. More conventional twice daily insulin regimes using mixtures of short and long-acting insulin require day-to-day consistency in carbohydrate intake, with three regular meals and snacks in between to balance the insulin action profile and prevent hypoglycemia. A bedtime snack is also required in patients on these regimes to prevent nocturnal hypoglycemia.[45-47]

AGE SPECIFIC NUTRITIONAL ADVICE

The nutrition education for children and adolescents with diabetes is often challenging and deem special consideration of nutritional and developmental needs of different age groups. The characteristics of different age groups must be considered when providing nutrition care to children and adolescents.

Toddlers

Toddlers have variable and unpredictable appetites. Regular small meals over the day may promote better glycemic control and nutritional adequacy. Insulin pump therapy may be effective in managing these eating patterns as it offers more flexibility as well as more precise delivery of small doses of insulin.[48,49] It is preferable to give preprandial insulin in toddlers. However, if it uncertain, if the toddler will eat all the food offered the insulin dose can be split and given as a combination of preprandial and during the meal. A variety of tastes, colors, and textures of foods should be encouraged. Since parental anxiety regarding food intake is a major concern in this age group; special consideration should be given when deciding on an insulin regimen.

School-aged children

Meal and snack routine should be incorporated into the school timetable. The school personnel should be informed and need understanding of the dietary management. The children should be explained and taught about carbohydrate contents of food under supervision and support.[50] Individual advice should be provided regarding carbohydrate intake to prevent hypoglycemia particularly for school events, such as sports days, excursions, and camps. However, it is not required for the child's usual active play. Importance of healthy food choices, food portion size, and physical activity to reduce the risks of inappropriate weight gain and cardiovascular disease should be emphasized. Sleepover and party advice should be discussed.

Adolescents

Adolescent period represents a critical stage in the development of a child. The nutritional management of diabetes needs special considerations. Various behaviors like staying out late, sleeping in, skipping insulin, missing meals and in some cultures, drinking alcohol pose more challenges. Adolescents should be educated and counseled for the healthy, family-based meals particularly during periods of rapid growth to prevent excessive afternoon or evening snacking. They require regular weight monitoring for early recognition of weight loss or inappropriate weight gain.
- Excessive weight gain requires careful review of insulin dosage, food intake, glycemic control, and physical activity.
- Weight loss or failure to gain weight may be associated with insulin omission for weight control and may be indicative of a disordered eating behavior or an eating disorder. In those with high HbA1c, irrespective of weight profile, further assessment of disordered eating thoughts and behaviors should be considered.

Parties, vacations, peer pressure to eat inappropriately, and healthy lifestyle advice all require discussion, problem-solving, and target setting. Advice on the safe consumption of alcohol and the risks of prolonged hypoglycemia is important in some societies.

CONCLUSION

Optimize glycemic control with improvements in clinical outcome in the form of maintaining ideal body weight and promoting health and growth is the goal of an effective dietary management of type 1 diabetes in children. Today the recommendation is use of intensive insulin regimes together with accurate and consistent carbohydrate counting, as well as low glycemic index food choices. Continuous glucose monitoring provides an insight into the effect of the composition of meals on glucose levels and the opportunity to tailor insulin therapy and dietary advice on an individual basis.

KEY LEARNING POINTS

- Dietary recommendations should be based on healthy eating principles individualized for children and families.
- The aim of dietary management is to promote growth and optimal body weight, maintain health, improve glycemic control and reduce cardiovascular risk.
- Intensive insulin regimes with matching of insulin doses to carbohydrate intake (ICR) provide the maximal potential for optimal glycemic control.
- Accurate carbohydrate counting, increased blood glucose monitoring and consumption of a low GI diet improve glycemic control.
- Dietary fat and protein intake impact on postprandial glucose excursions and insulin adjustment may be required on an individual basis according to meal composition.

REFERENCES

1. Escobar O, Drash AL, Becker DJ. Management of the child with Type 1 diabetes. In: Lifshitz F (Ed). *Pediatric Endocrinology* 5th edn. New York Informa Healthcare; 2007;101-121.
2. Delahanty LM, Nathan DM, Lachin JM, et al. Association of diet with glycated hemoglobin during intensive treatment of type 1 diabetes in the diabetes control and complications trial. *Am J Clin Nutr* 2009;89:518-524.
3. Franz MJ, Powers MA, Leontos C, et al. The evidence for medical nutrition therapy for type 1 and type 2 diabetes in adults. *J Am Diet Assoc* 2010;110:1852-1889.
4. Craig ME, Twigg SM, Donaghue K, Cheung NW, et al (for the Australian Type 1 Diabetes Guidelines Expert Advisory Group). *National Evidence-Based Clinical Care Guidelines for Type 1 Diabetes in Children, Adolescents and Adults.* Canberra:, Department of Health and Aging, Australian Government 2011.
5. National Institute for Clinical Excellence. Diagnosis and Management of Type 1 Diabetes in Children, Young People and Adults 2004. Available at: http://www.nice.org.uk/pdf/type1diabetes). Accessed on 10 February 2018.

6. Smart CE, Annan F, Bruno LP, Higgins LA, Acerini CL. ISPAD Clinical Practice Consensus Guidelines 2014. Nutritional management in children and adolescents with diabetes. International Society for Pediatric and Adolescent Diabetes. *Pediatr Diabetes.* 2014;15 Suppl 20:135-153. doi: 10.1111/pedi.12175.
7. Institute of Medicine of the National Academies: Dietary Reference Intakes for Energy, Carbohydrate, Fiber, Fat, Fatty Acids, Cholesterol, Protein, and Amino Acids (Macronutrients). Washington, DC: National Academy Press 2002:1–8 Available at: http://www.iom.edu/Object.File/Master/4/154/0.pdf Accessed on: 10 February 2018.
8. Perrotti N, Santoro D, Genovese S, et al. Effect of digestible carbohydrates on glucose control in insulin-dependent patients with diabetes. *Diabetes Care* 1984; 7:354-359.
9. Strychar IM, Blain E, Rivard M, et al. Association between dietary adherence measures and glycemic control in outpatients with type 1 diabetes mellitus and normal serum lipid levels. *J Am Diet Assoc* 1998;98:76-79.
10. Funnell MM, Anderson RM. Empowerment and self-management of diabetes. *Clin Diabetes* 2004;22:123-127.
11. Doherty Y, Dovey-Pearce G. Understanding the development and psychological needs of young people with diabetes. *Pract Diabetes Int* 2005;22:59-64.
12. Cameron FJ, de Beaufort C, Aanstoot H-J, et al. Lessons from the Hvidoere International Study Group on childhood diabetes: be dogmatic about outcome and flexible in approach. *Pediatr Diabetes* 2013:14:473-480.
13. Newfield RS, Cohen D, Capparelli EV, Shragg P. Rapid weight gain in children soon after diagnosis of type 1 diabetes: is there room for concern? *Pediatr Diabetes* 2009; 10:310-315.
14. Cole T, Bellizzi M, Flegal K, Dietz W. Establishing a standard definition for child overweight and obesity worldwide: international survey. *BMJ* 2000;320:1240-1243.
15. Davis NL, Bursell JDH, Evans WD, Warner JT, Gregory JW. Body composition in children with type 1 diabetes in the first year after diagnosis: relationship to glycaemic control and cardiovascular risk. *Arch Dis Child* 2012;97:312-315.
16. Silverstein J, Klingensmith G, Copeland K, et al. Care of children and adolescents with type 1 diabetes: a statement of the American Diabetes Association. *Diabetes Care* 2005;28:186-212.
17. Canadian Diabetes Association Clinical Practice Guidelines Expert Committee. Clinical practice guidelines. Nutrition therapy. *Can J Diabetes* 2013;37:S45-S55.
18. Spinks J, Guest S, Dietary management of children with type 1 diabetes, Pediatrics and Child Health (2017), Available at: http://dx.doi.org/10.1016/j.paed.2017.01.001 Accessed on: 11 February 2018.
19. Irani AJ, Menin PSN, Bhatia V. Type 1 Diabetes mellitus in children and adolescents in India. Clinical Practice Guidelines 2011 by Indian Society for Pediatric and Adolescent Endocrinology.
20. Ebbeling CB, Feldman HA, Chomitz VR, et al. A randomized trial of sugar-sweetened beverages and adolescent body weight. *N Engl J Med* 2012;367:1407-1416.
21. Kawamura T. The importance of carbohydrate counting in the treatment of children with diabetes. *Pediatr Diabetes* 2007;8:57-62.
22. Barclay AW, Petocz P, McMillan-Price J, et al. Glycemic index, glycemic load, and chronic disease risk – a meta-analysis of observational studies. *Am J Clin Nutr* 2008; 87:627-637.
23. Ryan R, King BR, Anderson D, Attia J, Collins CE. Influence of optimal insulin therapy for a low-glycemic index meal in children with type 1 diabetes receiving intensive insulin therapy. *Diabetes Care* 2008;31:1485-1490.

24. Foster-Powell K, Holt SH, Brand-Miller J. International table of glycemic index and glycemic load values: 2002. *Am J Clin Nutr* 2002;76:5-56.
25. National Health and Medical Research Council. *Australian Dietary Guidelines*. Canberra: National Health and Medical Research Council, 2013.
26. Svoren BM, Jospe N. Type 1 Diabetes Mellitus. In: Kliegman RM, Stanton BF, St Geme JW, Schor NF (Eds). *Nelson Textbook of Pediatrics* 20th edn. Philadelphia: Elsevier 2016;2763-2783.
27. Dyson PA, Kelly T, Deakin T, Duncan A, Frost G. Diabetes UK evidence based nutrition guidelines for the prevention and management of diabetes. *Diabet Med* 2011;28:1282-1288.
28. Margeirsdottir HD, Larsen JR, Brunborg C, Overby NC, Dahl-Jørgensen K. High prevalence of cardiovascular risk factors in children and adolescents with type 1 diabetes: a population-based study. *Diabetologia* 2008;51:554-561.
29. Cadario F, Prodam F, Pasqualicchio S, et al. Lipid profile and nutritional intake in children and adolescents with type 1 diabetes improve after a structured dietician training to a Mediterranean-style diet. *J Endocrinol Invest* 2012;35:160-168.
30. Dyson PA, Kelly T, Deakin T, Duncan A, Frost G. Diabetes UK evidence based nutrition guidelines for the prevention and management of diabetes. *Diabet Med* 2011:28:1282-1288.
31. Dewey K, Beaton G, Fjeld C, Lonnerdal B, Reeds P. Protein requirements of infants and children. *Eur J Clin Nutr* 1996;50:S119–S150.
32. Mann J, De Leeuw I, Hermansen K, et al. on behalf of the Diabetes and Nutrition Study Group of the European Association for the Study of Diabetes. Evidence based nutritional approaches to the treatment and prevention of diabetes mellitus. *Nutr Metab Cardiovasc Dis* 2004;14:373-394.
33. Wheeler ML, Dunbar SA, Jaacks LM, et al. Macronutrients, food groups, and eating patterns in the management of diabetes: a systematic review of the literature. *Diabetes Care* 2010;35:434-445.
34. Slavin JL. Position of the American Dietetic Association: health implications of dietary fiber. *J Acad Nutr Diet* 2008;108:1716-1731.
35. Institute of Medicine of the National Academies. *Dietary DRI Reference Intakes: The Essential Guide to Nutrient requirements*. Washington, DC: The National Academies Press, 2006.
36. Grober U, Spitz J, Reichrath J, Kisters K, Holick M. VitaminD: Update 2013. From rickets prophylaxis to general preventive healthcare. *Dermatoendocrinol* 2013;5: e2-331-e2-347.
37. World Health Organuization. *Evaluation of certain food additives and contaminants* (77th report of the Joint FAO/WHO Expert Committee on Food Additives) WHO Technical Report Series No. 983, 2013.
38. Knowles J, Waller H, EiserCet al. The development of an innovative education curriculum for 11-16 yr old children with type 1 diabetes mellitus. *Pediatr Diabetes* 2006;7:322-328.
39. Kawamura T. The importance of carbohydrate counting in the treatment of children with diabetes. *Pediatr Diabetes* 2007;8:57-62.
40. Burdick J, Chase HP, Slover RH, et al. Missed insulin meal boluses and elevated hemoglobin A1c levels in children receiving insulin pump therapy. *Pediatrics* 2004; 113:613-616.
41. Laurenzi A, Bolla A, Panigoni G, et al. Effects of carbohydrate counting on glucose control and quality of life over 24 weeks in adult patients with type 1 diabetes on

continuous subcutaneous insulin infusion. A randomized, prospective clinical trial (GIOCAR). *Diabetes Care* 2011;34:823-827.
42. Scavone G, Manto A, Pitocco D, et al. Effect of carbohydrate counting and medical nutritional therapy on glycemic control in type 1 diabetic subjects: a pilot study. *Diabet Med* 2010;27:477-479.
43. Anderson DG. Multiple daily injections in young patients using the ezy-BICC bolus insulin calculation card, compared to mixed insulin and CSII. *Pediatr Diabetes* 2009;10:304-309.
44. Shahbazi H, Ghofranipour F. The role of nutrition in children and adolescents with type 1 diabetes. *Austin J Nutri Food Sci* 2017;5:1084-1087.
45. Price K, Knowles J, Freeman J, Wales J, KICk-OFF Study Group. Improving outcomes for adolescents with type 1 diabetes: results from the Kids in Control OF Food (KICk-OFF) trial. *Pediatr Diabetes* 2013;14:19-49.
46. Hayes RL, Garnett SP, Clarke SL, Harkin NM, Chan AK. A flexible diet using an insulin to carbohydrate ratio for adolescents with type 1 diabetes—A pilot study. *Clin Nutr* 2012;31:705-709.
47. Enander R, Gundevall C, Stromgren A, Chaplin J, Hanas R. Carbohydrate counting with a bolus calculator improves post-prandial blood glucose levels in children and adolescents with type 1 diabetes using insulin pumps. *Pediatr Diabetes* 2012;13:545-551.
48. Patton S, Williams L, Dolan L, Chen M, Powers S. Feeding problems reported by parents of young children with type 1 diabetes on insulin pump therapy and their associations with children's glycemic control. *Pediatr Diabetes* 2009;10:455-460.
49. Phillip M, Battelino T, Rodriguez H, Danne T, Kaufman F. Use of insulin pump therapy in the pediatric age-group: consensus statement from the European Society for Paediatric Endocrinology, the Lawson Wilkins Pediatric Endocrine Society, and the International Society for Pediatric and Adolescent Diabetes, endorsed by the American Diabetes Association and the European Association for the Study of Diabetes. *Diabetes Care* 2007;30:1653-1662.
50. Smart CE, Ross K, Edge JA, King BR, McElduff P. Can children with type 1 diabetes and their caregivers estimate the carbohydrate content of meals and snacks? *Diabet Med* 2010;27:348-353.

25 Nutrition in Pediatric Irritable Bowel Syndrome

Yogesh Waikar

ABSTRACT
Pediatric irritable bowel syndrome (IBS) is one of the functional gastrointestinal disorders. Its prevalence is increasing. Abdominal pain, diarrhea and constipation are the common symptoms. Appropriate diagnosis with the help of Rome criteria is warranted. Management of these children with help of pediatric gastroenterologist, certified dietician and psychologist is now possible. Team efforts with dietary modifications are highlighted in this review.

Keywords: Abdominal pain, Constipation, Diarrhea, Diet, FODMAPS, Irritable bowel syndrome, Nutrition.

INTRODUCTION

Functional gastrointestinal disorders are increasingly diagnosed in Pediatric Gastroenterology practice according to the symptom based Rome IV criteria.[1] Irritable bowel syndrome (IBS) is one of the functional gastrointestinal diseases.

Proper diagnosis, appropriate management, avoiding cognitive bias to rule out organic etiologies, pharmacological add-ons and nutrition are the cornerstones in management of pediatric irritable bowel syndrome. Multifactorial involvement in pathophysiology of IBS is well-known.[1] Directing treatment at nutritional issues is one of the important aspects in management of these children.

Many factors in diet are involved in management. Age appropriate nutritional issues add to the complexity. Individualization of diet and food is sometimes necessary. Diet along with intestinal microbia[2,3] play a crucial role in threshold of phenotypic expression of functional gastrointestinal (GI) disorder. It is known that the fermented food products produced secondarily due to microorganisms in gut have a role in IBS.[4,5] Diets, such as low fermentable olio-di- and monosaccharides may provide benefit to patients with IBS.

Patients with mild symptoms in a diagnosed IBS would benefit from education regarding IBS and eliminating offending dietary substances causing symptoms from the diet. These symptoms should be noted in a food diary and clinically correlated. In kids with moderate to severe symptoms pharmacotherapy may be used. Cognitive behavioral therapy and other psychological treatment modalities are also considered to help these children.

DEFINITION OF PEDIATRIC IBS

According to Rome IV diagnostic criteria, irritable bowel syndrome must include all of the following criteria fulfilled for at **least 2 months** before diagnosis.
- Abdominal pain at **least 4 days per month** associated with one or more of the following:
  a. Related to defecation
  b. A change in frequency of stool
  c. A change in form (appearance) of stool.
- In children with constipation, the pain **does not resolve with resolution of the constipation** (children in whom the pain resolves have functional constipation, not irritable bowel syndrome)
- After appropriate evaluation, the symptoms **cannot be fully explained by another medical condition.**

DIETARY THERAPY FOR PEDIATRIC IBS

Reduction of dietary sugars like lactose and sorbitol or fructose is studied for pediatric IBS.[6] Low fermentable, oligo-di- and monosaccharides and polyols (FODMAP) diet is shown to be efficacious in school-age children with IBS.[7,8] There are very few double blind randomized pediatric studies. More studies are still needed.

Psyllium fiber 6 g for 7-11 years and 12 g for 12-18 years is studied in a randomized double blind trial. Kids with fibers experienced significantly greater reduction in abdominal pain episodes. Abdominal pain intensity but was unaffected. Fiber treatment did not alter the gut permeability. More studies with larger sample size are needed.[9]

WHAT ARE FODMAPS?

Fermentable oligo-di and monosaccharides and polyols are highly fermentable but poorly absorbed food products. They contain oligosaccharides like fructans, fructo-oligosaccharides, galacto-oligosaccharides. Fructose and polyols like sorbitol, mannitol, xylitol, polydextrose and isomalt. Thickened and sweetener used in food additives can also classified as FODMAPS.

Diet high in FODMAPS are considered to exacerbate the IBS symptoms. FODMAPS in normal kids help in increasing stool bulk, enhance calcium absorption and moderate immune function.[10] These beneficial effects are lost in low FODMAPS diet in IBS patients. Short chain fatty acid produced after fermentation in large intestine has trophic effects on colonocyte metabolism. This effect too is reduced in IBS patient on low FODMAPS diet.

A high dose of fructose or fructane significantly worsens IBS.[11] Low FODMAPS diet is studied in IBS patients only for short duration.[10] Long-term efficacy of low FODMAPS diet in kids of growing age is not known. Compliance variability to such modified IBS diet is uncertain. Low FODMAPS diet may impose indirect restriction of several nutrients. These diets reduce abdominal pain, bloating and diarrhea in IBS but their superiority to conventional IBS diet in long-term effect is unclear.[12]

INTERACTION OF MICROBIA WITH FODMAPS

The phenomenon is complex and difficult to extrapolate to the large and differential size of pediatric IBS patients. Kids with microbia of greater sacchrolytic capacity can serve as a biomarker for those[6] who may respond to FODMAPS avoidance.

One of the studies in adults compared diet suggested by National Institute for Health and Care Excellence for IBS-D with FODMAPS and found low FODMAPS better.[13] More studies are needed in children.

HIGH FODMAP DIET[10]

- Wheat, barley, rye
- Lentils, beans, chickpeas, soya, peas
- Artichokes, asparagus, cauliflower, garlic, leeks, mushroom, onion, scallions, shallots, snow peas
- Apple, apricot, pear, blackberry, cherry, figs, jackfruit, mangoes, nectarines, peach pear, persimmon, plums, prune, tamarillo, watermelon, white peach, grape
- Regular milk, ice cream, soft cheese, yogurt
- Sweeteners.

PRACTICAL TIPS OF DIET IN PEDIATRIC IBS

- Take diet history, ask specifically for food diary.
- Note high FODMAPS food like apple, pears, pumpkin, sweet potato, milk, yoghurt, wheat based pasta in diet.
- Try reducing your intake of resistant starches.
- Limit fizzy drinks.
- Restrict intake of caffeinated drinks (for example, tea, coffee or cola).
- Avoid foods high in fat, such as chips, fast foods, burgers and sausages, crisps and cakes.
- Ensure good fluid intake.
- Take help of pediatric gastroenterologist and certified dietician if pattern persist.

CONCLUSION

Diet is one of the important aspects in management of pediatric IBS. Judicious use of high FODMAP diet avoidance with education and pharmacotherapy is sometimes required. Long-term studies comparing one treatment modality with other are needed for IBS-constipation, IBS-diarrhea and IBS-abdominal pain. Differential dietary approach is possible. Individualization in each case makes dietary management in pediatric IBS interesting as well as difficult. Organic etiologies should be excluded if required with the help of pediatric gastroenterologist.

KEY LEARNING POINTS

- Use Rome IV criteria to diagnose pediatric IBS.
- Judicious avoidance of high FODMAPS in diet is desirable.
- Teamwork between Pediatric Gastroenterologist, Pediatrician, Certified dietician and Counselor is must in management of Pediatric IBS.

REFERENCES

1. Douglas A. Drossman. Functional Gastrointestinal Disorders: History, Pathophysiology, Clinical Features, and Rome IV. *Gastroenterology* 2016;150:1262–1279
2. Biedermann L, Rogler G. The intestinal microbiota: its role in health and disease. *Eur J Pediatr* 2015;174:151-167.
3. Shreiner AB, Kao JY, Young VB. The gut microbiome in health and in disease. *Curr Opin Gastroenterol* 2015;31:69-75.
4. Rajilic-Stojanovic M, Jonkers DM, Salonen A, et al. Intestinal microbiota and diet in IBS: causes, consequences, or epiphenomena? *Am J Gastroenterol* 2015;110:278-287.
5. Hyams JS, Di Lorenzo C, Saps M, Shulman RJ, Staiano A. Functional Disorders: Children and Adolescents. *Gastroenterology* 2016;150: 1456-1468.
6. Däbritz J, Mühlbauer M, Domagk D et al. Significance of hydrogen breath tests in children with suspected carbohydrate malabsorption. *BMC Pediatr* 2014;14(1)DOI: 10.1186/1471-2431-14-59
7. Chumpitazi BP, Cope JL, Hollister EB, et al. Randomised clinical trial: gut microbiome biomarkers are associated with clinical response to a low FODMAP diet in children with irritable bowel syndrome. Aliment. *Pharmacol* Ther 2015;42:418-27 DOI: 10.1111/ apt.13286:1-10.
8. Chumpitazi BP, Hollister EB, Oezguen N, et al. Gut microbiota influences low fermentable substrate diet efficacy in children with irritable bowel syndrome. *Gut Microbes* 2014;5:165-175.
9. Shulman RJ, Hollister EB, Cain K, Czyzewski DI, Self MM. Psyllium Fiber Reduces abdominal pain in children with irritable bowel syndrome in a randomized, double-blind trial. *Clin Gastroenterol Hepatol* 2016. doi: 10.1016/j.cgh.2016.03.04
10. Catassi G, Lionetti E, Gatti S, Catassi C. The Low FODMAP Diet: Many Question Marks for a Catchy Acronym. *Nutrients* 2017; 9: 292; doi:10.3390/nu9030292
11. Major G, Pritchard S, Murray K, et al. Colon hypersensitivity to distension, rather than excessive gas production, produces carbohydrate-related symptoms in individuals with irritable bowel syndrome. *Gastroenterology* 2017;152:124–133.

12. Altobelli E, Negro VD, Angeletti PM, LatellaG. Low-FODMAP diet improves irritable bowel syndrome symptoms: A meta-analysis. *Nutrients* 2017;9:940;doi:10.3390/nu9090940
13. Eswaran S, Chey WD, Jackson K, et al. A Diet low in fermentable oligo-, di-, and monosaccharides and polyols improves quality of life and reduces activity impairment in patients with irritable bowel syndrome and diarrhea. *Clin Gastroenterol Hepatol* 2017;15:1890-1899.

26 Nutritional Management of Diarrhea

Jatinder Singh, Harmesh S Bains, Vaneeta Bhardwar

ABSTRACT
Notwithstanding strides in the management of acute diarrheal disorders including oral rehydration therapy, it is estimated that diarrheal diseases still account for up to 30% of all hospital admissions in resource-poor countries. That diarrhea causes malnutrition is well-known. Diarrhea-related malnutrition is the result of erratic transport and impaired intestinal absorptive function causing reduced nutrient availability, increased metabolic needs, increased protein and other nutrient losses, and disturbed nutrient uptake. Reduction in the levels of essential amino acids and conditional amino acids (such as arginine and glutamine) and micronutrients, zinc and copper, may too develop. A focused attention to nutrition, especially continuing breastfeeding, and low lactose diet cause early weight gain and help in speedy recovery from diarrhea. In conclusion, varying type of dietary manipulation in acute, persistent and chronic diarrheas is warranted.

Keywords: Acute diarrhea, Breastfeeding, Celiac disease, Chronic diarrhea, Coconut water, Irritable bowel syndrome, Low FODMAPS diet, Gluten-free diet, Khichdi, Low lactose diet, Medium chain triglyceride, Oral rehydration salt (ORS), Pesistent diarrhea, Probiotics, Rice lentils.

INTRODUCTION

Diarrhea affect children globally, the morbidity and mortality being highest in the resource-poor countries.[1] It is estimated that 1 out of every 5 children who die of diarrhea worldwide is an Indian. In India, about 41 children lose their lives every hour due to diarrhea with reported point prevalence of 9–20% among children under 5 years. World Health Organization (WHO) estimated that there were approximately 700 million episodes of diarrhea annually among children under 5 years old in developing countries resulting in 4.6 million deaths. Despite vast improvement in the management of acute diarrheal disorders and oral rehydration therapy, it is estimated that diarrheal diseases still account for up to 30% of all hospital admissions in developing countries. Diarrhea cause malnutrition owing to transport, impaired intestinal absorptive function which reduced nutrient availability, increase metabolic needs, increase protein and other nutrient losses, disturb nutrient uptake and transport. Reduction in the level of essential amino acid, conditional amino acid (such as arginine and glutamine) and also in micronutrient levels of zinc and copper occurs.

Components of nutritional advice in diarrhea include breastfeeding, oral rehydration solution (ORS), low lactose diet, coconut water, *khichdi* (rice lentils), lactose formula, zinc supplements, medium-chain triglyceride, etc.

NUTRITION IN ACUTE DIARRHEA

In acute diarrhea, nutrients are lost directly from the intestinal tract. An increased stool clearance of α-1-antitrypsin, a serum protein marker present in the stools has been observed in about half of all rotavirus diarrheas and even more frequently in shigellosis infection in which tissue destruction is accompanied by losses of plasma, epithelia, and blood cells. Nearly two-third of patients with enterotoxigenic *Escherichia coli* also show an excessive loss of protein in the feces. Structural alterations in the mucosal epithelium is due to *spp. Shigella* rotavirus, and *Campylobacter spp.* infections also result in a "protein-losing enteropathy," similar to the measles-induced abrupt fall in plasma albumin through fecal losses. Losses of zinc and copper during early stages of acute diarrhea in children are well-known. These losses are greater when stool losses are larger. Nutritional management of acute diarrhea in infants involves administering low osmolarity ORS, continuation of breastfeeding, and supplementation with zinc. Prebiotics and probiotics may also have an important role.

Low Osmolarity ORS

In 2014, WHO and UNICEF recommended low osmolarity ORS to treat all type of diarrhea. It has a total osmolarity of 245 mmol/L and reduced level of glucose and sodium. Low osmolarity ORS has shown to reduce the stool output and vomiting by about 20 to 30%, respectively, in comparison to children using the original ORS formula. It was also shown to reduce the IV therapy by 33% among children with diarrhea. When osmolarity of some common fluids were compared, except coconut water, every other fluids seemed to have high osmolarity. It also seen that more efficacy in noncholera diarrhea. ORS should be given to infants with cup and spoon rather than bottles, in order not to interfere with suckling. When in a health system bottles are used for treatment, an implicit credibility is given to their role in modern treatment.

Breastfeeding

Breastfeeding is important in providing necessary calories and protein during a time when a loss of appetite for other foods is common. According to UNICEF survey 29% of children were not eating anything during diarrhea.

Limiting milk intake among young children can promote nutritional deficiency. Diarrheal disease control programs need to modify service delivery to ensure that breastfeeding mothers are not separated from their infants while being treated with oral rehydration therapy (ORT) as inpatients or outpatients. Breastfeeding has optimal balance of nutrients, such as carbohydrate, protein, fat and water. Although breast milk contains higher amount of lactose compared to cow's milk, it is better tolerated as compared to glucose-electrolyte feeds (when replaced for breast milk). WHO/UNICEF joint statement recommends continued breastfeeding during acute diarrhea in children.

Medium-chain Triglyceride

World Health Organization recommends feeding of fat or oil during diarrhea to enchance the nutrient density of foods, and provide maximum energy when there is limited absorptive capacity. It increases the caloric value, and improve palatability, digestibility, absorption, and transport of foodstuffs indicated for disease with maldigestion and malabsorption.

Role of Prebiotics and Probiotics

Approximately 70% of the immune system is localized in the gastrointestinal tract, i.e. its glands, mucosa, and mucosa-associated lymphoid system. Probiotics may mitigate the risk of diarrhea by several mechanism including barrier effect of mucosa, controlling intestinal motility, mucus production, and reducing the intestinal pH. The system influences health conditions because it produces large amounts of important gastrointestinal secretions as rich as breast milk in health-supporting and disease-preventing factors, and because of its rich gastrointestinal flora. The intestine normally contains 10 times more microbes than there are eukaryotic cells in the entire body. The optimal function of these microbes depends on the supply of food destined for the colonic bacteria (fermentable fibers, complex proteins, gastrointestinal secretions). The consideration of these functions influences outcome. Unfortunately, the conditions (supply of drugs—especially antibiotics, and reduced supply of food—especially fruits and vegetables) in the modern ICU are extremely poor both for optimal gastrointestinal secretion and for flora and need more attention. To improve treatment, a supply of new and effective flora (probiotics) and food for the flora (prebiotics) is needed, from which numerous health-supporting products (synbiotics) will be produced and absorbed at the level of the mucosa mainly in the lower gastrointestinal tract. A double-blind study reported that treatment with *Lactobacillus reuteri* DSM 17938 helps to reduce the frequency and duration of acute diarrhea and relapse rate of the disease.[2]

Zinc Supplementation[3-8]

Supplementary zinc benefits children with diarrhea because it is a vital micronutrient essential for protein synthesis, cell growth and differentiation, immune function, and intestinal transport of water and electrolytes. Zinc is also important for normal growth and development of children both with and without diarrhea. Zinc deficiency is associated with an increased risk of gastrointestinal infections, adverse effects on the structure and function of the gastrointestinal tract, and impaired immune function. Dietary deficiency of zinc is especially common in low-income countries because of a low dietary intake of zinc-rich foods (mainly foods of animal origin) or inadequate absorption caused by its binding to dietary fiber and phytates often found in cereals, nuts and legumes.

Although, the benefits of zinc supplementation in the management of diarrhea stand established, there remain a number of barriers to the widespread implementation of this treatment strategy. There is also concern that high zinc intakes may compete for absorption with other micronutrients, such as iron and calcium. This, in turn, can have unintended negative consequences for children's health and development. Studies are needed to help identify subpopulations that would benefit most in resource-limited settings and to ensure access to zinc supplementation, especially for those families whose children are most at risk of diarrhea but may not be able to afford treatments that include zinc supplements. However, zinc deficiency remains difficult to diagnose because measuring serum zinc levels is not necessarily accurate for this purpose.

Early Refeeding

Early refeeding helps in reducing the abnormal increase in intestinal permeability. It enchancing the enterocyte regeneration and promote the recovery of brush border membrane disaccharidases. The European Society for Pediatric Gastroenterology, Hepatology and Nutrition (ESPGHAN) recommends that children who require rehydration should continue to be fed. Food should not be withdrawn for longer than 4-6 hours after the onset of rehydration.

DIET IN PERSISTENT DIARRHEA

Diet in persistent diarrhea comprises of 3 plans:
1. Diet A (reduced lactose)
2. Diet B (lactose free)
3. Diet C (monosaccharide based).

Most of the patient respond to diet A and diet B plan.

In plan A, start with low lactose diet. If there is no improvement in 2 to 3 days, change to lactose-free diet (Plan B). If no response to even plan B, shift to plan C.

Criteria for changing the Plan A to B or B to C are:
- Tendency for dehydration/reappearance of dehydration at any time
- High purge volume, high purge rate seven or more stools/day at the end of 7 days.

Table 1: Three dietary plans in diarrhea.

Plan	Type of diet	Content of diet
A	Low lactose diet	Puffed rice, milk, sugar, oil, cereal + milk, mashed banana
B	Lactose free diet + low starch diet	Cereal based food (rice, wheat, ragi), sugar, oil, egg white + cereal + sugar + oil
C	Lactose and sucrose free diet	Glucose + oil + protein (egg/pureed chicken)

Ideal source of calories, protein, fat, and carbohydrates: Rice, Bengal gram, pulses groundnuts, chicken egg, white fat coconut oil due to high medium-chain triglyceride content.

Table 1 presents the salient features of the three dietary plans in persistent dirrhea.

The issue of lactose intolerance in persistent diarrhea deserves a special comment. Reduction in the surface area of the microvilli caused by infections is associated with reduced levels of enzymes (including lactase) that are vital for digestion and absorption of sugars. Lactase enzyme is located in the internal lining [brush border (microvilli) of the small intestine (enterocyte)]. A lactose restricted diet should be given during the period of secondary lactose intolerance. Lactase deficiency resolves once the diarrhea gradually diminishes with the disappearance of underlying inflammation. Secondary lactase intolerance is transient.

DIET IN CHRONIC DIARRHEA

Chronic diarrhea is defined as diarrhea that extends beyond 2 weeks and usually has a significant malabsorption.

Besides other therapeutic measures, varying types of nutritional adjustments depending on the merits of the case are important in treatment.

For instance, celiac disease needs exclusion of such foodstuffs as contain gluten in the form of wheat, barley and rye.[9]

For irritable bowel syndrome (IBS), the so-called "FODMAP diet"[10] is required. FODMAPS are naturally occurring carbohydrates found in foods (fruits, grains and legumes). These are supposed to be responsible for causing diarrhea and related digestive issues in sensitive subjects. This is discussed in details in Ch 25 (Nutrition in Pediatric Irritable Bowel Syndrome).

In case of IBD, recommendation is for the so-called IBD-AID which has 5 basic components:[11]

1. The modification of specific carbohydrates (e.g. refined or processed complex carbohydrates).
2. Emphasis on restoring the intestinal flora balance through ingestion of prebiotics and probiotics in the form of soluble fiber, such as leek, onion, and fermented foods.

3. Focus on decreasing total and saturated fats, eliminating hydrogenated oils, and encouraging the increase in food sources rich in omega-3 fatty acids.
4. Review of the overall dietary pattern, identification of food triggers and intolerances, and detection of missing nutrients; and
5. Food texture modification to enhance absorption and reduce intact fiber.

The so-called banana, rice, applesauce, toast "BRAT diet" may help to prevent overstimulation of the bowel, and slow down the frequency of bowel movements.

CONCLUSION

Diarrhea, if not controlled promptly, may lead to malnutrition. ORS, zinc supplementation and continued breastfeeding usually offer effective management of acute diarrhea. In persistent diarrhea, dietary manipulation starting with low lactose diet and then changing over to lactose-free diet and even carbohydrate-free diet, if the need plays a significant role. In chronic diarrhea, diet depends on the type of etiologic condition.

> **KEY LEARNING POINTS**
>
> ¤ Diarrhea in the presence of infection can cause a significant damage to intestinal barrier and might lead to malnutrition.
> ¤ ORS and zinc supplementation and continued breastfeeding may offer effective management of acute diarrhea in children.
> ¤ Although secondary lactase deficiency is common in diarrhea, studied have shown the benefits of continued breastfeeding.
> ¤ In persistent diarhea, dietary manipulation in the form of Plans A, B and C are important.
> ¤ In chronic diarrhea, diet depends on the etiologic factor, often warranting exclusion of certain foodstuffs as in the case of celiac disease and irritable bowel syndrome.

REFERENCES

1. Gupte S, Reddy A. Perspectives in pediatric diarrheal diseases: Experience from India. Proceedings, Asian-Oceanian Conference on Diarrhea, Hong Kong, 5-7 October 2012. Abstract No AOCoD/A-7.
2. Hillman GE, Gill P. Diarrhea: Changing trends in pediatric ractice. Proceedings, Asian-Oceanian Conference on Diarrhea, Hong Kong, 5-7 October 2012. Abstract No AOCoD/C-3.
3. Aggarwal R, Sentz J, Miller MA. Role of zinc administration in prevention of childhood diarrhea and respiratory illnesses: a meta-analysis. *Pediatrics* 2007; 119:1120-1130.
4. Haider BA, Bhutta ZA. The effect of therapeutic zinc supplementation among young children with selected infections: a review of the evidence. *Food and Nutr Bullet* 2009; 30(Suppl 1):S41-59.

5. Fischer Walker C, Kordas K, Stoltzfus RJ, Black RE. Interactive effects of iron and zinc on biochemical and functional outcomes in supplementation trials. *Am J Clin Nutr* 2005; 82:5-12.
6. Lutter CK, Dewey KG. Proposed nutrient composition for fortified complementary foods. *J Nutr* 2003; 133:3011S-3020S.
7. Fischer Walker CL, Fontaine O, Young MW, Black RE. Zinc and low osmolarity oral rehydration salts for diarrhoea: a renewed call to action. *Bullet WHO* 2009; 87:780-786.
8. Winch PJ, Gilroy KE, Doumbia S, et al. Operational issues and trends associated with the pilot introduction of zinc for childhood diarrhoea in Bougouni district, Mali. *J Health Popul Nutr* 2008; 2615:151-156.
9. Patwari A, Gupte S, Anderson RA. Pediatric gastroenterology. In: Gupte S (Ed): *The Short Textbook of Pediatrics*, 12th edn. New Delhi: Jaypee 2016:549-587.
10. WebMed. Irritable bowel syndrome: Controlling symtoms with diet. Available at: https://www.webmd.com/ibs/controlling-irritable-bowel-syndrome-with-diet. Accessed on: 30 January 2018.
11. Crohn and Colitis Foundation. Relationship between food and IBD. In: *Diet, Nutrition and Inflammatopry Bowel Disease*. Available at: http://www.crohnscolitisfoundation.org/resources/diet-nutrition-ibd-2013.pdf Accessed on: 29 December 2018.

27 Nutrition in Cystic Fibrosis

Thomas L Ratchford, Jeffrey H Teckman, Dhiren R Patel

ABSTRACT

Cystic fibrosis (CF), a severe, progressive genetic disease affecting many organs of the body, is caused by mutations in the *CF transmembrane conductance regulator (CFTR)* gene. Optimizing nutrition is critical in this disorder, as higher growth parameters are associated with better pulmonary function and outcomes. These patients are prone to malnutrition, growth failure, and vitamin deficiencies due to the malabsorption inherent to the pathophysiology of the disease. Hence, they require serial assessments of growth parameters as well as clinical and biochemical evaluation for malnutrition. Patients with CF have a large differential diagnosis for poor growth, and multidisciplinary evaluation for this problem is essential. Effective nutritional management generally includes the provision of sufficient pancreatic enzyme replacement therapy (PERT), adequate calories for growth, fat-soluble vitamins, and minerals, though many factors must be considered for the individual patient. Many patients require enteral feedings via gastrostomy tube in order to achieve enough caloric input for growth, and this therapy should be pursued without hesitation if it is needed. There are many recent and ongoing developments occurring regarding novel nutritional treatments in CF, and several new therapies are in clinical trials.

Keywords: Cystic fibrosis transmembrane conductance regulator, Cystic fibrosis, Enteral Nutrition, Failure to thrive, Growth failure, Malabsorption, Malnutrition, Nutrition, Pancreatic enzyme replacement therapy, Pancreatic insufficiency vitamin deficiency.

INTRODUCTION

Cystic fibrosis (CF) is a progressive, autosomal recessive genetic disorder that causes shortened lifespans in those afflicted.[1,2] Though mainly diagnosed in Caucasians, it is also seen in patients of other ethnic and racial backgrounds. In the United States, the mean prevalence is 0.74 in 10,000 persons. It is caused by mutations in the *cystic fibrosis transmembrane conductance regulator (CFTR) gene* which encodes CFTR protein. The lack of adequately functioning CFTR protein causes disruption of transport of sodium and chloride ions across cell membranes leading to thickened mucus secretions throughout the body including lungs, pancreas, liver, gallbladder, and intestines.[1,3] The combination of impaired intestinal absorption and increased metabolic demand to achieve homeostasis leads to challenges in providing adequate nutritional intake, and these patients are prone to malnutrition and vitamin deficiencies.[4] In recent years, the major focus to limit morbidity and mortality in CF has been on lung disease. However, optimizing growth and nutrition is paramount in patients with CF, especially children, as the medical literature is clear that undernourished CF patients, whether children or adults are more likely to experience poorer clinical outcomes including reduced lung function.[3-6] This chapter will review the significance, pathogenesis, evaluation, and management of the nutritional aspects of CF.

BACKGROUND: GROWTH AND OUTCOMES IN CYSTIC FIBROSIS

Improved outcomes in pediatric and adult CF patients with higher objective body measurement parameters, at multiple stages of life are demonstrated in several studies. Young children with CF and CF-related pancreatic insufficiency (PI) who regained their weight-for-age z-score at birth within 2 years of their CF diagnosis had better pulmonary function at age 6 years than those who did not regain their birth weight z-score within 2 years.[7] Konstan, et al. showed that children with CF whose weight-for-age measurement at age 3 years was below the 5th percentile had significantly decreased lung function at age 6 compared to children with CF whose weight-for-age measurement was over the 75th percentile at age 3 years.[8] In an observational, prospective study of over 3000 CF patients enrolled in the Cystic Fibrosis Foundation (CFF) Registry, higher weight-for-age percentile at age 4 years was correlated with higher rates of survival, fewer complications, improved pulmonary function, higher body mass index (BMI) and greater height at 18 years of age.[9] Data from the CFF Registry from 1994-2003 showed that in patients with CF and PI, higher BMI was associated with higher objective pulmonary function in children aged 6-12 and 13-20 years, as well as adults aged 21-40 years.[10] Studies have shown that in addition to achievement of growth, maintenance of growth is also important, as a more severe rate of decline in BMI in adolescence in CF patients was significantly associated with a substantial decline in lung function in young adulthood.[11] Furthermore, in subgroups of both school-aged children and adolescents of a large German cohort with data obtained over 1996-1997, improvement in lung function was correlated with gains in weight-for-height measurements, and worsening lung function was correlated with loss or stasis in weight-for-height measurements.[12] Because of the unambiguous body of data correlating weight gain with improved outcomes in CF, much attention should be directed toward optimizing growth and nutrition in these patients. Malnutrition must be not only aggressively treated, but also closely monitored for and avoided.

Pathogenesis of Malnutrition in Cystic Fibrosis

Dysfunction of the CFTR membrane protein is caused by mutations in the *CFTR* gene, located at 7q31.2. Currently, over 1900 CFTR mutations have been identified, the most common being a deletion at position 508, annotated as F508del.[13] In the United States, this mutation is homozygous in 48% of patients, and heterozygous in 40%.[14] Any of the hundreds of other mutant CFTR alleles can pair with each other or F508del to cause the disease. Specific mutations cause dysfunction in the CFTR protein in different ways, and six different classes have been defined to categorize the nature of the protein's dysfunction. The cause of dysfunction has been identified as defective protein production, defective processing, defective regulation, defective conduction, reduced amounts of functional protein, and enhanced turnover of protein, in classes I, II, III, IV, V, and VI, respectively. Classes I, II, and III have more severe disease phenotypes and are more strongly associated with pancreatic insufficiency. Of note, the F508del mutant is included as a class II mutation and correlates with the high prevalence of PI in CF patients in the United States.[13-15]

The CFTR protein, a cyclic adenosine monophosphate-regulated chloride channel is located on the apical surface of epithelial cells in many organs of the body and regulates the secretion and absorption of several other ions in addition to chloride including sodium, bicarbonate, and potassium.[14] When this channel is dysfunctional as seen in CF, secretions from the affected organs are abnormal.[3] Loss of excess sodium and chloride in the skin leads to increased need for replenishment.[1,6] Mucus secreted in the lung, pancreas, hepatobiliary system, and GI tract is much thicker than normal, as water, which follows the chloride ions into the lumen does not flow as usual.[13,14] This has drastic, wide-ranging consequences, as the thickened secretions cause significant damage to secretory ducts and organs.[16] In the lungs, the abnormally thick and adherent mucus is difficult for cilia to clear, colonization of pathogenic bacteria occurs as a result, and neutrophil-released elastase cause damage to lung parenchyma.[13,17] The result is a proinflammatory milieu, an increased frequency and severity of pulmonary infections, bronchiectasis and decreased lung function.[17] The pancreas is also severely affected, as thickened secretions cause obstructions in the pancreatic ducts and thus impair the transport of digestive enzymes and pancreatic bicarbonate to the intestinal lumen leading to exocrine pancreatic insufficiency, poor absorption of fat-soluble vitamins (A, D, E, and K), and an acidified intestinal tract.[2,4,15] The intestines of CF patients are further altered by the abnormal functioning of Brunner's glands where CFTR is highly expressed.[2,18] Acidification of the intestinal lumen impairs pancreatic enzyme function, whether the enzymes are endogenous or provided as exogenous supplements, and also likely impairs micelle formation and other luminal biochemical events critical to absorption.[18,19] In an attempt to neutralize the acidified digestive tract to a more physiologic state, multiple studies have been performed measuring the clinical benefits of acid suppression in CF patients, but results have been mixed with no definite conclusions made regarding efficacy, and so trialing proton pump inhibitors in individual patients may be considered with caution especially in patients prone to small bowel bacterial overgrowth (SBBO).[19] The accumulation of abnormally thick mucus in the intestines is widely thought to play a major role in the anomalous intestinal milieu, though the exact mechanisms in digestion and intestinal transit time has not yet been well-defined.[2,18,19] One set of views proposes that thickened, CF intestinal mucus overlies the epithelium and leads to an abnormal chyme-epithelium interface causing decreased absorption of nutrients.[2,20,21] Another hypothesis proposes that the abnormal mucus leads to intestinal stasis and serves as a biofilm, the combination of which leads to dysbiosis and frequent SBBO.[18,20,22] Interestingly, De Lisle, et al. showed that CF-mutant mice hydrated with polyethylene glycol-based laxative instead of water had a significant reduction in both intestinal mucus accumulation and bacterial load compared to the CF-mutant mice hydrated only with water.[22] While not carefully evaluated in controlled human studies, in the authors' experience, some symptoms (e.g. abdominal pain, bloating) theoretically derived from thick mucus in the small bowel may be relieved with a daily dose of a polyethylene glycol-based stool softener, and on occasion, a limited, empiric course of oral metronidazole for presumed SBBO when suggestive symptoms are present.

All of these factors together lead to the marked malabsorption of nutrients and bile acids, the latter of which further contributes to poor absorption of the fats and fat-soluble vitamins.[18] Patients with CF-related liver disease (CFLD) are also at a higher risk of fat-soluble vitamin deficiency due to cholestasis.[4,5,14] Thus, the combination of increased metabolic demands to maintain respiratory function, abnormal electrolyte losses throughout the body, and malabsorption form the backbone of malnutrition in CF patients.

NUTRITIONAL EVALUATION

Estimated Energy Requirements

Because of the pathogenesis of disease as detailed above, children and adults with CF are thought to require additional caloric intake compared to their nonaffected counterparts. Historically, the standard of care in regards to nutrition in CF has been a high-fat, high-calorie diet with pancreatic enzyme replacement therapy (PERT) and supplementation of fat-soluble vitamins.[3] Though individual energy needs can vary based on multiple factors (e.g. frequency of pulmonary exacerbations, degree of malabsorption, presence/absence of CFLD and/or CF-related diabetes (CFRD), individual compliance with therapies), guidelines from both Europe and United States advise higher caloric intake in patients with CF.[3] European guidelines recommend energy intake for CF patients be 120–150% of the daily caloric load taken by unaffected individuals, and the CFF recommends intakes of 110–200% of that of the standards for unaffected individuals.[10,23]

Growth Parameters

Because of the outcomes evaluated in the studies mentioned in the background section, as well as overall feasibility, different anthropomorphic benchmark measures should be utilized based on the age to assess nutritional status in CF patients. In CF patients with adequate nutritional status, routine nutritional assessment including weight and length measurement (as well as head circumference measurements in children below 24 months of age) should occur every 3 months. However, closer attention to growth and nutritional status is essential in the first year of life, during the first year of diagnosis, during the peripubertal period, and whenever nutritional status is judged to be suboptimal.[5,6] For this reason, the European Society for Clinical Nutrition and Metabolism (ESPEN) recommends evaluation and measurements every 1–2 weeks then monthly for the first year of life, until clear establishment of adequate nutrition, after which visits can be spaced to every 3 months.[3]

For children under 2 years of age, weight, height, and weight-for-length percentiles should be utilized in nutritional assessment. CF patients in this age group should achieve a weight-for-length percentile greater than or equal to the 50th percentile on Centers for Disease Control and Prevention (CDC) growth charts. CDC growth charts are preferred to World Health Organization (WHO) growth charts, as WHO charts assign a higher percentile for the same weight, and CF patients at the 50th percentile for weight-for-length by WHO definition were found to have lower forced expiratory volumes than those at 50th percentile by CDC definition.[6] For children 2–18 years of age, maintaining a BMI percentile equal to or greater than the 50th percentile for age should be the desired target. For adults over the age of 18 years, CF patients should have a BMI equal to or greater than 22 kg/m^2 and 23 kg/m^2, for females and males, respectively.[3,6] Patients not meeting these criteria, and those who fail to gain weight between visits should be identified as having an at-risk nutritional status, evaluation and management of their poor growth should begin. If at any time weight-for-length or BMI (depending on the age of the patient) crosses below the 10th percentile for age, or if their growth curve inappropriately flattens or declines over multiple visits, they should be more aggressively evaluated and managed for failure to thrive.[3]

Other Measures

In addition to growth parameters, periodic monitoring of biochemical nutritional markers, bone mineral density, and dietary history should occur. ESPEN recommends consideration of yearly analysis of blood electrolytes, serum transaminases, albumin, bilirubin, blood cell counts, iron status, plasma fat-soluble vitamin levels, plasma or serum phospholipid fatty acid patterns, and to evaluate for exocrine pancreatic function, an annual fecal pancreatic elastase-1 measurement.[3] Obtaining annual coagulation factors including prothrombin time, to assess for coagulopathy due to vitamin K deficiency is also advisable. The fecal pancreatic elastase-1 measurement may need to be repeated more frequently during the first year of life, as pancreatic insufficiency frequently develops in infancy, and PERT should be initiated when this laboratory measurement is abnormally low even in the absence of symptoms.[24] Dual-energy X-ray absorptiometry (DEXA) is recommended every 1–5 years (interval depending on multiple factors) starting at 8–10 years of age to assess bone health. Lastly, a dietary review, including questions related to recommended dietary plans is recommended every 3 months in children and every 6 months in adults.[3]

EVALUATION AND MANAGEMENT OF POOR GROWTH AND MALNUTRITION IN CYSTIC FIBROSIS

Because of the association of poorer overall outcomes with malnutrition in CF, both patient-specific and CF-related factors of poor growth and nutritional deficiencies should be investigated without delay in patients with at-risk or failing nutritional status.[3,5,6] Initially, immediately identifiable factors should be recognized and promptly corrected. These include inadequate diet by patient/parent history, clinically obvious malabsorption (frequent steatorrhea or poor adherence to (PERT), and current pulmonary exacerbations).[6]

Thorough multidisciplinary assessment is warranted if an immediately obvious cause of poor growth is not identified, the degree of malnutrition is severe, or if suboptimal growth continues over multiple time points. Interventions to correct the patient's nutritional status should occur in concert as the nature of the patient's malnutrition is investigated.[5,6]

Diagnostic Considerations

The differential diagnosis of poor growth is broad, as it includes etiologies of failure to thrive generalizable to all children as well as those specific to CF and the individual patient. As malnutrition in CF patients is often multifactorial with one or several comorbid diagnoses contributing to the poor nutritional status, evaluation by a multidisciplinary team is needed. This group should include a pulmonologist, gastroenterologist, endocrinologist, dietician, social worker, psychologist, clinical nurse, and the patient's primary care provider.[6,25] The differential diagnosis may be age-specific, and there are multiple subspecialty considerations with some diagnoses having more clinical impact than others. Potential etiologies are gastrointestinal [pancreatic insufficiency, celiac disease, gastroesophageal reflux disease (GERD), constipation, dysmotility, inflammatory bowel disease (IBD), CF-associated liver disease, SBBO, insufficient caloric intake, eosinophilic gastrointestinal disease, enteral infectious disease], pulmonary (CF pulmonary exacerbation), endocrine (CFRD), psychological/psychiatric (mood disorders, body image disorders, eating disorders), socioeconomic (food insecurity, economic stressors), and patient-specific (lack of compliance to medications, PERT, and/or dietary recommendations).[1,4-6,14,18,25]

While these etiologies are being investigated, initial interventions to manage the suboptimal or poor weight gain should begin.[6] Nutritional interventions in the nutritionally-failing patient focus on three main tenets: Correcting any identified medical co-diagnoses as mentioned above, optimizing PERT, and increasing caloric intake.[3,5,6,24]

Pancreatic Enzyme Replacement Therapy

The PERT involves the delivery of multiple exogenous (porcine), enterically-coated, pancreatic enzymes especially lipase, amylase, and protease to the lumen of the duodenum in order to facilitate digestion of fat and protein.[1,3,15] This therapy is indicated for exocrine pancreatic insufficiency which usually presents during early infancy but may develop later in life.[15,24] Currently, there are multiple methods to evaluate for PI including measurements of pancreatic fluid in the duodenum as well as 72-hour fecal fat collection, but given its accuracy and convenience, fecal pancreatic elastase-1 is most practical particularly for screening purposes.[15,26] In CF patients under the age of 2 years, PERT should be initiated in those who have two CFTR mutations known to cause PI in those whose fecal pancreatic elastase-1 is less than 200 µg/g in a formed stool in those under 6 months of age whose fecal coefficient of fat absorption is less than 85%, and in those who have clear signs and symptoms of PI (while awaiting results of confirmatory testing).[24] Multiple PERT dosing guidelines have been published for infants, children, and adults.[1,3,10,23,24] Despite this, Calvo-Lerma, et al. demonstrated much variability of PERT dosing between patients and centers, as PERT efficacy is affected by multiple factors including disease state, diet composition, and patient compliance.[1,27] Proper administration of PERT is important to prevent inactivation of the enzymes before delivery to the duodenum, so proper teaching of PERT administration should occur with the patient and caretakers.[28] Overall response to PERT should be assessed regularly, and signs of malabsorption (e.g. steatorrhea, abdominal bloating) or poor weight gain despite appropriate caloric intake should cause the clinician to consider increasing the dose.[1] However, increasing the dose of PERT should be done carefully, as excessive dosing of PERT above the daily maximum value increases the risk of fibrosing colonopathy.[4,23]

Dietary and Behavioral Evaluations

Optimizing caloric intake is critical in the poorly growing CF patient, and this entails the enhancement of both feeding behaviors and feeding content. Baseline intake should be well-determined. A 24-hour dietary recall is a practical, in office first step in this endeavor, though a prospective, 3-5 days dietary log is advised for a more accurate assessment of intake.[3,5] If caloric intake is low, behavioral evaluation toward food intake should occur.[5] Targeted behavioral therapy can be helpful in young children, and is recommended in young children who are not meeting caloric needs or have identified behavioral challenges at mealtime.[25] In adolescents and adults, concerns about body image should be addressed if negatively impacting food intake.[6]

Oral Nutritional Supplementation

In addition to addressing feeding behaviors, nutritional substance should be appropriately adjusted. In infants, human breast milk is the initial form of nutrition recommended by the CFF, but standard (nonhydrolyzed) infant formulas are also appropriate and are recommended by the CFF if human breast milk is not utilized.[24] In the setting of suboptimal weight gain in infancy, trialing a hydrolyzed or elemental formula can be considered, especially if a diagnosis of milk protein intolerance or another allergic disorder is suspected, though there is no recommendation for the routine use of specialized formulas in infants with CF.[3,24] Caloric concentration of the infant's feed, whether human milk or formula should be increased in the setting of suboptimal weight gain in addition to the initiation or increasing of PERT as mentioned previously.[24] In older children and adults, dietary interventions start with the maximization of high-calorie, high-fat foods in the patient's diet, and the initiation of oral nutritional supplements in addition to (rather than replacing) these foods.[4-6] Medications to stimulate appetite including cyproheptadine, megestrol acetate, and dronabinol may be considered in this setting with the risks of the potential medication side effects taken into account for each patient.[1,4,6] While these medications are commonly used in the authors' experience they are seldom able to restore normal growth when used alone in undernourished patients.

Enteral Nutritional Supplementation

Despite best efforts by patients and providers, maintenance of adequate growth via the oral route is often unable to be achieved, and initiation of supplemental enteral feeding is required. The CFF advises starting enteral tube feeds when oral caloric intake is insufficient in meeting anthropomorphic benchmarks despite treatment by a multidisciplinary team.[6,29] Because of the frequency of this necessity, as well as its beneficial effects, information regarding enteral tube feeds should be presented to the patient and family early in life, and it should be introduced as a positive tool utilized to bring about better outcomes.[5,6] The gastrostomy tube, whether placed via laparoscopic surgical technique, percutaneous endoscopic technique, or radiologic technique, are the most commonly utilized enteral feeding medium used for long-term enteral feeding.[6,29] Due to an increased association with complications, the CFF recommends against the open surgical technique for gastrostomy tube placement in CF patients, unless there is a clear contraindication against the aforementioned, less invasive techniques.[29] Nasogastric tubes are recommended when supplemental tube feeds are anticipated to last 3 months or less.[29] If a comorbidity, such as pancreatitis, severe gastroesophageal reflux or gastroparesis, prevents tolerance of gastric feeding, gastrojejunal or jejunal tube feeds may be employed.[6,29] While supplemental enteral nutrition can be given in boluses or at a longer, continuous rate, CFF recommends supplementation in the form of continuous nocturnal infusions, as this may prevent decreases in oral nutritional consumption while the patient is awake during the daytime.[5,29] There is no consensus for CF patients over 2 years of age regarding the type of enteral formula given (polymeric, semi-elemental, or elemental), and patient-specific factors should be considered by the multidisciplinary care team.[3,6,24,29] In authors' experience, formulas closer to isotonic osmolality are better tolerated than the concentrated and hypertonic ones. Even if a larger volume of the isotonic formula is needed to provide the same caloric load, as it seems to the authors that hypertonic feeds tend to exacerbate symptoms of bloating, abdominal pain and diarrhea. The authors hypothesize that this observation may be explained by the previously described CF intestinal environment that already contains abnormally thickened, concentrated mucus.

Parenteral Nutrition

Parenteral nutrition is not typically advised as a nutritional support for patients with CF because of its substantial burden (i.e. need for central access, cost, and maintenance), risk of infection, and risk of parenteral nutrition-associated liver disease (PNALD). Recommended use is limited to exceptional instances when enteral feeding is not possible, such as in the postoperative period of a major gastrointestinal surgery, in an infant with meconium ileus, or in intestinal failure (IF) or short bowel syndrome (SBS).[3,6]

Vitamins, Minerals and Micronutrients

Cystic fibrosis patients are at increased risk for micronutrient deficiency, and they require monitoring and supplementation of multiple vitamins and minerals.[5] Although fat malabsorption in patients with PI and cholestasis in patients with CFLD puts them at high-risk of fat-soluble vitamin deficiency, all CF patients are at risk of this complication, and obtaining serum levels of vitamins A, D, E, and K are recommended at diagnosis as well as annually.[3,5] Though less sensitive, prothrombin time is commonly obtained as a surrogate marker for vitamin K.[1,3] Additionally, in patients with PI, ESPEN recommends checking fat-soluble vitamin levels 3-6 months after initiation of vitamin and enzyme supplementation or a change in vitamin dosing.[3] Multiple formulations of fat-soluble vitamins tailored to CF patients are commercially available, and these supplements should be given with PERT and fat-containing food to maximize absorption.[1] Dosing of these vitamins is guided by obtained serum levels, and CF patients often require doses above the upper recommended dietary reference intake for unaffected individuals.[1] However, when deficiencies are detected, lack of absorption and lack of patient adherence should be ruled out before increasing the dosage.[3] Deficiencies in water-soluble vitamins are usually uncommon except in atypical circumstances, such as vitamin B12 deficiency following a large ileal resection for meconium ileus.[3]

In addition to vitamin deficiencies, CF patients are at risk for insufficient amounts of minerals due to losses from sweat, malabsorption, and chronic inflammation.[3] Sodium deficiency is of particular concern especially during infancy (partially due to relatively low sodium content in breast milk and infant formulas) and during times of excessive fluid loss, such as when exercising or experiencing vomiting or diarrhea from an illness. Because of this, CFF recommends providing infants with CF 1/8 teaspoon of table salt per day from diagnosis until 6 months of age, and then ¼ teaspoon of table salt per day from 6 months of age until 2 years of age not to exceed 4 mEq/kg/day.[24] In older patients eating a Western diet with traditionally high sodium content, additional sodium supplementation is usually only needed in times of excessive losses, such as in hot weather, when exercising, or when experiencing symptoms of illness (fever, vomiting, diarrhea). In these times, small amounts of salt can be added to sports drinks, or salt tablets can be consumed.[1] Iron deficiency is frequent in CF patients and should be screened for annually with serum iron levels, and if low, iron deficiency anemia must be differentiated from anemia of chronic disease before providing iron supplementation, per ESPEN guidelines.[3] Though CF-specific multivitamins are known to contain zinc, additional supplementation may be needed for patients in whom zinc deficiency is suspected particularly in breastfed infants who are not fed meat by 6 months of age and develop poor growth, or in patients with inexplicable growth arrest, severe malabsorption, eye problems, increased susceptibility to infections, or prolonged diarrhea.[1,3] The CFF recommends empiric zinc supplementation for up to 6 months in CF patients with failure to thrive if caloric intake and PERT are otherwise appropriate.[5,24] Because of its importance in bone health, both CFF and ESPEN recommends calcium intake and levels be, at a minimum, kept at the recommended amounts for the unaffected, healthy populations of the same age.[3,5] ESPEN does not recommend routine supplementation of selenium in CF patients.[3] Deficiencies of essential fatty acids (EFA) including linoleic and alpha-linolenic acids can occur in CF (particularly those with PI) but there is currently insufficient data for the CFF to recommend routine EFA supplementation.[5,24] In the small percentage of CF patients who develop cirrhosis, portal hypertension, and end-stage liver disease, there are additional nutritional considerations beyond the scope of this discussion. In such a situation, careful attention to liver disease related wasting, limited bile flow, and the risk of bleeding is essential. These patients should undergo consultation with a liver specialist and will sometimes require specialized administration of D-alpha-tocopheryl polyethylene glycol 1000 succinate (TPGS) fat-soluble vitamin preparations for improved absorption.[30,31]

NOVEL NUTRITIONAL THERAPIES IN CYSTIC FIBROSIS

Much research is directed toward novel therapies for CF, and some developments have impact on nutrition and growth in this disease.[32,33]

The CFTR modulators, drugs that modify the function of the defective CFTR protein in CF are major recent advances.[32,34] The first CFTR modulator, ivacaftor was approved by the US Food and Drug Administration (FDA) in 2012.[34] Over a 48-week period, this drug compared to placebo, improved z-scores for weight and BMI in CF patients over 6 years of age having at least one G551D-CFTR mutation.[6,35] A second CFTR modulator, lumacaftor/ivacaftor was approved by the FDA in 2015 for patients 12 years of age and over who have a homozygous F508del mutation.[34] This newer drug compared to placebo, improved BMI in patients with this mutation and demographic in a randomized controlled trial (RCT) over 24 weeks.[36] Lumacaftor/ivacaftor was later shown to improve BMI z-score over 24 weeks in patients from 6–11 years of age with the homozygous F508del mutation.[37] At the present time, it is estimated that CFTR modulators are available for approximately half of CF patients in the United States.[32,34] Multiple other promising drugs targeting the CFTR protein are currently in various phases of clinical trials, and with wider use, growth and nutrition in the CF population may improve.[6,32]

Due to malnutrition and growth failure often seen in CF, recombinant human growth hormone (GH) has attracted clinical interest as a potential therapy. A 2015 Cochrane Review examined four studies involving this therapy in CF patients and found improvements in some anthropomorphic parameters when compared to no treatment. However, the authors concluded that long-term, RCTs in patients with CF were needed before a recommendation could be made for routine utilization.[38]

Relizorb™, a single-use, in-line cartridge designed to improve delivery of lipase during enteral tube feeds was shown to increase plasma omega-3 fatty acid levels (a surrogate marker for fat absorption) 2.8-fold over placebo in a RCT of patients with CF, though the study population was relatively small.[39]

CONCLUSION

Cystic fibrosis is a severe, progressive genetic disease that affects many organs of the body. It is caused by mutations in the *CFTR* gene, and numerous CFTR mutations exist. Higher growth parameters are associated with better pulmonary function and outcomes. Therefore, optimizing nutrition is critical in CF patients, especially in children. Patients with CF are prone to malnutrition, growth failure, and vitamin deficiencies because of the malabsorption inherent to the pathophysiology of the disorder, and they require serial assessments of growth parameters as well as clinical and biochemical evaluation for malnutrition. Patients with CF have a large differential diagnosis for poor growth, and multidisciplinary evaluation for this problem is essential. Effective nutritional management generally includes the provision of sufficient pancreatic enzyme replacement therapy, adequate calories for growth, fat-soluble vitamins, and minerals, though numerous factors must be considered for the individual patient. Many patients require enteral feedings via gastrostomy tube in order to achieve enough caloric input for growth, and this therapy should be pursued without hesitation if it is needed. There are several recent developments in novel treatments for CF that affect nutrition, and multiple new therapies are in clinical trials.

> **KEY LEARNING POINTS**
>
> - Cystic fibrosis is a multisystemic disease. The effects of its gastrointestinal manifestations are wide-ranging, and a multidisciplinary approach involving a pulmonologist, gastroenterologist, endocrinologist, dietitian, psychologist, and social worker is very important in both evaluation and management of the disorder.
> - Early identification and prompt management of CF and its nutritional complications are critical, as malnutrition is a consequence of the disease, and improved outcomes and lung function are associated with better growth parameters. PERT is an essential therapy in CF patients.
> - Enteral supplemental nutrition should be discussed early in the patient's course and should be facilitated by the involvement of a gastroenterologist and dietitian experienced in CF-related nutritional issues. Gastrostomy tube feeds should be utilized when long-term supplementation is warranted.
> - The clinician should evaluate for deficiencies in macro- and micronutrients in CF patients, and fat-soluble vitamins, as well as minerals including sodium chloride should be provided in a timely manner to prevent macro- and micronutrient deficiency.
> - New therapies including CFTR modulators are becoming increasingly available, and it is hoped that with new discoveries, nutritional outcomes will be improved.

REFERENCES

1. Schindler T, Michel S, Wilson AW. Nutrition Management of Cystic Fibrosis in the 21st Century. *Nutr Clin Practice* 2015;30:488-500.
2. Li L, Somerset S. Digestive system dysfunction in cystic fibrosis: challenges for nutrition therapy. *Digest liver Dis* 2014;46:865-874.
3. Turck D, Braegger CP, Colombo C, et al. ESPEN-ESPGHAN-ECFS guidelines on nutrition care for infants, children, and adults with cystic fibrosis. *Clin Nutr* 2016;35:557-577.
4. Solomon M, Bozic M, Mascarenhas MR. Nutritional issues in cystic fibrosis. *Clin Chest Med* 2016;37:97-107.
5. Borowitz D, Baker RD, Stallings V. Consensus report on nutrition for pediatric patients with cystic fibrosis. *J Pediatr Gastroenterol Nutr* 2002;35:246-259.
6. Sullivan JS, Mascarenhas MR. Nutrition: Prevention and management of nutritional failure in Cystic Fibrosis. *J Cystic Fibrosis* 2017;16(Suppl 2):S87-s93.
7. Lai HJ, Shoff SM, Farrell PM. Recovery of birth weight z score within 2 years of diagnosis is positively associated with pulmonary status at 6 years of age in children with cystic fibrosis. *Pediatric* 2009;123:714-722.
8. Konstan MW, Butler SM, Wohl ME, et al. Growth and nutritional indexes in early life predict pulmonary function in cystic fibrosis. *J Pediatr* 2003;142:624-630.
9. Yen EH, Quinton H, Borowitz D. Better nutritional status in early childhood is associated with improved clinical outcomes and survival in patients with cystic fibrosis. *J Pediatr* 2013;162:530-535.e531.

10. Stallings VA, Stark LJ, Robinson KA, Feranchak AP, Quinton H. Evidence-based practice recommendations for nutrition-related management of children and adults with cystic fibrosis and pancreatic insufficiency: results of a systematic review. *J Am Dietet Assoc* 2008;108:832-839.
11. Vandenbranden SL, McMullen A, Schechter MS, et al. Lung function decline from adolescence to young adulthood in cystic fibrosis. *Pediat Pulmonol* 2012;47:135-143.
12. Steinkamp G, Wiedemann B. Relationship between nutritional status and lung function in cystic fibrosis: cross sectional and longitudinal analyses from the German CF quality assurance (CFQA) project. *Thorax* 2002;57:596-601.
13. Rafeeq MM, Murad HAS. Cystic fibrosis: current therapeutic targets and future approaches. *J Translat Med* 2017;15:84.
14. Gelfond D, Borowitz D. Gastrointestinal complications of cystic fibrosis. *Clin Gastroenterol Hepatol* 2013;11:333-342; quiz e330-331.
15. Uc A, Fishman DS. Pancreatic Disorders. *Pediatr Clin North Am.* 2017;64:685-706.
16. Wilschanski M, Durie PR. Patterns of GI disease in adulthood associated with mutations in the CFTR gene. *Gu* 2007;56:1153-1163.
17. Bhagirath AY, Li Y, Somayajula D, Dadashi M, Badr S. Cystic fibrosis lung environment and Pseudomonas aeruginosa infection. *BMC Pulmon Med* 2016;16:174.
18. De Lisle RC, Borowitz D. The cystic fibrosis intestine. *Cold Spring Harbor Perspec Med* 2013;3:a009753.
19. Wouthuyzen-Bakker M, Bodewes FA, Verkade HJ. Persistent fat malabsorption in cystic fibrosis; lessons from patients and mice. *JC cystic Fibrosis* 2011;10:150-158.
20. Borowitz D, Durie PR, Clarke LL, et al. Gastrointestinal outcomes and confounders in cystic fibrosis. *J Pediatr Gastroenterol Nutr* 2005;41:273-285.
21. Jakab RL, Collaco AM, Ameen NA. Characterization of CFTR High Expresser cells in the intestine. *Am J Physiol Gastrointest Liver physiology* 2013;305:G453-465.
22. De Lisle RC, Roach E, Jansson K. Effects of laxative and N-acetylcysteine on mucus accumulation, bacterial load, transit, and inflammation in the cystic fibrosis mouse small intestine. *Am J Physiol Gastrointest Liver Physio* 2007;293:G577-584.
23. Sinaasappel M, Stern M, Littlewood J, et al. Nutrition in patients with cystic fibrosis: a European Consensus. *J Cystic Fibrosis* 2002;1:51-75.
24. Borowitz D, Robinson KA, Rosenfeld M, et al. Cystic Fibrosis Foundation evidence-based guidelines for management of infants with cystic fibrosis. *J Pediatr* 2009;155(6 Suppl):S73-93.
25. Lahiri T, Hempstead SE, Brady C, et al. Clinical Practice Guidelines from the Cystic Fibrosis Foundation for Preschoolers With Cystic Fibrosis. *Pediatrics* 2016;137(4). pii: e20151784.
26. Dominguez-Munoz JE, P DH, Lerch MM, Lohr MJ. Potential for screening for pancreatic exocrine insufficiency using the fecal elastase-1 test. *Dig Dis Sci* 2017;62:1119-1130.
27. Calvo-Lerma J, Hulst JM, Asseiceira I, et al. Nutritional status, nutrient intake and use of enzyme supplements in paediatric patients with cystic fibrosis:A European multicentre study with reference to current guidelines. *J Cystic Fibrosis* 2017;16:510-518.
28. Giuliano CA, Dehoorne-Smith ML, Kale-Pradhan PB. Pancreatic enzyme products: digesting the changes. *Ann Pharmacother* 2011;45:658-666.
29. Schwarzenberg SJ, Hempstead SE, McDonald CM, et al. Enteral tube feeding for individuals with cystic fibrosis: Cystic Fibrosis Foundation evidence-informed

guidelines. *J Cystic fibrosis : official journal of the European Cystic Fibrosis Society* 2016;15(6):724-735.
30. Sokol RJ. A New Old Treatment for Vitamin E Deficiency in Cholestasis. *Journal of pediatric gastroenterology and nutrition* 2016;63(6):577-578.
31. Leung DH, Narkewicz MR. Cystic Fibrosis-related cirrhosis. *Journal of cystic Fibrosis* 2017;16(Suppl 2):S50-S61.
32. Zemanick ET, Daines CL, Dellon EP, et al. Highlights from the 2016 North American Cystic Fibrosis Conference. *Pediatr Pulmonol* 2017;52(8):1103-1110.
33. Shawcross A, Barry PJ. Highlights from the 30th North American Cystic Fibrosis Conference, Orlando 2016. *Paediatr Respir Rev* 2017, Mar 14. pii: S1526-0542(17)30033-7.
34. Martiniano SL, Sagel SD, Zemanick ET. Cystic fibrosis: a model system for precision medicine. *Currt Opin Pediatr* 2016;28:312-317.
35. Borowitz D, Lubarsky B, Wilschanski M, et al. Nutritional status improved in cystic fibrosis patients with the g551d mutation after treatment with ivacaftor. *Digest Dis Sci* 2016;61:198-207.
36. Wainwright CE, Elborn JS, Ramsey BW, et al. Lumacaftor-ivacaftor in patients with cystic fibrosis homozygous for phe508del CFTR. *N Engl J Med* 2015;373:220-231.
37. Milla CE, Ratjen F, Marigowda G, Liu F, Waltz D, Rosenfeld M. Lumacaftor/Ivacaftor in Patients Aged 6-11 Years with Cystic Fibrosis and Homozygous for F508del-CFTR. *Am J Respir Crit Care Med* 2017;195:912-920.
38. Thaker V, Haagensen AL, Carter B, Fedorowicz Z, Houston BW. Recombinant growth hormone therapy for cystic fibrosis in children and young adults. *Cochrane Database system Rev* 2015;(5):Cd008901.
39. Freedman S, Orenstein D, Black P, et al. Increased fat absorption from enteral formula through an in-line digestive cartridge in patients with cystic fibrosis. *J Pediatr Gastroenterol Nutr* 2017;65:97-101.

28 Nutrition in Celiac Disease

Shaveta Kundra

ABSTRACT

Gluten-free diet (GFD) is the cornerstone treatment for celiac disease (CD). GFD implies a strict and lifelong elimination from the diet of gluten, the storage protein found in wheat, barley, rye and hybrids of these grains, such as kamut and triticale. The nutritional adequacy of GFD is particularly important in children, this the age being of maximal energy and nutrient requirements for growth, development and activity. Strict adherence to gluten-free diet is mandatory. Exposure to even small amounts of gluten is sufficient to maintain the disease. Patient and caregivers should be counseled in detail about the nature and lifelong treatment of the disease. Counseling should be provided by an experienced dietician to patient and family at periodic intervals. Majority patients respond to GFD within weeks to months after starting GFD. Patients should be followed at regular intervals and should be monitored for compliance to GFD, their clinical parameters, such as weight, height, resolution of symptoms and rise in hemoglobin.

Keywords: Barley, Celiac disease, Diet, Gliadin, Gluten-free diet (GFD), Malabsorption, Nutrition, Rye, Steatorrhea, Wheat.

INTRODUCTION

Celiac disease (CD) is a chronic systemic autoimmune disorder caused by a permanent intolerance to gluten proteins in genetically susceptible individuals.[1-3] Samuel Gee first described the classic presentation with malabsorption in 1888: "The celiac affection",[4] but it was not until the late 1940s that Dicke, a Dutch pediatrician, first recognized that the ingestion of wheat was responsible for manifestation of the disease.[5] CD is strongly associated with the human leukocyte antigen (HLA)-DQ2 and DQ8 haplotypes.[6] Although presumed to be a rare disease earlier with a prevalence of about 0.02% recent studies done in Europe, India, South America, Australia and USA using serology and biopsy, have shown the prevalence of 0.33 and 1.06% in children and between 0.18–1.2% in adults.[7-10] The highest prevalence (5.66%)

in childhood has been observed in Sahrawi.[11] The clinical presentation of CD differ greatly and depend on age of the patient, duration and extent of extra-intestinal manifestations.[12-14] The usual clinical manifestations resemble chronic protein-energy malnutrition with predominant features of chronic diarrhea, abdominal distension, anemia, growth failure and loss of appetite.[15] Although symptomatic forms seem to be more common in developing countries, serological screening studies in these regions have shown many cases are asymptomatic or present with mild complaints.[16]

PATHOPHYSIOLOGY

Celiac disease occurs as a result of interplay of several environmental, genetic and immunologic factors.[1,17] Proteins in the dietary cereal grains, wheat, rye, and barley are the major known environmental factors that are required for disease activation.[18] Collectively, the disease-activating proteins in wheat, rye, and barley are widely termed "gluten." Gluten is actually the scientific name for only the disease-activating proteins in wheat. It itself contains 2 major protein fractions, gliadins and glutenins, both of which contain disease-activating proteins.[19,20] The closely related proteins in barley and rye that activate disease are termed *hordeins* and *secalins,* respectively.[21,22] Wheat, rye, and barley have a common ancestral origin in the grass family. Oats are distantly related to wheat, barley and rice and hence only rarely activates celiac disease that too in a small fraction of patients.[23,24] Proteins in rice, maize, sorghum, and millet are still more distantly related and do not activate celiac disease.[21,22]

The very high glutamine and proline content in the gliadins and glutenins of wheat, as well as in hordeins and secalins, plays a key role in disease pathogenesis. The high proline content renders these proteins relatively resistant to proteolytic digestion by gastric, pancreatic, and brush border enzymes in the human intestine. This results in generation and presence of relatively large peptides with a high proline and glutamine content in the small intestine which plays role in disease causation. This process is more exaggerated in the small intestine of individuals with active disease, i.e. with marked epithelial cell brush border injury and/or accompanying pancreatic dysfunction. Interestingly, prolyl endopeptidases produced by bacteria can digest these proline-rich gluten peptides, and treatment with such enzymes has been suggested as a possible therapeutic adjunct to the standard "gluten" free diet.[25,26]

NUTRITIONAL STATUS OF CELIAC SUBJECTS

Since CD is a chronic systemic gastrointestinal (GI) disease, small intestinal mucosal damage leads to malabsorption of nutrients which are normally absorbed in the proximal small bowel like iron, folate and calcium. Depending upon the severity of small intestinal damage, celiac patients have variable nutritional deficiencies, such as calorie/protein, dietary fiber, minerals (iron, calcium, magnesium and zinc) and vitamins (vitamin D, folate, niacin, vitamin B_{12} and riboflavin)[26-35] at the time of diagnosis. Incidence of iron deficiency in celiac disease varies from 12% to 69% and incidence of vitamin B_{12} deficiency in untreated patients ranges from 8% to 41%, though there is a relative sparing of villous atrophy in the ileum where vitamin B_{12} is absorbed.[34,35] Deficiency of calcium, phosphorus, and vitamin D may occur due to malabsorption or decreased intake of milk and dairy products. The severity of the nutritional deficiencies is modulated by different factors: Duration of illness prior to diagnosis, extent of small intestinal villous involvement and the degree of malabsorption.

Although most of these nutritional deficiencies in CD disappear following strict gluten-free diet (GFD) some of the deficiencies persist despite gluten-free diet; since GFD does not guarantee adequate nutritional intake.[36] Nutritional deficiency of fiber, folate, niacin and vitamin B_{12} have been described after treatment with a long-term GFD for about 8-12 years.[36] The long-term dietary fiber deficiency is likely due to the composition of many gluten-free (GF) foods which are made with starches and/or refined flours with low fiber content.[36,37] In fact during refining, the outer layer of grain containing most of the fiber is removed leaving only the starchy inner layer.

GLUTEN-FREE DIET

The only accepted treatment for CD involves the lifelong elimination of gluten in the diet, i.e. GFD.[38-41] Once the diagnosis of CD has been made, it is important to effectively motivate and educate the patient about the need for a stringent GFD. Patient needs thorough clinical evaluation for the presence of deficiencies or complications of malabsorption. The National Institutes of Health consensus development conference identified 6 elements required for the management of CD (Table 1).[42] The overall goal of the treatment plan is to relieve symptoms, heal the intestine, and reverse the consequences of malabsorption while enabling the patient to maintain a healthy, interesting, practical GFD.

The GFD is based on 2 fundamental premises[40,41,43-45]:
1. The elimination of all products that contain prolamines from wheat or any triticum species, such as wheat, barley, spelt, rye, or their crossbred varieties.

Table 1: Management of celiac disease (CD): Six key elements (CELIAC).

Consultation with a skilled dietitian
Education about CD
Lifelong adherence to a gluten-free diet
Identification and treatment of nutrition deficiencies
Access to a support group
Continuous long-term follow-up

2. The elimination of any products deriving from these cereals (starch, flour, semolina, bread, pasta, pastries, and cakes) and all of the byproducts of these grains in food products, beverages, and medication.

The inclusion of oats is controversial. As already stated oats are usually well tolerated by most patients with celiac disease and it improves the nutritional content of the diet and overall quality of life. However, oats are not uniformly recommended because most commercially available oats are contaminated with gluten-containing grains during growing, transportation, and milling processes.[45]

GFD should be offered to:
- All symptomatic children with characteristic histology
- Asymptomatic children with a condition associated with CD and characteristic histology
- Patient presenting with celiac crisis when treatment cannot safely be delayed without prior complete diagnostic evaluation.

Benefits of Gluten-free diet

- Resolution of clinical symptoms
- Reversal of anemia and bone demineralization
- Improved height velocity
- Resolution of micronutrient deficiencies
- Decreased rate of delayed puberty, menstrual problems, infertility, spontaneous abortions and low birth weight babies
- Decreased rate of some intestinal cancers to normal population levels.

While planning gluten-free diet, all patients should be counseled for a balanced diet as per their nutritional requirement. The amount of the nutrients required by an individual varies with his/her age, gender and level of activities which he/she does in his/her day-to-day life. A balanced diet should comprise of 45–65% carbohydrate, 20–35% fat and 10–30% proteins.[46] The diet should be planned by using right combination of five food groups, such as cereal products; pulses and legumes; milk, egg and flesh foods; fruits and vegetable; and fats and sugar as suggested by the Nutrition Expert Group of Indian Council of Medical Research.[47]

During initial phase of the treatment, patients with CD should be given supplements of vitamins, minerals, and extra protein supplement to overcome deficiencies and replenish nutrient stores.[48,49] Up to 80% of patients with CD in India have anemia.[49-51] Anemia should be treated with iron, folate, or vitamin B_{12} depending on the type of anemia. Bone disease is frequent in patients with CD resulting from malabsorption of calcium and/or vitamin D, with subsequent osteopenia, osteoporosis, or osteomalacia. All patients with CD should receive elemental calcium and vitamin D_3 supplementation.[38,41] Secondary lactose intolerance may occur in some patients with CD, a low lactose diet may be useful in controlling symptoms at least during initial few months of treatment.[41] Certain authors suggest that exocrine pancreatic insufficiency is responsible for relative lactase deficiency to the extent that trypsin is required for the enzymatic activation of lactase.[45]

Gluten-free Foods

Vegetables, fruits, rice, pulses, nuts, vegetable oils, milk and dairy products, fish, eggs, butter and plain meats are inherently GF as long as they are prepared without gluten-containing ingredients. In the past decade, there has been a vast improvement in the availability and quality of foods specifically manufactured using GF alternative flours. In the Food Safety and Standards (Food Products Standards and Food Additives) Regulations, 2011 the FSSAI proposes to add a new regulation called *Gluten-Free Food*. FSSAI has published Draft Food Products Standards cum Packaging and Labeling (Amendment) Regulations, 2015 to set maximum limits and labeling requirements for gluten and nongluten foods.[46]

Gluten-free foods:
- These foods consist of or are made from one or more ingredients which may contain rice, rye, barley, oats and millets or ragi, pulses and legumes, where the inherent gluten has been reduced and the gluten level does not exceed 20 milligram (mg)/kilogram (kg) in total based on the food as sold or distributed to the consumer.
- The product does not contain wheat or any of its ingredients.
- A food which, by its nature, is suitable for use as part of a gluten-free diet shall not be named as "special dietary"/"special dietetic" or any other equivalent term. However, such a food may bear a statement on the label that "this food is by its nature gluten-free".

Foods specially processed to reduce gluten content to a level above 20 up to 100 mg/kg: These foods consist of one or more ingredients from rice, rye, barley, oats, millet, or ragi, pulses and legumes which have been specially processed to reduce the inherent gluten present in them to a level between 20 and 100 mg/kg in total.

The gluten-free food products are easily available in the markets albeit at a greater expense than gluten-containing foods. Premade gluten-free breads, buns, rolls, pizza crusts, donuts, pastas, cereals, and desserts can be purchased. The availability of gluten-free foods increases a patient's food choices and improves diet variety while allowing patients to feel "normal" when eating among their peers.[43]

The common ingredients used in gluten-free breads and baking mixes are cornstarch, potato flour/starch, tapioca flour/starch, and brown/white rice flour. Although flours from wheat, rye, and barley are fortified with vitamins and minerals, such as vitamins B and iron, gluten-free flours are not fortified. Gluten-free baked goods tend to be high in fat and calories to enhance flavor, texture, appearance and overall acceptability of the gluten-free products and hence leads to reciprocal increase in fat consumption.[45,52]

Monitoring Response to Gluten-free Dite

In confirmed cases, GFD will be required lifelong with regular support of dietician. Strict dietary adherence to GFD is mandatory. In majority of patients response to GFD is remarkable within weeks in most patients. Improvement in overall well-being is one of the early symptoms to recover because of improvement in energy supply, correction of deficiencies of micronutrients and improvement in hemoglobin.[38,41,44,53] Serologic titers fall soon after initiating a GFD with substantially lower antibody levels at 1 year with ongoing decline to negative/normal by 2 years.[54,55] Although antibody levels will decline in partially adherent patients, the rate of decline is less than with strict compliance. However, negative serology does not guarantee strict adherence to GFD; in addition, many patients have ongoing villous abnormalities despite negative serology.

Mucosal recovery is faster and more complete in children with 95% recovery in 2 years and 100% recovery long-term in children following a GFD.[46] Persistent injury is more likely in those who are nonadherent to GFD. Follow-up visits can be scheduled after 1–3 months according to clinical presentation, and serology should be repeated minimum 6 months after the commencement of gluten-free diet. Subsequently, patients may be followed at one yearly interval. At follow-up visits, patients should be assessed for clinical symptoms, dietary adherence and monitor for growth or any delay in onset and progress of puberty, as well as the development of other autoimmune conditions, such as type 1 diabetes and hypothyroidism. The clinician should be alert to signs and symptoms that may suggest poor adherence to a GFD or development of other autoimmune associations during routine clinic visits including:

- Increased lethargy/polyuria/polydipsia/weight loss (diabetes)
- Excessive weight gain/deterioration in school performance/new-onset constipation/failure to gain (hypothyroidism).[56]

Patients can be assessed, if necessary, for histological improvement after 2 years on a GFD. Patients should be reinforced for avoiding consumption of gluten once they start to gain weight and feel better because even small amounts of gluten can lead to mucosal alterations after several weeks with modifications in the intestinal biopsy.[57]

A key to the success of the GFD is adherence to GFD. Dietician-led evaluation by direct history taking, food records, and cross-check questioning is very useful for assessing the adherence to GFD.[38,41,44] The range of adherence to a strict GFD as reported by patients is 45–81%. These may be overestimates, as some patients reporting strict adherence have abnormal intestinal histopathology.[58] The range of reported complete lack of adherence is 6–37%.

Four targets of therapy have been proposed. The traditional target—relief of symptoms is readily assessable and important, especially because symptom avoidance is a major motivation for adherence to the GFD and is directly related to quality of life. The second target is correction of nutritional deficiencies.[46,59] This is of paramount importance in children because physical growth, rapid catch-up in height, and normalization of body mass index is associated with institution of GFD in a child with newly diagnosed CD. The third potential target is to normalize immunological abnormalities, such as normalization of serological titer. The final target is to achieve mucosal healing which is an excellent surrogate for correction of immunological activation and is associated with improved outcomes in terms of morbidity and mortality.[59]

Nonfood Sources of Gluten

Because of its viscoelastic properties, gluten is used extensively in the food and other industry, and may be found in many items used daily, such as lipsticks, postage stamps, beer, ice creams, sweets, confectionary and excipients.[38-41] Topical products, such as shampoos, lotions, or other toiletries are not a concern. Both over-the-counter and prescription medications and vitamin and mineral supplements may contain gluten in the inert ingredients, excipients, coatings, or capsules.[60] These inactive ingredients can be changed by the manufacturers without warning because there are no regulations on the formulation of inactive drug components. Nebulous (questionable) ingredients, such as vegetable gum and modified food starch can contain gluten. All medications should be checked for nebulous ingredients, especially if they must be taken for a long period.[61]

TREATMENT ALTERNATIVES TO THE GLUTEN-FREE DIET

A GFD is currently the only available treatment for CD. Any alternative treatment in the future must have a safety and effective profile equivalent to that of the GFD, but with the advantage of increased compliance, quality of life, and feasibility in developing countries in which implementation of a GFD is complicated by formidable economical, cultural, and distribution difficulties.

Enzyme Therapy

Gluten peptides are resistant to digestion by pancreatic and brush border proteases.
- Enzyme supplement therapy with bacterial prolyl endopeptidases has been proposed to promote digestion of cereal proteins and thus destroy T cell multipotent epitopes.
- An alternative approach is based on a pretreatment of gluten-containing food with bacterial derived peptidase.[62]
- Another approach to produce nontoxic, wheat-based products is transamidation of gluten peptides by tTG, because it has been shown that these peptides inhibit interferon gamma expression in intestinal T-cell lines.[63]

- Engineered Grains and Inhibitory Gliadin Peptides Breeding programs and/or transgenic technology may lead to the production of wheat that is devoid of biologically active peptide sequences.

Immunomodulatory Strategies

The autoantigenic tTG is mainly expressed in the lamina propria and catalyzes transamidation of gluten peptides (glutamine to glutamic acid), increasing their rate of phagocytosis by antigen-presenting cells. Selective inhibition of tTG in the small intestine may represent a useful therapeutic strategy in CD.[64]

Correction of the Intestinal Barrier Defect

The correction of the intestinal barrier defects may represent an innovative therapeutic alternative in CD, because small intestinal permeability abnormalities are seen in untreated CD patients which return to normal on a GFD.[65,66]

EDUCATION AND COUNSELING

The management of CD is truly different and unique from the treatment of other medical or surgical diseases. The cornerstone of treatment of CD is GFD; dietary counseling and regular reinforcement for adherence by a nutrition specialist/dietician plays a very important role.[38-41,46] The fact that the child must never eat wheat products makes the caregivers restless. They are likely to resort to alternative medicine. It is therefore, extremely important that patients and their families are counseled well about the disease and the treatment.[40,41,44]

An expert nutritionist or dietician should be involved in counseling of a patient and their family. A detailed diet chart mentioning list of allowed and restricted food should be provided to all patients and their families. Caregivers should have an ability to identify (cross contamination and hidden sources) gluten in food enable them to make appropriate choice of food items. Nutrition expert should discuss topics, such as how to avoid contamination at home (using an electric or manual chakki at home for grinding flour in order to avoid contamination with wheat at commercial facilities) and school/workplace. Travel and restaurant tips should be discussed with patients and their families. Sufficient time should be spent in counseling and reinforcing messages periodically.[41,43,44] Various studies have shown that repeated counseling is associated with better rate of adherence to GFD.[38,41,43,67] Patients with excellent and good adherence to GFD show significantly higher improvement not only in the celiac-related symptoms but also in the level of hemoglobin and weight after 6-months of follow-up in comparison to those with poor adherence to GFD.[68] (Table 2)

Most common cause of partial or nonresponse to GFD in India is poor adherence to GFD.[38,41,46] There are many barriers to adherence to GFD in India, such as inappropriate counseling, nonavailability of gluten-free food,

Table 2: Dos and don'ts in using gluten-free foods.

Do's	Dont's
Use home prepared foods in which you can monitor the presence of gluten	Avoid eating outside homes or in places where wheat contamination of foods may be common
Buy foods that are labeled as gluten-free	Do not buy foods that do not have label and may be contaminated with wheat
Use a separate grinder or chakki for preparing flour for a CD patient	Do not buy flour from local mills where wheat may also be grounded and can contaminate
Reinforce the message of GFD to the patient periodically	
Educate the child's teachers about the importance of GFD for the child with CD in order to avoid compulsion to eat wheat products in school	
Ensure that medication administered to the patient do not contain wheat flour as filler	

and lack of labeling for GF food. Nonresponse in symptoms of CD even after 6 months of GFD despite compliance should raise the possibility of small intestinal bacterial overgrowth, autoimmune enteropathy, tropical sprue, drug-associated enteropathy (such as olmesartan), microscopic colitis, and eosinophilic gastroenteritis.[63] A persistent or recurrent elevation of serologic titers suggests ingestion of gluten either voluntary or adventitious.[38,41,44,46] There may be gluten exposure in nonfood items, such as medications, supplements, cosmetics, and glues.

CONCLUSION

Gluten-free diet, the cornerstone treatment for celiac disease is a strict and lifelong elimination of gluten-containing foods, i.e. wheat, barley, rye and hybrids of these grains, such as kamut and triticale. Exposure to even small amounts of gluten is sufficient to maintain the disease. As a rule, patients respond to GFD within weeks to months. A follow-up at regular intervals is mandatory for monitoring compliance to GFD and the clinical parameters, such as weight, height, resolution of symptoms and rise in hemoglobin.

KEY LEARNING POINTS

- ¤ Lifelong and complete avoidance of gluten or gluten containing dietary items is the most effective and the main stay of treatment of CD. While planning gluten-free diet, all patients should be counseled for a balanced diet as per their nutritional requirement.

Contd...

Contd...

- ¤ Patient and family including caregivers should be counseled in detail about the nature and lifelong treatment of the disease.
- ¤ A nutritionist or dietician should be involved in counseling of a patient and their family.
- ¤ Exposure to even small amounts of gluten is sufficient to maintain the disease.
- ¤ Patients with CD are likely to have nutritional deficiencies and should receive appropriate nutritional supplementation. This may include vitamin D, calcium, iron, zinc, vitamin B_{12} and other macro- and micronutrients.
- ¤ Most patients respond to gluten-free diet within weeks to months. CD patients should be followed at regular intervals and should be monitored for compliance to gluten-free diet, their clinical parameters, such as weight, height, resolution of symptoms and rise in hemoglobin.
- ¤ Dietary counseling is an ongoing process and should be periodically reinforced.
- ¤ The most common cause of either partial response or nonresponse is poor compliance to the dietary restrictions.
- ¤ Serological tests at 6 months and 1 year can be used to monitor adherence.

REFERENCES

1. Saturni L, Ferretti G, Bacchetti T. The gluten-free diet: Safety and nutritional quality. nutrients 2010; 2:16-34; doi:10.3390/nu2010016.
2. Green PH, Rostami K, Marsh MN. Diagnosis of celiac disease. *Best Pract Res Clin Gastroenterol* 2005;19: 389-400.
3. Murray JA, Van Dyke C, Plevak MF, et al. Trends in the identification and clinical features of celiac disease in a North American community, 1950-2001. *Clin. Gastroenterol Hepatol* 2003;1: 9-27.
4. Goddard CJR, Gillett HR. Complications of coeliac disease: are all patients at risk? *Postgrad Med J* 2006;82:705–712. doi: 10.1136/pgmj.2006.048876.
5. Dicke WK, Weijers HA, van de Kamer JH. Celiac disease II: the presence in wheat of a factor having deleterious effect in cases of celiac disease. *Acta Paediatr Scand* 1953;42:34 42.
6. Murch S, Jenkins H, Auth M, et al. Joint BSPGHAN and Celiac UK guidelines for the diagnosis and management of celiac disease in children. *Arch Dis Child* 2013; 98: 806-811 doi: 10.1136/archdischild-2013-303996. Available at: http://adc.bmj.com/content/98/10/806.full.html Accessed on: 7 March 2018.
7. Barker JM, Liu E. Celiac disease: pathophysiology, clinical manifestations, and associated autoimmune conditions. *Adv. Pediatr* 2008;55:349-365.
8. Fasano A, Berti I, Gerarduzzi T, et al. Prevalence of celiac disease in at-risk and not-at-risk groups in the United States: A large multicenter study. *Arch Intern Med* 2003;163:286-292.
9. Dube C, Rostom A, Sy R, et al. The prevalence of celiac disease in average-risk and at-risk Western European populations: A systematic review. *Gastroenterology* 2005;128:S57-S67.
10. Sood A, Midha V, Sood N, Malhotra V. Adult celiac disease in northern India. *Indian J. Gastroenterol* 2003;22:124-126.
11. Catassi C, Rätschl M, Gandolfi L, Pratesi R, Fabiani E. Why is coeliac disease endemic in the people of the Sahara? *Lancet* 1999,354:647-648.

12. Van Heel DA, Franke L, Hunt KA, et al. A genome-wide association study for celiac disease identifies risk variants in the region harboring IL2 and IL21. *Nat Genet* 2007;39:827–829.
13. Van Heel DA, Hunt K, Greco L, et al. Genetics in celiac disease. *Best Pract Res Clin Gastroenterol* 2005;19:323–339.
14. Catassi C, Ratsch IM, Fabiani E, et al. Coeliac disease in the year 2000: exploring the iceberg. *Lancet* 1994;343:200–203.
15. Fasano A, Araya YM, Bhatnagar S, et al. Federation of International Societies of Pediatric Gastroenterology, Hepatology, and Nutrition Consensus Report on Celiac Disease. *J Pediatr Gastroenterol Nutr* 2008;47:214–219.
16. White LE, Bannerman E, McGrogan P, et al. Childhood coeliac disease diagnoses in Scotland 2009-2010: the SPSU project. *Arch Dis Child* 2013;98:52–56.
17. Shan L, Molberg O, Parrot I, et al. Structural basis for gluten intolerance in celiac sprue. *Science* 2002;297:2275-2279.
18. Kagnoff MF. Overview and pathogenesis of celiac disease. *Gastroenterology* 2005;128:S10–S18
19. van de Wal Y, Kooy YM, van Veelen P, et al. Glutenin is involved in the gluten-driven mucosal T cell response. *Eur J Immunol* 1999. pp.29:3133–3139.
20. Shewry PR, Tatham AS, Kasarda DD. Cereal proteins and celiac disease. In: Marsh MN (Ed):. *Celiac disease*. London: Blackwell 1992:305–342.
21. Kasarda DD. Gluten and gliadin: precipitating factors in celiac disease. In: Maki M, Collin P, Visakorpi JK (Eds): *Celiac disease*. Tampere, Finland: Celiac Study Group , Institute of Medical Technology 1997:195–212.
22. Janatuinen EK, Kemppainen TA, Julkunen RJ, et al. No harm from five-year ingestion of oats in celiac disease. *Gut* 2002;50:332–335.
23. Hogberg L, Laurin P, Falth MK, Grant C, Grodzinsky E. Oats to children with newly diagnosed coeliac disease: a randomised double blind study. *Gut* 2004;53: 649–654.
24. Hausch F, Shan L, Santiago NA, Gray GM, Khosla C. Intestinal digestive resistance of immunodominant gliadin peptides. *Am J Physiol Gastrointest Liver Physiol* 2002;283:G996–G1003.
25. Inian Council of Medical Research. *ICMR Guideline on Diagnosis and Management of Celiac Disease in India*. New Delhi: Division of Noncommunicable Diseases, ICMR 2016.
26. Kemppainen T, Uusitupa M., Janatuinen E, et al. Intakes of nutrients and nutritional status in coeliac patients. *Scand J Gastroenterol* 1995;30:575-579.
27. Kinsey L, Burden ST, Bannerman EA. Dietary survey to determine if patients with celiac disease are meeting current healthy eating guidelines and how their diet compares to that of British general population. *Eur J Clin Nutr* 2008;62:1333-1342.
28. Barton, SH, Kelly, DG, Murray JA. Nutritional deficiencies in celiac disease, *Gastroenterol Clin North Am* 2007;36:93-108.
29. See J, Murray JA. Gluten-free diet: The medical and nutrition management of celiac disease, *Nutr Clin Pract* 2006;21:1-15.
30. Halfdanarson TR, Litzow MR, Murray JA. Hematological manifestations of celiac disease, *Blood* 2006;109:412-421.
31. Farrell RJ, Kelly CP. Celiac sprue. *N Eng J Med* 2002;346:180-188.
32. Scott EM, Gaywood I, Scott BB. Guidelines for osteoporosis in celiac disease and inflammatory bowel disease: British Society of Gastroenterology. *Gut* 2000;46:1-8.
33. Penagini F , Dilillo D, Meneghin F, Mameli C, Fabiano V, Zuccotti GV. Gluten-free diet in children: An approach to a nutritionally adequate and balanced diet. Nutrients 2013;5:4553-4565; doi:10.3390/nu5114553

34. Halfdanarson TR, Litzow, MR, Murray JA. Hematological manifestations of celiac disease. *Blood* 2006;109:412-421.
35. Dahele, B.; Ghosh, S. Vitamin B12 deficiency in untreated celiac disease. *Am J. Gastroenterol.* 2001;96:745-750.
36. Thompson, T. Folate, iron, and dietary fiber contents of the gluten free diet. *J Am. Dietetic Assoc.* 2000;100:1389-1396.
37. Thompson, T. Thiamin, riboflavin, and niacin contents of the gluten-free diet: Is there cause for concern? *J Am Dietetic Assoc.* 1999;99:858-862.
38. Kupper C. Dietary guidelines and implementation for celiac disease. *Gastroenterology.* 2005;128:S121-127.
39. Kelly CP, Bai JC, Liu E, Leffler DA. Advances in diagnosis and management of celiac disease. *Gastroenterology* 2015;148:1175-1186.
40. Fasano A, Catassi C. Clinical practice: Celiac disease. *N Engl J Med.* 2012;367:2419-2426.
41. See JA, Kaukinen K, Makharia GK, Gibson PR, Murray JA. Practical insights into gluten-free diets. *Nat Rev Gastroenterol Hepatol* 2015;12:580-591.
42. James SP. National Institutes of Health Consensus development conference statement on celiac disease, June 28–30, 2004. *Gastroenterology.*2005;128:S1–S9.
43. Niewinski MM. Advances in celiac disease and gluten-free diet. *J Am Diet Assoc.* 2008;108:661-672.
44. Case S. The gluten-free diet: how to provide effective education and resources. *Gastroenterology* 2005;128(4 Suppl 1):S128-134.
45. Manzanares AG, Lucendo AJ. Nutritional and dietary aspects of celiac disease. *Nutr Clin Pract* 2011;26:163-173. DOI: 10.1177/0884533611399773.
46. Indian Council of Medical Research. Indian balanced diet: Dietary guidelines. In: Gopalan C, Rama BV, Balasubramanian SC (Eds): *Nutritive Value of Indian Foods.* Hyderabad: National Institute of Nutrition, Indian Council of Medical Research 2004. pp. 40-41.
47. Shrivastav RK, Tiwari BK, Aggrawal Y, Calorie count and diet plan. In: *Current Nutritional Therapy Guideline.* New Delhi: Director General of Health Services, Ministry of Health and Family Welfare, Government of India 2008. pp. 49-58.
48. Theethira TG, Dennis M, Leffler DA. Nutritional consequences of celiac disease and the gluten free diet. *Expert Rev Gastroenterol Hepatol.* 2014;8:123-129.
49. Snyder J, Butzner JD, DeFelice AR, et al. Evidence-Informed expert recommendations for the management of celiac disease in children. *Pediatrics* 2016;138:e20153147
50. Singh P, Arora S, Makharia GK. Presence of anemia in patients with celiac disease suggests more severe disease. *Indian J Gastroenterol* 2014;33:161-164.
51. Poddar U, Thapa BR, Nain CK, Singh K. Is tissue transglutaminase autoantibody the best for diagnosing celiac disease in children of developing countries? *J Clin Gastroenterol* 2008;42:147-151.
52. Ferrara P, Cicala M, Tiberi E, et al. High fat consumption in children with celiac disease. *Acta Gastroenterol Belg* 2009;72:296-300.
53. Oxentenko AS, Murray JA. Celiac disease: Ten things that every gastroenterologist should know. *Clin Gastroenterol Hepatol* 2015;13:1396-404.
54. Nachman F, Sugai E, Vázquez H, González A, Andrenacci P. Serological tests for celiac disease as indicators of long-term compliance with the gluten-free diet 2011;23:473-480.
55. Husby S, Koletzko S, Korponay-Szabó IR, et al European Society for Pediatric Gastroenterology, Hepatology, and Nutrition guidelines for the diagnosis of coeliac disease. *J Pediatr Gastroenterol Nutr* 2012;54:136-160.

56. Paul SP, Kirkham EN, Pidgeon S, et al. Celiac disease in children. *Nus Standard* 2015; 29, 49, 36-41.
57. Clinical Guideline for the Diagnosis and Treatment of Celiac Disease in Children: Recommendations of the North American Society for Pediatric Gastroenterology, Hepatology and Nutrition. *J Pediatr Gastroenterol Nutr* 2005;40:1-19.
58. Niewinski MM. Advances in Celiac Disease and Gluten-Free Diet. J Am Diet Assoc. 2008;108:661-672.
59. Makharia GK, Mulder CJ, Goh KL, Ahuja V, Bai JC. (For World Gastroenterology Organization-Asia Pacific Association of Gastroenterology Working Party on Celiac Disease). Issues associated with the emergence of celiac disease in the Asia–Pacific region: a working party report of the World Gastroenterology Organization and the Asian Pacific Association of Gastroenterology. *J Gastroenterol Hepatol* 2014;29:666-677.
60. See J, Murray JA. Gluten-Free Diet: The Medical and Nutrition Management of Celiac Disease. Nutr Clin Pract 2006 21: 1 DOI: 10.1177/011542650602100101. Available at: http://ncp.sagepub.com/content/21/1/1 Accessed on: 7 March 2018.
61. Fasano A, Catassi C. Current approaches to diagnosis and treatment of celiac disease: an evolving spectrum. *Gastroenterology* 2001;120:636-651.
62. Rose C, Howard R. Living with coeliac disease: a grounded theory study. *J Hum Nutr Diet* 2014;27:30-40.
63. Rajpoot P, Sharma S, Harikrishna S, Baruah BJ, Ahuja V. Adherence to glutenfree diet and barriers to adherence in patients with celiac disease. *Indian J Gastroenterol.* 2015;34:380-386.
64. Di Cagno R, De Angelis M, Auricchio S, et al. Sourdough bread made from wheat and nontoxic flours and started with selected lactobacilli is tolerated in celiac sprue patients. *Appl Envison Microbiol* 2004;70:1088-1096.
65. Di Cagno R, De Angelis M, Lavermicocca P, et al. Proteolysis by sourdough lactic acid bacteria: effects on wheat flour protein fractions and gliadin peptides involved in human cereal intolerance. *Appl Environ Microbiol* 2002;68:623-633.
66. Gianfrani C, Siciliano RA, Facchiano AM, et al. Transamidation of wheat flour inhibits the response to gliadin of intestinal T cells in celiac disease. *Gastroenterology* 2007;133:780-789.
67. Piacentini M, Colizzi V. Tissue transglutaminase: apoptosis versus autoimmunity. *Immunol Today* 1999;20:130-134.
68. Fasano A, Shea-Donohue T. Mechanisms of disease: the role of intestinal barrier function in the pathogenesis of gastrointestinal autoimmune diseases. *Nat Clin Pract Gastroenterol Hepatol* 2005;2:416-422.

29 Diet in Inflammatory Bowel Disease

Pankaj C Vaidya

ABSTRACT

Crohn's disease (CD) and ulcerative colitis (UC) are the two broad phenotypes of inflammatory bowel disease (IBD) characterized by chronic mucosal inflammation. CD is characterized by its ability to involve any part of the gastrointestinal tract in a discontinuous fashion. Nutritional complications are common in patients with IBD, and include growth failure, osteopenia/osteoporosis, anemia, and vitamin malabsorption. Poor growth is one of the presenting features in pediatric IBDs especially CD and also in severe or complicated UC. The pathogenesis of growth failure in IBD is multifactorial. However, delayed puberty, corticosteroids, and proinflammatory cytokines, such as TNF-α and interleukin 6 are also responsible for the growth failure in this patient population. The goal of caring for patients with IBD is to ensure that clinical remission occurs concurrently with good nutrition intake and optimal growth. Children with IBD are prone to deficiencies in energy, protein, multivitamins and fat. Exclusive enteral nutrition (EEN) is recommended as first-line therapy to induce remission in pediatric CD but only few studies have analyzed the effect of dietary interventions for IBD maintenance of remission.

Keywords: Diet, Enteral nutrition, Exclusive enteral nutrition, Inflammatory bowel disease (IBD), Nutrition, Crohn's disease, Ulcerative colitis.

INTRODUCTION

Inflammatory bowel disease (IBD) is a perplexing disease characterized by chronic mucosal inflammation. It results from a complex interplay of various factors including genetic and environmental, and adaptive immunity of the host. Crohn's disease (CD) and ulcerative colitis (UC) are the two broad phenotypes of IBD. CD is characterized by its ability to involve any part of the gastrointestinal tract in a discontinuous fashion. The inflammation associated with CD is often transmural and granulomatous. UC on the other hand tends to involve the rectum and the adjoining colonic mucosa to a variable extent; albeit in a continuous fashion. The inflammation in UC is usually superficial when compared with CD. Inflammatory bowel disease in pediatric age group is being increasingly detected. In fact, it is one of the important disease entities seen by general pediatricians as well as pediatric gastroenterologists.[1] In the pediatric age group unlike adults, the prime concern in those suffering from IBD lies in growth and nutrition of these children. Many of the factors that affect quality of life in these patients are also directly related to nutrition. In children with UC, rectal bleeding, chronic diarrhea and abdominal pain are more common; while weight loss is a prominent feature of CD (58% vs. 35%). The classic triad of pediatric CD, i.e. abdominal pain, chronic diarrhea and weight loss are seen in only one-fourth of the cases; 25% of the children may present with only nonspecific symptoms like vague abdominal discomfort, lethargy and anorexia.

Nutrition has a significant role in pediatric IBD. A systematic review of studies on preillness diet and the risk of development of IBD revealed that high intakes of total fat, polyunsaturated fatty acid (PUFA), omega-6 fatty acids, and meat were consistently associated with increased risk of developing UC as well as CD. High vegetable intake was consistently associated with decreased risk of UC, whereas fiber and fruit intake was consistently associated with reduced risk of CD.[2]

Poor growth is one of the presenting features in pediatric IBDs, especially CD and also in severe or complicated UC. Overall linear growth impairment in pediatrics IBD is 35% with 60–70% in CD and 10–12% in UC. The reflection is basically in weight for age, height for age and body mass index (BMI) which are more affected in CD than UC. In the latter group, growth failure almost always is due to the prolonged use of high-dose corticosteroids.[3] In many cases, it could be the presentation before the onset of luminal symptoms and could be dismissed or misdiagnosed as other causes like primary malnutrition or familial/constitutional growth delay. The outcomes are also reflected in the psychosocial and sexual development of the child.

ETIOPATHOGENESIS

The causes of poor appetite and growth impairment in IBD are as follows:
- Cytokines produced by direct role of inflammatory cytokines in linear growth inhibition (IGF-1 inhibition; interference with kinetics, chronically inflamed intestine, of bone growth)
- Insufficient caloric intake due to anorexia
- Food avoidance because of exacerbation of gastrointestinal symptoms by eating
- Mucosal inflammation leading to protein-losing enteropathy and steatorrhea
- Malabsorption due to IBD, bowel resection, bile salt depletion and bacterial overgrowth
- Increased nutritional needs in fever
- Corticosteroid treatment leading to inhibition of IGF-1.

The pathogenesis of growth failure in IBD is multifactorial (Fig. 1). However, delayed puberty, corticosteroids, and proinflammatory cytokines, such as TNF-α and interleukin 6 are also responsible for growth failure in this patient population. Weight loss may precede reduced height velocity.

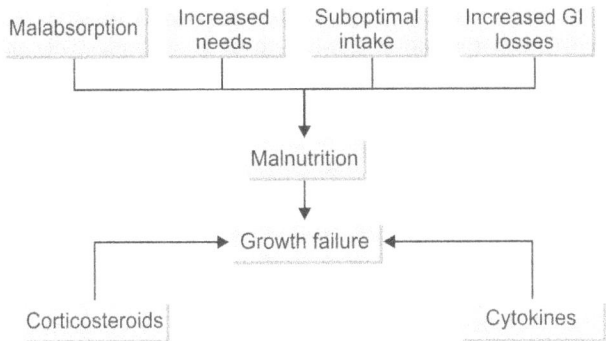

Fig. 1: Pathogenesis of growth failure in IBD.
(GI: gastrointestinal)

In CD, where there is involvement of small bowel, malabsorption is an important cause of malnutrition. Moreover, these patients have transmural involvement which leads to intestinal obstruction causing pain abdomen further causing food aversion and/or feed intolerance. The inflammatory cytokines which are related to inflamed gut lead to a central effect by acting on the satiety center causing loss of appetite. Many of the micronutrient deficiencies (like zinc deficiency) lead to altered taste sensation. Intestinal fistulas in CD can lead to bowel bypass and malabsorption. Also, since these patients are prone to recurrent exacerbations of the disease due to various infectious agents, these contribute to poor intake and malnutrition.[4] Steroid therapy causes early fusion of growth plates and suppression of insulin-like growth factor (IGF-1) causing stunting.

NUTRITIONAL ASSESSMENT

The goal of caring for patients with IBD is to ensure that clinical remission occurs concurrently with good nutritional intake and optimal growth. Nutritional complications in pediatric IBD are:[5]
- Growth failure
- Delayed puberty
- Osteopenia and osteoporosis
- Anemia
- Micronutrient deficiencies: Iron, folate, vitamin B_{12}, vitamin E, vitamin A, beta-carotene, magnesium, selenium, and zinc.

History: The assessment of nutrition during follow-up starts with dietary intake assessment. A meticulous history should include the appetite status, the choice of food and concurrent abdominal symptoms needs to be asked for. It is known that IBD patients tend to consume fewer amounts of cereals, milk and vegetables which implies that these children are usually deficient in calories, calcium and iron followed by other dietary components. The European Society for Paediatric Gastroenterology, Hepatology and Nutrition

(ESPGHAN) recommends a 3–5 days dietary record method to assess the intake in these patients and it should be done at least twice in a year in children <5 years of age.

Examination of specific vitamin or mineral deficiencies, such as iron, calcium, vitamin D, vitamin K, folate, and vitamin B_{12} are usually based upon clinical presumption of deficiency and may help to guide a clinician about treatment.

Growth monitoring: The indicators for proper nutrition are growth parameters that include trends in weight-for-age, weight-for-height, and height-for-age measurements. Body mass index can help to identify overweight and obese adolescents, and measurements of mid-arm circumference and triceps skinfold thickness can be used to assess lean muscle mass and fat stores. Monitoring of growth and treatment in case of growth retardation forms the cornerstone of therapy in pediatric IBD patients. Both lean body mass and linear impairment of growth are markers of disease severity and tend to improve with therapy; they can be the presenting features in up to 46% of pediatric CD patients even before the onset of luminal symptoms and may even persist in a fraction of patients with successful therapeutic responses, unlike in UC where the children tend to completely catch-up the expected nomograms. In the modern era, obesity is also coming up as an important comorbidity in these patients.

Monitoring of nutritional status in children with IBD: These patients should be routinely monitored for growth retardation during follow up with weight, height and BMI z-scores; the height velocity over 6–12 months corroborates maximum with the disease course. Individual appropriate growth charts should be kept and during each follow-up should be plotted for analyzing the catch-up of growth. It is also known that IBD is associated with pubertal delay and the yearly screening should be started at the age of 10 years.

DIETARY REQUIREMENTS IN IBD

Children with IBD have been found to have normal resting energy expenditure (REE) and hence have normal dietary requirement as healthy children of the same age and sex. This is contrary to the initial adult studies which showed a higher REE in these patients. The major contributory factor is rather a poor dietary intake and hence counseling and properly tailored diet chart needs to be given to these patients.[6]

Dietary macronutrients: Carbohydrate intake should be providing 60% of the calories for these patients. The levels of serum leptin as an indirect measure of fat stores is conflicting in these patients. However, the percentage of fat intake contributing to the total calories varies widely 40% in infants, 35–40% in toddlers and 20–25% in older children. Protein intake should be increased during the episodes of active disease as the catabolism and protein loss is found to be higher during this time. Indirect measurements of muscle protein can be made using urinary creatinine: Height ratio or a

3-methylhistidine level. The catabolism can be quantified using 24-hour urine urea nitrogen. The recommendation is to increase the intake by at least 25% during active disease, until the height velocity is adequate.

Vitamin deficiencies: Mucosal inflammation in IBD and consequent malabsorption leads to multiple vitamin deficiencies; though patients with IBD usually do not present with overt symptoms of vitamins or micronutrient deficiency.[7]

Fat-soluble vitamins: Vitamin D is found to be low in up to 35% patients with IBD. A serum value less than 20 ng/mL indicates severe deficiency and should be treated with megadoses of vitamin D followed by a maintenance dose as per protocol. A daily dose of 2,000 IU or weekly 50,000 IU may be needed to maintain sufficiency.[8] Even though isolated studies have demonstrated deficiencies of vitamin A, E and K in children with IBD, routine serum monitoring or supplementation is not recommended unless frank clinical features are present or in case of a coexisting liver disease.

Water-soluble vitamins: Special mention is needed for supplementing folic acid and vitamin B_{12} in these patients. Folate supplements are to be given at 1 mg per day for at least 3 weeks to abate the deficiency and annual folate measurement is recommended by the European Crohn's and Colitis Organization (ECCO) guideline to supplement further. In case of ileal CD or UC undergoing ileal pouch surgery, vitamin B_{12} should be given 1,000 micrograms intramuscularly every other day till 1 week followed by single weekly dose until clinical improvement; followed by periodic monitoring of MethylMalonic acid levels. Lifelong supplementation is needed for those who undergo >60 cm ileal resection. Other water-soluble vitamins are to be supplemented as per the deficiency signs.

Minerals: Iron supplementation: Apart from the villous atrophy and GI bleed that happens in IBD, abnormality in the hepcidin-ferroportin axis and also reduced erythropoietin contributes to iron deficiency anemia. Oral supplementation is adequate in the case of mild anemia >10 mg/dL but parenteral iron carboxymethylcellulose is the preparation of choice in cases of moderate to severe anemia. The incidence of hypersensitivity is reported to be as low as 4% from the newer iron preparations. Iron deficiency anemia is known to correlate with the disease activity in both CD and UC.

Magnesium levels are not routinely monitored in patients with IBD and when deficiency is encountered, it should be supplemented daily for 2 to 4 weeks orally. Refractory hypocalcemia can be a manifestation of hypomagnesemia. There is no recommendation to supplement calcium in these patients and doses ranging from 450 mcg to 1,150 mcg per day as per the age group are recommended. Contrary to the logical sense, reduced bone mineral density (BMD) has lesser correlation with calcium and vitamin D levels in these patient and supplements are not shown to improve the same. Even though a low BMI is seen in approximately 2/3rd of these patients, routine screening is not recommended with DEXA scan unless the patient is on steroid therapy or in those with higher risk of osteoporosis.

Micronutrients: Zinc deficiency is common in children with malnutrition especially in tropics and can be an independent contributor to stunting. It can be seen in up to 40% of the patients with IBD. ESPGHAN recommends daily intake of zinc 20-40 mg in case of IBD with chronic diarrhea for a short period of 4 weeks.[9] The applicability of this in tropical countries needs to be redefined. Selenium supplementation is not routinely done in these patients.

THERAPEUTIC ASPECTS OF NUTRITION IN IBD

Parental nutrition (PN): PN as a modality for nutritional rehabilitation of IBD is very uncommonly used in children especially in UC patients. It is used in intestinal failure or when the patient has ischemia or in case of a high output fistulae. It can also be used during perioperative period. It has its inherent risks including the risk of infections as a major concern. It is not used as a method for inducing remission in these patients. Early and aggressive medical intervention using immunomodulators alone or in combination with biologic agents targeting tumor necrosis factor α (TNF-α) shows promise in altering the natural history of CD in the future. This improvement in the available therapies has enabled clinicians to achieve disease remission in severe phenotypes of CD.[10]

Exclusive Enteral Nutrition (EEN): Voitk in 1973 first used elemental diet for providing nutritional support in a patient with CD who was posted for surgical intervention. Subsequently, many trials have demonstrated equal efficacy of EEN with respect to steroids for inducing remission in patients with CD. This was first demonstrated in the pediatric age group by Sanderson, et al. EEN is recommended as the first-line therapy to induce remission in pediatric CD patients but only a few studies have analyzed the effect of dietary intervention for IBD maintenance of remission.[11] There are multiple formulas which are available of which the polymeric formula has the maximum palatability and acceptance. Parenteral nutrition has demonstrated significant benefits in inducing remission in patients with active Crohn's disease; however, similar to enteral nutrition, when it is withdrawn, relapse is often immediate. Patients with gut failure from extensive disease or bowel resection represent one of the largest adult populations of those who receive home parenteral nutrition. The enteral nutrition approach is as rapid, in onset of response and as effective as the other treatments.[12] Pediatric studies have suggested similar efficacy to prednisone for improvement in clinical symptoms, but enteral nutritional therapy is superior to steroids for actual healing of mucosa. Because the affected patients have a poor appetite and these formulas are relatively unpalatable, they are often administered via a nasogastric or gastrostomy infusion usually overnight. The advantages are that it is relatively free of side effects, avoids the problems associated with corticosteroid therapy, and simultaneously addresses the nutritional rehabilitation therapy with home parenteral nutrition resulting in nutritional repletion, a reduced requirement for steroid treatment, and a general improvement in quality of life. This therapy, however, is associated with significant morbidity from complications, such as catheter blockage, catheter-related sepsis, dehydration, and electrolyte imbalance.

The possible mechanisms by which EEN acts are:
- **Anti-inflammatory activities:** From experimental models, it has been demonstrated that elemental or polymeric formulae decreases the pro-inflammatory cytokines and increase anti-inflammatory cytokines, hence reflecting in the clinical response.
- **Alteration in intestinal microbiota:** It is seen from experimental models that administration of elemental diet decreases both number and variety of gut flora in patients with IBD and the effect is sustained. Since intestinal flora plays an important role in the pathogenesis of IBD, this is the most probable mechanism by which EEN acts to maintain remission.
- **Epithelial barrier function:** It is now being increasingly recognized that increased mucosal permeability is a primary event triggering inflammation in IBD rather than a result of the same. EEN is known to induce complete reversal of permeability in animal models and hence decreases the associated inflammatory response.

In active luminal Crohn's disease, North American Society for Pediatric Gastroenterology, Hepatology and Nutrition (NASPGHAN) recommends use of EEN as the first-line therapy for induction of remission as the efficacy is comparable not only to steroids but also to biologicals. There are recommendations to use EEN in relapse in CD, but with a lesser response rate (73% vs. 58%). It is known to induce mucosal healing and even a transmural healing in patients with CD. The duration of therapy should be at least 8 weeks and gradual introduction of conventional food with a concomitant decrease in the EEN volume over 2-3 weeks is the usual practice that is adopted. The response to EEN does not depend on the disease location. There is no response in cases of oral and anal CD or in patients who have extra intestinal manifestations.

A dietary polymeric formula is recommended as the EEN of choice unless the patient has other coexisting food allergies. Post induction, relapse rate of 40 to 70% is seen in the first 2 years and median time of relapse ranges from 6 to 12 months.

Common adverse effects of EEN includes bloating, pain abdomen and vomiting, but the major effect often encountered is the re-feeding syndrome secondary to hyperinsulinemia in these children chronically starving due to malabsorption. This is characterized by the onset of anasarca and dyelectrolytemia which can be life-threatening. Once detected, a slower increase of EEN is warranted from a baseline calorie of 50% and stepwise increase is adopted once the dyselectrolytemia and edema gets corrected.

Apart from induction, there is no role of EEN for maintaining remission in CD. It is also ineffective in induction of remission in UC patients. It is inferred from multiple studies that EEN increases the lean body mass and quality of life in these patients but the effects on height and BMD has been conflicting.

Partial enteral nutrition (PEN): It as an induction therapy in CD is done in selected cases of mild disease severity and the optimum duration of therapy needs to be established. In case of maintenance of remission, a long-term course of PEN along with normal diet may be used to prolong remission in cases where no other agents are used for the same. Studies have thrown light on improvement in linear growth in such cases. Recent meta-analysis show that corticosteroid therapy is more effective than enteral nutrition for inducing remission of active CD as was also found in previous systematic reviews. Protein composition does not influence the effectiveness of EN in the treatment of active CD.[13]

DIET RESTRICTIONS IN PEDIATRIC IBD

Special diets like ova- lacto vegetarian, vegan, palaeolithic, low Fermentable Olig- Di- Monosaccharides, and Polyols (FODMAPS) have been advocated in patients with IBD to improve symptoms. In children, the specific carbohydrate diet has been found to improve luminal symptoms. It mainly consists of monosaccharides with eliminated di- and polysaccharides. However, the level of evidence is poor to recommend these currently. A low lactose diet or a lactase enzyme supplementation is recommended in patients suffering from symptoms of lactose intolerance like bloating and diarrhea. Dairy products are advised not to be avoided. Low FODMAPS diet which can induce symptom relief in patients with IBS should not be given in IBD as the nutrition can get compromised more.[14] Some sets of diet which should be avoided because of their possible association with IBD includes emulsifiers, high saturated fat diet and high-calorie low-fiber westernized food.

Probiotics are not used for induction of remission in pediatric CD but VSL#3 (a probiotic) is used as an alternative to 5-aminosalicylic acid (5-ASA) therapy in maintaining remission in mild to moderate UC where the ASA compounds are contraindicated or are intolerable. They are also used in maintenance of remission in pouchitis in IBD. Fiber supplementation may have an effective role in managing UC or pouchitis but not CD.[15]

CONCLUSION

Nutritional complications are common in patients with IBD, and include growth failure, osteopenia/osteoporosis, anemia, and vitamins malabsorption. Nutritional management in IBD is of utmost importance especially in the pediatric age group. The general principles for managing nutritional complications include:
- Pharmacologic and/or surgical intervention to reduce or remove chronic intestinal inflammation
- Minimization of corticosteroid use

- Supplementation of macronutrients to reduce protein–energy malnutrition, and
- Supplementation of micronutrients when appropriate.

The final outcome including the overall quality of life depends on the adequacy of nutritional rehabilitation of these patients. The use of EEN has revolutionized the therapy of CD as it is one of the diseases where diet modification is known to bring about remission. A combination of immunomodulators with EEN may be a better option but needs to be substantiated in future studies.

> **KEY LEARNING POINTS**
>
> ¤ Since malnutrition and growth failure are the integral complications of IBD in children, the afflicted child needs a special attention in terms of growth and nutrition care.
> ¤ Proper nutrition care and diet can prevent many complications in IBD.
> ¤ Supplements of vitamin, minerals, and calories in adequate amounts are needed in children with IBD.
> ¤ Exclusive enteral nutrition can induce remission in IBD children and should always be tried.

REFERENCES

1. Kapoor A, Bhatia V, Sibal A. Pediatric inflammatory bowel disease. *Indian Pediatr* 2016;53:993-1002.
2. Kappelman MD, Bousvaros A. Nutritional concerns in pediatric inflammatory bowel disease patients. *Mol Nutr Food Res* 2008;52:867-874. doi: 10.1002/mnfr.200700156.
3. Hyams JS. Inflammatory bowel disease. *Pediatr Rev* 2005;26:314-320.
4. Hou JK, Abraham B, El-Serag H. Dietary intake and risk of developing inflammatory bowel disease: a systematic review of the literature. *Am J Gastroenterol* 2011;106:563-573. doi: 10.1038/ajg.2011.44.
5. Wędrychowicz A, Zając A, Tomasik P. Advances in nutritional therapy in inflammatory bowel diseases: Review. *World J Gastroenterol* 2016;22:1045-66. doi: 10.3748/wjg.v22.i3.1045.
6. Hyams JS. Crohn's disease. In: Wyllie R, Hyams JS (Eds): *Pediatric Gastrointestinal Disease: Pathophysiology, Diagnosis, and Management*, 2nd edn. Philadelphia, Pa: WB Saunder1999:408-418.
7. Gerasimidis K, McGrogan P, Edwards CA. The aetiology and impact of malnutrition in paediatric inflammatory bowel disease. *J Hum Nutr Diet* 2011;24:313-326. doi: 10.1111/j.1365-277X.2011.01171.x.
8. Veit LE, Maranda L, Fong J, Nwosu BU. The vitamin D status in inflammatory bowel disease. PLoS One. 2014;9:e101583. doi: 10.1371/journal.pone.0101583. eCollection 2014. Available at: http://journals.plos.org/plosone/article?id=10.1371/journal.pone.0101583. Accessed on: 3 May 2018.
9. Sikora SK, Spady D, Prosser C, El-Matary W. Trace elements and vitamins at diagnosis in pediatric-onset inflammatory bowel disease. *Clin Pediatr (Phila)* 2011;50:488-492. doi: 10.1177/0009922810397041.
10. Issa M, Binion DG. Bowel rest and nutrition therapy in the management of active Crohn's disease. *Nutr Clin Pract* 2008;23:299-308. doi: 10.1177/0884533608318675.

11. Young RJ, Vanderhoof JA. Nutrition in pediatric inflammatory bowel disease. *Nutrition* 2000;16:78-80.
12. Tighe MP, Cummings JR, Afzal NA. Nutrition and inflammatory bowel disease: primary or adjuvant therapy. *Curr Opin Clin Nutr Metab Care* 2011;14:491-496. doi: 10.1097/MCO.0b013e328349eb4d.
13. Zachos M, Tondeur M, Griffiths AM. Enteral nutritional therapy for induction of remission in Crohn's disease. *Cochrane Database Syst Rev* 2007;(1):CD000542.
14. Mallon DP, Suskind DL. Nutrition in pediatric inflammatory bowel disease. *Nutr Clin Pract* 2010;25:335-339. doi: 10.1177/0884533610373773.
15. Penagini F, Dilillo D, Borsani B, Cococcioni L, Galli E. Nutrition in pediatric inflammatory bowel disease: from etiology to treatment. a systematic review. *Nutrients* 2016;8. pii: E334. doi: 10.3390/nu8060334.

30 Diet in Chronic Liver Disease

Aditi, Pankaj C Vaidya, Vibhor V Borkar

ABSTRACT

Chronic liver disease (CLD) in children is commonly seen in specialist clinics as well as general outpatient department (OPD). The evaluation of underlying etiology, specific treatment and complications overshadows the time spent in the nutritional assessment and management of these children. It is now increasingly being realized that nutrition in children with CLD is of paramount importance and one of the prognostic marker for both pre-and post-transplantation status of CLD patients. Disease morbidity as well as reduced reserve per se increases the susceptibility of CLD patients to multiple nutrient deficiencies as well as protein-energy malnutrition. This chapter deals with multifactorial nature of malnutrition, nutritional assessment and management in children with CLD.

Keywords: Chronic liver disease, Hepatic encephalopathy, Liver disease, Malnutrition, Multiple nutrient deficiencies, Nutritional status, Protein-energy malnutrition.

INTRODUCTION

Chronic liver disease (CLD) is a broad diagnosis which includes two major subgroups, mainly cirrhotic and noncirrhotic. The precise duration of 6 months for defining CLD has now been questioned.[1] In the early stages, symptoms of CLD are subtle and the disease may remain undiagnosed for months to years. Children with CLD commonly present with jaundice followed by hepatosplenomegaly and abdominal distention. One-fourth of CLD patients however, have no jaundice.[2] Diagnosis is made on variable combinations of clinical, radiological, endoscopic and histological features. The incidence of CLD in the pediatric age group reported by an Indian study is 1.1% of the total admissions (55 out of 5,146) and the need for a high index of suspicion for diagnosis cannot be under-emphasized.[3.]

Malnutrition in CLD is common to all stages of the disease with 65–90% of patients with advanced disease having undernutrition and also seen to have a direct relationship with the severity of liver disease.[4] Children are particularly susceptible to malnutrition due to their higher energy needs especially for their growth. There is also higher risk of micronutrient deficiencies. Early identification and correction of micro- and macronutrient deficiencies lessens the chances of morbidity and mortality associated with CLD.[5] Even in the postliver transplantation patients, malnourishment is associated, not only with increased morbidity and mortality but also poorer growth and neurocognitive outcomes.

ETIOLOGY AND PATHOPHYSIOLOGY

Malnutrition in CLD is multifactorial, the causes being enumerated in Table 1. These are divided predominantly into three main groups viz, decreased intake, impaired metabolism and increased requirement. Decreased intake is secondary to anorexia and nausea which are associated with liver disease. Anorexia is attributed to changes in the amino acid metabolism which results in increased tryptophan levels and subsequent increase in brain serotonergic activity.

Tryptophan is the amino acid precursor to serotonin which regulates eating behavior.[6] Dysgeusia is associated with zinc and magnesium micronutrient deficiencies. Presence of splenomegaly, gastroparesis and ascites lead to early satiety. Further, iatrogenic causes like restrictive diets (salt restriction) and drugs like diuretics, binders like cholestyramine, frequent paracentesis and laxatives like lactulose hamper food metabolism and cause increased losses.

Impaired metabolism in CLD is mainly because of portal hypertension causing chronic mesenteric ischemia and mucosal edema leading to portal hypertensive enteropathy, increased mucosal permeability and villous atrophy. Deficiency of bile salts affects absorption of fat and fat-soluble vitamins. Cholestatic liver disease which is the most common cause of cirrhosis in children accentuates malnutrition by affecting bile salts metabolism and causing secondary steatorrhea. Up to 50% of long-chain

Table 1: Causes of malnutrition in chronic liver disease.

Decreased energy intake	• Anorexia • Dysgeusia • Early satiety
Increased energy needs	• Increased energy needs 150% estimated average requirement (EAR) • Catabolic state
Endocrine dysfunction	• Impaired growth hormone (GH)/insulin-like growth factors (IGF) axis • GH resistance
Malabsorption/ disordered metabolism	• Hypoglycemia due to glycogen deficit • Impaired protein synthesis with increased degradation • Fat malabsorption due to bile salt deficiency with bacterial overgrowth and portal hypertensive enteropathy • Pancreatic insufficiency in cystic fibrosis, progressive familial intrahepatic cholestasis (PFIC-1), Alagille syndrome

triglycerides (LCTs), fat-soluble vitamins and essential polyunsaturated fatty acids (PUFAs) may not be absorbed well in children with CLD. Deficiencies in long-chain polyunsaturated fatty acids (LcPUFAS), such as arachidonic acid and docosahexaenoic acid (DHA) are critical to neurologic growth and development and can develop within 8–12 weeks.[7]

Presence of growth hormone resistance [deficiency of insulin-like growth factors (IGF) and IGF-binding proteins (IGFBP)] further exacerbates growth hormone deficiency, commonly seen in noncirrhotic liver diseases. Energy utilization is also disorganized as hepatic and muscle glycogen stores are decreased leading to reduced availability of glucose as energy substrate, which results in increased degradation of proteins and fats through gluconeogenesis and ketosis, respectively. Also, in CLD there occurs a decrease in branched chain amino acids/aromatic amino acids (BCAA/AAA) ratio as observed in sepsis or major trauma.[8] Thus, sarcopenia is the most common complication of cirrhosis (up to 60% of patients).[9] Increased demand is because of catabolic state of the body with up to 34% of adult patients having a resting energy expenditure (REE) of 120% above the expected value.[10] Portal hypertension may cause chronic blood loss and iron deficiency anemia.

Deficiency of water- and fat-soluble vitamins and other micronutrients is prevalent in CLD.[11] The mechanisms of common deficiencies are detailed in Table 2.

NUTRITIONAL STATUS ASSESSMENT

Nutritional assessment is predominantly based on dietary history, anthropometric parameters and biochemical parameters (Table 3). It is well proven that nutritional status assessment is important in prognostication of CLD patients. However, there is no consensus about a simple well validated

Table 2: Micronutrient deficits in CLD: Etiopathogenesis and symptomatology.

Micronutrient deficient	Etiopathogenesis	Symptomatology
Thiamine	• Deceased Intake • Decreased absorption • Reduction of hepatic reserves	• Wernicke encephalopathy • Korsakoff dementia
Vitamin B_{12}	• Decreased intake • Decreased absorption • Reduction of hepatic reserves	• Anemia • Glossitis • Neurological symptoms
Folic acid	• Decreased intake • Decreased absorption • Reduction of hepatic reserves	
Retinol	• Decreased absorption • Impaired hepatic mobilization	• Dermatitis • Night blindness or photophobia • Increased risk of neoplastic disorders including HCC

Contd...

Contd...

Micronutrient deficient	Etiopathogenesis	Symptomatology
Vitamin K	• Decreased absorption • Reduction of the hepatic reserves	• Increased risk of bleeding
Vitamin D	• Decreased intake • Decreased absorption • Reduction of the exposure to UV light • Impaired liver hydroxylation in its active metabolite in liver	• Osteomalacia
Zinc	• Decreased intake • Diets with restriction of animal origin protein • Decreased absorption • Treatment with diuretics	• Dyguesia • Growth retardation • Dermatitis • Dysfunction of immune system • Increased ammonia genesis, risk of HE
Selenium	• Decreased intake • Decreased absorption	
Magnesium	• Decreased intake • Treatment with diuretics	• Rickets/osteomalcia

(HCC: hepatocellular carcinoma; HE: hepatic encephalopathy).

Table 3: Nutritional assessment in CLD patients.

Dietary record	24 hour recall method/7 days recall method (diary of food intake)
Biochemical assessment	• Serum proteins relate to liver disease severity than with the level of malnutrition • Albumin, prealbumin and retinol binding protein affected by hepatic dysfunction, use unreliable • Immunological parameters, such as lymphocytes levels, hypersensitivity skin test or complement levels—low sensitivity and specificity • Creatinine/height index is a reliable method if the patient's renal function is normal
Anthropometric parameters	• Weight and body mass index (BMI): Altered by electrolyte disturbances, renal failure and the presence of edema or ascites; low sensitivity and reliability • Skinfold thickness (tricep, bicep and subscapular) is less affected by hydropic changes—best methods for indirect assessment; low interobserver reproducibility
Bioelectrical impedance analysis (BIA)	Noninvasive, safe, easy to perform and relatively inexpensive and sensitive method that may provide prognostic information
Dynamometry (handgrip strength)	Most sensitive methods; follow-up possible; less available, difficult in small children; overestimates malnutrition severity
Indirect calorimetry	REE through Weir equation, by measuring oxygen consumption and carbon dioxide production, complicated, expensive
Subjective global assessment (SGA)	Elements of the clinical history and physical examination (weight, food intake, gastrointestinal symptoms, functional capacity, nutritional requirements, metabolic requirements and physical examination). Validated for the assessment of nutritional status in cirrhotic patients and may provide prognostic information

and reproducible method for quantification and classification of malnutrition in children or adults with liver disease.

TREATMENT

The goal of treatment is improvement of protein energy deficits with correction of micronutrient deficiencies and maintenance of positive nitrogen balance.

Cooking method: Food should be well cooked, given the patient's increased susceptibility to infections and should be distributed into 5-7 small daily meals in order to prevent protein overload and nausea/vomiting.[12] It is recommended to minimize overnight fasting period in order to avoid fasting periods longer than 6 hours and reduce the catabolism rate.

Energy: Carbohydrates form the base of most calories (approximately 50-60% of nonprotein calories) in all individuals. An energy content of 35-40 kcal/kg/day is usually sufficient to restore nutritional status and enhance liver regeneration. Complex carbohydrates, such as maltodextrin and glucose polymers can be particularly useful, as their use restricts the osmolality of feeds, while maintaining a high energy density greater than 1 kcal/mL.

Protein: Children with CLD require 2-3 g/kg/day of protein, but can tolerate up to 4 g/kg/day without developing encephalopathy.[13] Protein needs are higher in stress situations (such as bleeding, infection or surgery) provided that there is no renal dysfunction or encephalopathy. Children with CLD usually do not require protein restriction due to their increased growth needs. European Society for Clinical Nutrition and Metabolism (ESPEN) does not recommend regular use of BCAA enriched formula, given the higher cost and oral intolerance; instead recommends, in general, a diet rich in a whole protein formula.[14] Even in encephalopathy, the protein supplementation should not be stopped and may be restricted to 1-2 g/kg/day limited to the duration of encephalopathy.

Fat : In patients with steatorrhea, the diet content of long-chain fatty acids must be reduced at the expense of medium and short-chain fatty acid.[15] Medium chain triglycerides (MCTs), unlike LCTs do not require micellar solubilization to be transported into the enterocyte, and are transferred directly into the enterocyte and to the portal circulation without re-esterification. About 95% of MCTs are absorbed even in very cholestatic children, thus MCTs are critical in managing nutrition in children with CLD, where absorption of LCTs is highly compromised.[16] Although 30-50% of total fat should be provided as MCTs, care should be taken, not to eliminate LCTs from the diet, as they provide essential fatty acids.[17] In infant formulas, up to 70% of the total fat requirements can be given through MCTs.

Micronutrients: There is little consensus regarding the empirical use of multivitamin or other micronutrient supplements vs. cost-effectiveness of evaluation of nutritional deficiencies and for providing these supplements.

ESPEN suggests that empirical daily supplementation should be considered in all patients with CLD. In cholestatic disease, fat-soluble vitamins supplementation should be considered. Sodium restriction may be required in patients with ascites/edema unresponsive to diuretics, however making food more unpalatable for children. Fluid restriction should only be recommended in severe hyponatremia (Na$^+$ <120 mEq/mL) and is not indicated in compensated liver disease.

Alternative methods of feeding: Cirrhotic patients who cannot meet their nutritional requirements from oral food should be considered for starting enteral nutrition (EN) in order to prevent progression of malnutrition. Overnight nasogastric feeding plus daytime oral food ad libitum is also an alternative. The use of percutaneous endoscopic gastrostomy (PEG)/percutaneous endoscopic jejunostomy (PEJ) is associated with a higher risk of complications (due to ascites or varices) and is not recommended. Parenteral nutrition (PN) is a second choice in comparison to EN, but should be initiated if the patient cannot be fed orally or enterally.[18] This can occur in cases of severe hepatic encephalopathy (III/IV) and in the absence of cough reflex or impaired swallowing. The risk of infection is due to PN versus the risk of aspiration due to EN should always be weighed.

CONCLUSION

Malnutrition in CLD patients is omnipresent and multifactorial. Diagnosis is further challenging because of associated comorbidities and the routine anthropometric methods become ineffective. Most patients with CLD can have a practically normal diet with addition of supplements as necessary. Restrictions may be harmful and should be individualized. The treatment should be based on maintaining adequate protein and caloric intake and to correct micronutrient deficiencies.

REFERENCES

1. Mieli-Vergani G, Vergani D. Autoimmune liver disease. *Indian J Pediatr* 2002;69:93-98.
2. Arora NK, Lodha R, Mathur P, Arora N. Child with chronic liver disease. *Pediatr Today* 1998;1:207-211.
3. Dhole SD, Kher AS, Ghildiyal RG, Tambse MP. Chronic Liver Diseases in children: Clinical profile and histology. *J Clin Diagn Res* 2015;9:SC04-SC07.
4. Campillo B, Richardet JP, Scherman E, Bories PN. Evaluation of nutritional practice in hospitalized cirrhotic patients: results of a prospective study. *Nutrition* 2003;19:515-521.
5. Møller S, Bendtsen F, Christensen E, Henriksen JH. Prognostic variables in patients with cirrhosis and oesophageal varices without prior bleeding. *J Hepatol* 1994;21:940-946.
6. Laviano A, Cangiano C, Preziosa I, Riggio O, Conversano L. Plasma tryptophan levels and anorexia in liver cirrhosis. *Int J Eat Disord* 1997; 21:181-186.

7. Kelly DA, Proteroe S, Clarke S. Acute and chronic liver disease. In: Duggan C, Watkins JB, Koletzko B, Walker WA Eds):*Nutrition in Pediatrics*, 5th edn. Shelton: People's Medical Publishing House 2016:851-863.
8. McCullough AJ, Tavill AS. Disordered energy and protein metabolism in liver disease. *Semin Liver Dis* 1991;11:265-277.
9. Rivera Irigoin R, Abilés J. Nutritional support in patients with liver cirrhosis. *Gastroenterol Hepatol* 2012;35:594-601. Spanish.
10. Müller MJ, Böttcher J, Selberg O, Weselmann S, Böker KH. Hypermetabolism in clinically stable patients with liver cirrhosis. *Am J Clin Nutr.* 1999;69:1194-1201.
11. Silva M, Gomes S, Peixoto A, Torres-Ramalho P, Cardoso H. Nutrition in chronic liver disease. *GE Port J Gastroenterol* 2015; 31;22:268-276.
12. Mesejo A, Juan M, Serrano A. Liver cirrhosis and encephalopathy: clinical and metabolic consequences and nutritional support. *Nutr Hosp* 2008;23 Suppl:8-18. Spanish.
13. Charlton CP, Buchanan E, Holden CE, Preece MA, Green A. Intensive enteral feeding in advanced cirrhosis: reversal of malnutrition without precipitation of hepatic encephalopathy. *Arch Dis Child* 1992;67:603-607.
14. Plauth M, Cabré E, Riggio O, Assis-Camilo M, Pirlich M, Kondrup J. ESPEN Guidelines on Enteral Nutrition: Liver disease. *Clin Nutr* 2006;25:285-294.
15. O'Brien A, Williams R. Nutrition in end-stage liver disease: principles and practice. *Gastroenterology*. 2008;134:1729-1740.
16. Beath SV, Booth IW, Kelly DA. Nutritional support in liver disease. *Arch Dis Child*. 1993;69:545-547.
17. Nightingale S, Ng VL. Optimizing nutritional management in children with chronic liver disease. *Pediatr Clin North Am*. 2009;56:1161-1183.
18. Plauth M, Cabré E, Campillo B, Kondrup J, Marchesini G. ESPEN. ESPEN Guidelines on Parenteral Nutrition: *Hepatology. Clin Nutr* 2009;28:436-444.

31 Nutrition in Acute Kidney Injury

Sumantra Kumar Raut, Rajiv Sinha

ABSTRACT

Children suffering from acute kidney injury (AKI) are prone to develop undernutrition which can adversely affect outcome. Decrease intake of nutrition, increase energy and protein expenditure due to acute stress and loss of nutrients from hypercatabolism and loss in dialysate are the prime reasons for this prevalent under nutrition in children with acute kidney injury (AKI). Diagnosis of undernutrition in this setting is based on certain anthropometric and biochemical parameters keeping in mind that many of the convention tools will not correctly reflect the nutrition status in the presence of fluid retention. Nutritional support by the enteral and/or parenteral route seems to be clinically helpful. Unfortunately studies have shown that nutritional needs of critically ill children with AKI are not covered by nutrition support practices currently followed in most of the centers. There is no evidence based controlled trials of the effect of undernutrition or its therapy on the outcome of AKI. Better nutritional assessment and providing adequate nutrition by rational calculation of protein, calorie and other nutrients are the keys to success in managing malnutrition in sick child with AKI.
Keywords: Acute kidney injury, Nutrition, Protein energy wasting, Protein catabolic rate, Renal replacement therapy, Urea nitrogen appearance.

INTRODUCTION

Nutritional assessment is a valuable tool to monitor and follow-up children with acute kidney injury (AKI). Patients suffering from AKI are prone to develop malnutrition irrespective of their premorbid nutritional status. It can adversely affect the outcome especially in critically ill child.[1] Nutritional support by the enteral and/or parenteral route seems to be clinically helpful in most cases of AKI admitted in hospital and probably more complicated than that of chronic care hemodialysis patients as AKI patients have more significant protein catabolism, insulin resistance, altered fat metabolism, and AKI patients on continuous renal replacement therapy (CRRT) are at much greater risk of protein and micronutrient losses. There is no evidence based on controlled trials of the effect of malnutrition or its therapy on the outcome of AKI as it seems intrinsically unethical to starve a catabolic patient as control group. AKI is a inflammatory stress condition and the goal of nutritional support are the same as for any other critically ill patients with normal renal function [grade E recommendation, level IV evidence (nonrandomized study or historical controls)], such as adequate nutrition, prevent protein energy wasting, promote wound healing and tissue repair, support immune system function and to reduce morbidity and mortality.[2] Altered renal handling of the protein/electrolytes load due to AKI makes this more challenging.

PATHOGENESIS OF PROTEIN WASTING IN AKI

Acute kidney injury is a proinflammatory, pro-oxidative, and hypercatabolic states. It alters the water, electrolytes and acid-base balance of the body as also the metabolism of macronutrients responsible for inflammatory state. The major factors contributing towards altered nutrition in AKI patients are:

- **Decrease intake**: In critically ill children, nutrition support is often deferred until patients are medically stabilized which may delay adequate nutrition support for several days. This may be due to fluid restriction, digestive intolerance or need for interruption of feeding for diagnostic and therapeutic procedures. Pediatric patients are highly dependent on nutritional support due to their intrinsic high anabolic drive and lower nutrient reserves compared with adults. One also needs to remember that children with AKI may also have decrease appetite due to uremic toxins.
- **Increase need:** Demand of calorie may increase during AKI due to multiple factors like insulin resistance, increased secretion of catabolic hormones (glucagon, catecholamines, glucocorticoids), resistance to and/or suppressed secretion of growth/anabolic factors, critical illness/acute phase reaction/systemic inflammatory response (cytokines), metabolic acidosis and different proteases (like ubiquitine).[3]
- **Loss of nutrients:** Loss of nutritional substrates may occur due to hypercatabolism and also during renal replacement therapy. Amino acids have a small molecular weight (average 140 Daltons). Dialysis can be associated with the loss of up to 10–20 g amino acids in each session, depending on the modality and filter type.[2] With CRRT 10 to 15% of infused amino acids are lost everyday. Hypercatabolic state results in circulation of inflammatory mediators and increased secretion of catabolic hormones that leads to marked loss of lean body mass through the activation of muscle-protein catabolism, gluconeogenesis and changes in amino acid metabolism. Valencia et al. (Table 1) have classified AKI in three categories as per loss of urine urea nitrogen (UUN).[4] Patients with lower catabolism [loss of urine urea nitrogen (UUN) <5 g of the dietary nitrogen] have a low mortality rate (20%), nephrotoxicity is a useful example of this status, and they rarely need dialysis. Patients with moderate catabolism (nitrogen losses 5–10 g/day) have higher mortality rates (approximately 60%), surgery or infections are good examples and they may need dialysis. Finally, patients with marked catabolism (nitrogen losses >10 g/day) are those with sepsis or severe injuries and they have high mortality rate (80%) and they frequently need dialysis.

Table 1: Classification of AKI as per Urine nitrogen appearance (UNA).

Category	UUN loss as compare to dietary nitrogen (per day)	Nutrition management	Renal replacement requirement
Group 1	<5 g	Enteral	
Group 2	5–10 g	Enteral with parenteral	RRT to limit waste product accumulation
Group 3	>10 g	Parenteral	RRT/CRRT to limit waste product accumulation

(UUN: urine urea nitrogen; RRT: renal replaement therapy; CRRT: continuous renal replacement therapy; AKI: acute kidney injury).

METABOLIC ALTERATIONS IN AKI

In AKI there is a general disruption of the 'internal milieu' with specific changes in protein, carbohydrate and lipid metabolism (Table 2).[5,6] Kidneys are important site of gluconeogenesis and insulin metabolism, thus AKI leads to altered glucose homeostatis and insulin resistance. Hyperglycemia correlates with mortality in AKI. Hypoglycemia may be even more common and is often due to overzealous control of hyperglycemia. Dialysis is also an independent risk factor for the development of hypoglycemia. Protein catabolism is increased in AKI and its degradation/release from skeletal muscle is increased along with decreased protein synthesis. Amino acid extraction from plasma, hepatic gluconeogenesis and urea production are increased, while the synthesis of protein, apart from visceral and acute phase proteins is inhibited. Inflammation redirects protein utilization toward hepatic acute phase protein synthesis rather than anabolism.

Plasma levels of triglycerides (TGs) and very low-density lipoprotein (VLDL) levels are increased while those of total cholesterol, high-density lipoprotein (HDL) and low-density lipoprotein (LDL) are decreased owing to impaired lipolysis.[7] Fat clearance following parenteral administration of lipids is reduced in AKI particularly if the administration rate is high. Incidentally fatty acid oxidation is preserved in AKI, and lipids are a key energy substrate in AKI, as suggested by the low respiratory quotient measured in this setting.

BURDEN OF MALNUTRITION IN AKI

Almost half of critically sick patients with AKI may already have severe malnutrition on admission.[8] In-hospital mortality according to nutritional status as assessed by subjective global assessment (SGA) tool in 309 AKI patient by Fiaccadori et al. showed 80/129 in class C (severe malnutrition) vs. 24/132 in class A (normal nutrition) ($p < 0.001$).[9] A retrospective chart review of 167 pediatric patients admitted to the pediatric intensive care unit (ICU) of Texas children hospital with 39% having various degrees of AKI (as defined by RIFLE staging, Table 3)[10] showed I/F patients were more likely to be fasted versus receiving enteral/parenteral nutrition ($n = 813$ patient days) and to receive <90% of basal metabolic rate, i.e. BMR ($n = 832$ patient days).[11]

Table 2: Metabolic abnormalities in AKI.

Renal	Hepatic	Sketelal muscle	Fat tissue
Decrease gluconeogenesis	Increase gluconeogenesis	Decrease glucose uptake	Decrease glucose uptake
Increase glutamine metabolism	Decrease glycolysis	Increase glycolysis	Increase glycolysis
Decrease insulin metabolism	Increase urea synthesis	Increase lactate and alanine synthesis	Increase lactate synthesis
	Increase acute phase protein synthesis	Increase protein breakdown	Increase glycerol and fatty acid release
	Decrease albumin synthesis	Decrease protein synthesis	Reduced peripheral lipoprotein lipase by 50%
	Decrease hepatic triglyceride lipase level		Elevated TGs and VLDL; Decreased cholesterol, LDL and HDL

(TGS: triglycerides; VLDL: very low-density lipoprotein; LDL: low-density lipoprotein; HDL: high-density lipoprotein).

Table 3: RIFLE classification of renal failure.

Class	Serum creatinine/GFR	Urine output
Risk	↑ by 1.5 times/↓ 25–50%	<0.5 mL/kg/hour for 6 hours
Injury	↑ by 2 times/↓ >50%	0.5 mL/kg/hour for 12 hours
Failure	↑ by 3 times or absolute ↑ of 0.5mg/dL if baseline >4 mg/dL/↓ 75%	<0.3 mL/kg/hour for 24 hours, or anuria for 12 hours
Loss	Complete loss of kidney function (>4 weeks)	
End-stage kidney disease	Complete loss of kidney function (>3 months)	

The actual energy intake was significantly lower in I/F group compared with the no AKI/R group on day 3 (p <0.03). The actual median 5-day energy intake was lower relative to estimated BMR across all groups (no AKI/R: 24.9 kcal/kg/day versus 48.5 kcal/kg/day; I/F: 16.0 kcal/kg/day versus 46.3 kcal/kg/day; all p <0.001). Protein underfeeding was significantly greater than energy underfeeding in critically sick children with AKI (<68% of energy needs and <35% of protein needs were covered) by the nutrition practises. The study also revealed that patients with an R classification (HR, 2.7; CI 1.2–5.9; p = 0.02), but not I/F patients (HR, 1.5; CI, 0.5–4.5; p = 0.51) were significantly more likely to show chronic malnutrition (growth stunting) than patients with no AKI.

HOW TO ASSESS NUTRITION IN AKI

The lean body mass wasting and fat mass depletion occurring in AKI is best characterized by the term 'protein energy wasting' (PEW).[12]

As per current recommendation PEW is assessed on four categories of diagnostic criteria:
1. Biochemical (such as albumin or prealbumin)
2. Body weight loss
3. Decrease in muscle mass
4. Low energy and protein intakes

Diagnosis can be affirmed when at least one parameter is detected in three of the four nutritional variables (Table 4).[12]

PEW seems to be a frequent problem in AKI: As a matter of fact, severe malnutrition, as defined by SGA, can be observed in 40% of critically sick patients with AKI. Severe PEW adversely affects patient's outcome, such as length of hospital stay, risk of complications (sepsis, bleeding, arrhythmia, respiratory failure) and mortality. PEW is a consequence of low ingestion of nutrients, anorexia, prescription of restrictive diets, acidosis, action of uremic toxins, increased inflammatory cytokine production, oxidative stress, hypercatabolism, endocrine disorders, and presence of comorbidities and also due to loss of nutrients during dialysis.

A major problem in AKI is the lack of adequate tools for nutritional status evaluation at the individual level, and for monitoring of the effects of nutritional support. Various parameters and their utility as well as pitfalls in assessing nutrition in children with AKI are shown in Table 5.[9]

ANTHROPOMETRY

Evaluation of nutritional status in AKI based on anthropometry faces challenges due to alterations in body water distribution and external fluid balance from continuous flux in the hydration status.[9] Hence, different tools for nutritional assessment need to be standardized before using in critically ill

Table 4: Readily utilizable criteria for the clinical diagnosis of protein energy wasting in AKI/CKD.

Criteria	Variable	Value
Serum chemistry	Albumin Prealbumin Cholesterol	<3.8 g/dL <30 mg/dL (patient on RRT) <100 mg/dL
Body mass	BMI Total body fat	<23 <10%
Muscle mass	Reduced muscle mass Reduced mid arm circumference	>5% over 3 months >10% of 50th percentile of reference
Dietary intake	Low daily protein intake Low daily energy intake	<0.8 g/kg/day for 2 months <25 kcal/kg/day for 2 months

(AKI: acute kidney injury; CKD: chronic kidney disease; BMI: body mass index; RRT: renal replacement therapy).

Table 5: Nutritional markers of AKI and their limitations.

Markers	Limitations
White cell count	Lacks specificity
Albumin, prealbumin, cholesterol	Reduced regardless of protein wasting due to negative acute phase reactant
Change in body weight	Hypervolemia can mask muscle mass
Triceps skin fold, arm circumference	Mask by edema
Protein catabolic rate, protein nitrogen appearance	Calculation based on urea kinetics + collection in dialysate
Energy expenditure	Not accurate in critically ill child with altered body weight due to fluid retention
SGA, growth hormone/IGF-1, bioelectrical impedance	SGA is laborious and overall there is lack of substantiate data in AKI

(SGA: subjective global assessment; IGF-1: insulin like growth factor 1).

patients because of interference of factors related to changes in the hydration status.

Body mass index (BMI): Contrary to increase in body mass classically leading to increased mortality and worse prognosis in the general population, data analysis of 5,232 AKI patients on dialysis showed that patients with a higher BMI between 30 and 35 kg/m^2 had a 20% reduction in the survival.[13]

Bioelectrical impedance analysis (BIA): Bioelectrical impedance analysis is a noninvasive method, easy to use, and low cost. Unfortunately, it is not of much use in AKI as BIA assumes the concept that hydration of bodily tissues is constant in all individuals which is actually not in AKI patients due to changes in tissue hydration due to edema or diuretics usage.

Subjective global assessment (SGA): It is a simple but elaborative method based on loss of body weight, changes in food ingestion, gastrointestinal symptoms, functional capacity, and physical examination for loss of fat and body mass. Fiaccadori, et al. applied this evaluation in 309 AKI patients, of which 67% needed dialysis.[9] The study identified 58% who were malnourished, of which 16% were moderately malnourished (B class) and 42% severely malnourished (C class).

Calorimetry: With indirect calorimetry, Metha, et al. found that >50% AKI patients were hypometabolic, about 25% were normometabolic, and 17% were hypermetabolic.[14]

Urea nitrogen appearance (UNA) and protein catabolic rate (PCR): The standard nitrogen balance calculation method usually utilized for critically ill patients requires a creatinine clearance of 50 mL/minute/1.73 m^2, and is hence not reliable for AKI. In AKI, UNA and PCR are more accurate. Weighing scale beds or Bluetooth bed scales are required to accurately measure body weight which is required to accurately determine fluid and nitrogen balance which in turn is required for the calculation of the appropriate prescription of protein.[15]

UNA (g/day) = UUN + [(BUN2 − BUN1) × 0.6 x BW1] + (BW2 − BW1) × BUN2]
PCR g/day = UNA × 6.25
[BUN1: Initial collection of blood urea nitrogen, postdialysis (g/L)
BUN2: Final collection of blood urea nitrogen, predialysis (g/L)
BW1: Postdialysis weight (kg)
BW2: Predialysis weight (kg) of subsequent session
UUN: Urinary urea nitrogen (g/day)].[16]

BIOCHEMICAL PARAMETERS

Biochemical parameters [such as albumin, cholesterol, prealbumin, insulin-like growth factor 1 (IGF-1)] are commonly used in clinical practice and are also influenced by non-nutritional factors like loss of liver function and ongoing inflammatory status. Subjective global assessment and calculation of the nitrogen balance seem to be useful as screening parameters for worse prognosis and higher mortality in AKI patients but is laborious and often not feasible in a busy pediatric intensive care unit (PICU).

Visceral proteins (albumin, transferrin, prealbumin) are useful tool to monitor the metabolic response to nutritional support but one need to remember that factors like disruption of liver function, and inflammatory status can also result in reduction in the levels of these proteins. Albumin, the classic malnutrition marker can lose its accuracy in AKI patients, since the reduction in its levels is not always a consequence of the limited energy and protein substrate intake. Acute inflammation prioritizes the production of acute-phase proteins leading to less albumin production and making albumin of little value as a nutritional marker. Despite this it is still used as a predictor of mortality in AKI. Each 1 g/dL increase in serum albumin levels reduced the mortality by 44%. More recently, International Society of Renal Nutrition and Metabolism (ISRNM) recommended that levels below 3.8 g/dL of albumin can be used as a diagnostic parameter of PEW in AKI and chronic kidney disease.[12]

Low cholesterol level is also a predictor of complications and mortality. Extremely low cholesterol and LDL-cholesterol levels is seen in critically, ill patients with trauma, sepsis, dilution secondary to bleeding, and liver dysfunction.[17] Cholesterol level below 100 mg/dL is one of the criteria of clinical diagnosis of PEW in AKI as per the ISRNM.

Prealbumin (transthyretin) is a nutritional marker and a negative phase reactant as well. It has a half-life of about 2 days which is much shorter than albumin and hence reflects acute changes in nutrition more nicely. Although its interpretation can also be hindered by the presence of infection and inflammation it can be used as a predictor of survival and marker of nutritional support. In a longitudinal study evaluating 161 AKI patients, Perez, et al. showed that level below 11 mg/dL of prealbumin was associated with greater mortality in AKI.[18]

Insulin-like growth factor 1 is a peptide analogous to insulin whose synthesis is influenced by hormonal and nutritional factors. Its reduction is associated with a lower survival in AKI patients. Guimaraes, et al. showed that IGF-1 levels lower than 50.6 ng/mL had a significant association with decreased survival regardless of the presence of sepsis in 56 AKI patients.[19]

INDICATIONS FOR NUTRITIONAL SUPPORT AND ROUTE OF FEEDING IN AKI

The indications for nutritional support in AKI are similar as in other critically ill patients. The route of feeding depends on whether we have a functional gastrointestinal tract (GIT). Thus, in AKI the enteral route (EN) should be preferable for nutritional support if the GIT is functioning, or else parenteral route (PN) should be used when GIT cannot be used, or when EN appears inadequate to reach nutrient intake goals (Flowchart 1). Gastrointestinal motility can be impaired by AKI, dyselectrolytemia, medications, such as sedatives, opiates or catecholamines, mechanical ventilation, etc. AKI also leads to upper gastrointestinal bleeding. Although standard enteral formulae are adequate for the majority of critically ill patients with AKI, the use of disease-specific (renal) formulae designed for patients with chronic kidney disease may be preferred due to their high energy (2 kcal/mL) and protein content (70 g/L) and low electrolytes contents. Many a time parenteral supplementation of amino acids is likely to be required to meet the targeted nitrogen requirement. In sick patients with AKI, the combination of enteral and parenteral feeding allows successful nutritional support.[20] In most cases, the two routes can be considered complementary rather than mutually exclusive.[20] Standard formulae for parenteral nutrition (commercial three-in-one nutrient admixtures) containing both essential and nonessential amino acids are preferred in AKI needing RRT.

Flowchart 1: Decision tree for nutritional support in AKI patients with PEW or at risk of PEW.

(AKI: acute kidney disease; PEW: protein energy wasting; GI: gastrointestinal).

GOALS OF NUTRITIONAL SUPPORT IN AKI

As in other critically sick patient poor nutrient intakes and high catabolic rates put the patients with AKI in negative nitrogen balance which leads to negative outcomes associated with severe PEW. Attaining a positive nitrogen balance with gain in lean mass though ideal is often not practical in real world scenario in such patients. Optimum target may be considered to minimize muscle wasting and to preserve as much lean mass as possible by nutritional support. Regain of lean mass with positive nitrogen balance can be planned in due course during convalescence. Kyle UG, et al. showed that the nutritional needs of critically ill children with AKI were not covered by nutrition support practices and adequate nutrition support did not occur until 4–5 days after PICU admission.[11]

THERAPY

Enteral nutrition should be the initial modality for artificial nutrition in AKI; in most cases it should be integrated with PN. More intensive nutritional support is required with daily RRT (Table 6).[6]

Energy: In AKI energy expenditure measured by indirect calorimetry rarely exceeds 1.3 times the basal/resting energy expenditure (BEE/REE) calculated by the Harris-Benedict equation.[21] Optimum intake includes 20–25 nonprotein kcal/kg/day and intake of protein from 1.4 to 1.8 g/kg/day.[22] Study shows that with a same protein intake of 1.5 g/kg/day, an increase in energy provision up to 40 kcal/g/day did not improve nitrogen balance compared with lower energy intakes (30 kcal/kg/day); instead there was increase in metabolic complications (hypertriglyceridemia, hyperglycemia).[23] Similarly an intake of >2 g/kg/day protein is unlikely to contributes anything additional to protein synthesis, simply increasing urea production. The European Society of Clinical Nutrition and Metabolism (ESPEN) guideline suggests provision of energy not more than 25 kcal/kg/day (nonprotein), two-third

Table 6: Various nutritional parameters in AKI.

Parameters	Recommendations
Route of feeding	• Enteral route is preferred if gut is healthy • Parenteral route till full enteral nutrition is achieved
Timings	Within 24–48 hours of admission
Energy	20 to 30% above resting energy expenditure (REE) 40–50% protein 25–30% carbohydrate 20–25% lipids
Carbohydrate	50–60% of nonprotein calorie; 2–5 g/kg/day of glucose
Protein	1.5–2 g/kg/day; increase if on RRT
Lipids	30–40% of nonprotein calorie; 0.7–1.5 g/kg/day
Electrolytes	Monitor hyperkalemia; hypophosphatemia during continuous RRT

RRT: renal replacement therapy; AKI: acute kidney injury).

of nonprotein calories as glucose (not >5 g/kg/day) and one-third as lipids (1-1.5 g/kg/day).

Protein: Both essential amino acids (EAA) and non-EAA are recommended in AKI, since a higher provision of only EEA does not appear to be advantageous.[2] Amino acid losses through HD can be as much as 0.2 g amino acids/liter of ultra filtrate (5-10 g/day of protein), especially when high-flux filters and/or highly efficient modalities, such as CRRT or sustained low efficiency daily dialysis (SLEDD) are used. So the protein intake should be increased by at least 0.2 g/kg/day in these children. For patients with the milder nonoliguric AKI which are less catabolic and not needing RRT and who are likely to regain renal function in a few days, such as contrast nephropathy and drug toxicity, lower protein intakes (up to 0.8 g/kg/day) with adequate calorie intakes (30 kcal/kg/day) will be sufficient for short periods. The optimal energy to nitrogen ratio has not been clearly defined in patients with AKI. The resting energy expenditure (REE) in AKI patients is around 1,835 kcal/69 kg, i.e. 27 kcal/kg/day which is similar to other critical points. So the target intake for optimum nitrogen balance may be 25-30 kcal/kg of energy and 1.5 g/kg of proteins. Study on total parenteral nutrition with 30 vs. 40 kcal/day of energy with 0.25 g/kg nitrogen showed more problems with high calorie regimens in AKI patients related to increased fluid administration, increased insulin needs and high glucose levels. The protein intake also depends on the RRT modality being used, such as 0.8 g/kg/day on conservative management, 1-1.5 g/kg/day if on extracorporeal therapy and 1.5-2.0 g/kg/day if on continuous therapy.[24, 25]

Case example of the protein requirements for a child (weight 30 kg) with acute kidney injury either not on renal replacement therapy, or on intermittent hemodialysis or on continuous renal replacement therapy:

The calculation of protein requirements for a patient weighing 30 kg:
- Not on RRT: 0.6-1 g × 30 kg = 18-30 g protein/day
- Intermittent dialysis: 1.2 1.5 g (1.3 g) × 30 kg = 36-45 g protein/day
- CRRT: 1.7-2 g × 30 kg = 51-60 g protein/day

Carbohydrates: Recommendations suggest that two-third of total nonprotein calories (2-5 g/kg/day of glucose) should be administered. AKI patients on peritoneal dialysis can absorb approximately 40 to 50% of the total prescribed glucose in the dialysate and this contribution to be considered when calculating total requirements.

Lipids: European directives recommend lipids intake of 0.7-1.5 g/kg/day.[26] Some authors recommend the use of about 30% or one-third of total nonprotein calories, both using lipid emulsions composed of medium- and long-chain triglycerides. Since hepatic triglyceride lipase is decreased in AKI, serum triglycerides should be closely monitored and lipid administration in diet/total parenteral nutrition (TPN) should be discontinued whenever their levels exceed 400 mg/dL. To achieve the target of 30-35% of total nonprotein energy supply from lipids in the case of parenteral nutrition 0.8-1.2 g/kg/day of lipid from 10 to 30% lipid emulsions or as a part of the commercially available three-in-one total nutrient mixtures can be provided as infusion over 18-24 hours. Lipid losses through the filters do not occur during dialysis or filtration.

Micronutrients: There is scarcity of study on the requirements of minerals and vitamins in AKI patients as most of the studies are on patients with chronic kidney disease. In AKI patients micronutrients are lost mostly during dialysis (Table 7).[27] Serum levels of thiamine, folic acid and other water soluble vitamins are low in AKI patients on RRT. Approximately 265 μg of folic acid per/day is lost in the ultrafiltrate during CRRT. Supplementation with 1 mg/day of folic acid is recommended in CRRT. Some of the specialized renal enteral feeds contain 1 mg folic acid per liter and hence additional supplementation is unnecessary. Excessive amounts of vitamin C and retinol supplementation may be deleterious to AKI patients as vitamin C is converted to oxalate and in renal failure oxalate is not adequately removed by RRT which accumulates in the renal tubules and exacerbates the existing AKI and potentially limits renal recovery.[28] Hence, vitamin C supplementation is limited to 100 mg in intermittent HD and 100-200 mg for CRRT. The 1,25 (OH)D levels may remain within the normal range until a severe degree of vitamin D deficiency is reached. Vitamin D therapy [60 000 IU × two doses] administered to critically ill children, demonstrated significant increases in serum 25 (OH) D but 25-hydroxy vitamin D supplementation for prolong period can cause hypercalcemia, hypercalciuria. Levels of trace elements are also low due to acute phase reaction/critical illness, variable protein binding, redistribution of elements between plasma and tissues, dilution and varying concentrations of trace elements in dialysis/hemofiltration fluids. Selenium, chromium, copper and zinc can be removed from plasma by convective/diffusive RRTs.[29] Continuous venovenous filtration (CVVH) is associated with reduced plasma selenium, chromium and copper levels and zinc was detected in effluent fluid in continuous venovenous hemo diafiltration (CVVHDF), but zinc balance was surprisingly not negative owing to the zinc content of PN and replacement fluid solutions, and its presence as a contaminant of the anticoagulant solution (trisodium citrate).[30] In AKI plasma retinol levels should be maintained with supplementation especially if continuous modalities of RRT are used. No supplementation of other fat-soluble vitamins is usually necessary in AKI.

Table 7: Dialysate losses of micronutrients and recommended replacement.

Micronutrients	Mean dialysate losses/day	Recommendations (parenteral)
Vitamin B_1	4.1 mg	3 mg
Vitamin C	10 mg	100 mg
Vitamin E	No data	10 IU
Zinc	0.2 mg	6.5 mg
Chromium	25 μmol	15 μmol
Selenium	110 μg	60 μg
Copper	0.41 mg	1 mg

Highly efficient modalities of RRT often induce hypophosphatemia and hypomagnesemia.

Parenteral nutrition solutions should be compounded using 20% amino acids, 50% to 60% dextrose, and 20% to 30% lipids to reduce volume. Parenteral nutrition should not be used to correct electrolyte abnormalities, and additional intravenous supplementation may be needed for electrolyte abnormalities. Trace elements are administered 2-3 times per week.

A standard nutrition prescription of a child with AKI is shown in Table 8.

Table 8: Example of nutrition chart for a 30 kg child with AKI on hemodialysis.

An 8 year-old boy weighing 30 kg who is admitted with a diagnosis of hemolytic uremic syndrome and presently undergoing alternate day hemodialysis with an ultrafiltrate of 1 liter per session and having an urine output of 350 mL/day with mild edema. His investigations show—Na: 140 meq/L, K: 5.2 meq/L, Ca: 8.8 mg/dL, PO_4: 5.5 mg/dL. He has stable vitals and is able to take orally.

Nutrient parameter	Quantity	Comments
Energy	30 kcal/kg/day = 900 kcal (non protein)	REE + moderate catabolism
Volume	1250 mL/day (urine output + insensible loss + daily basis ultrafiltrate)	Energy dense nutrition is required, insensible loss 350–400 mL/m², ultrafiltrate 1 L for 2 days
Protein	1.5 mg/kg/day = 45 g	Moderate catabolism (UNA of 5–10 mg/day) + RRT losses
Carbohydrate	Two-third of nonprotein energy = 120 g/day	<5 g/kg/day
Lipids	One-third of nonprotein energy = 353 g/day	<1.5 g/kg/day
Vitamin K	4 mg/week	Specially if on antibiotics
Vitamin E	10 IU/day	
Niacin	20 mg/day	
Thiamine	1.5 mg/day	
Riboflavin	1.5–1.7 mg/day	
Pantothenic acid (B_6)	5–10 mg/day	
Vitamin C	60–125 mg/day	Excess supplements can cause oxalosis
Biotin	150–300 µg/day	
Folic acid	1 mg/day	
Vitamin B_{12}	4 µg/day	
Zinc	20 mg	
Vitamin A		Avoid
Sodium	2.0–3.0 g/day	Based on blood pressure, edema; to replaced the loss in diuretic phase
Potassium	2.0–3.0 g/day	Avoid initially as he is having high K; replace loss in diuretic phase
Phosphorus	100 mg	Protein in g × 15 = PO_4 in mg (approx) avoid during low flux dialysis
Calcium		Maintain serum value within normal limits

OUTCOME

Studies on effects of nutritional support on patient outcome in AKI are largely underpowered and in pediatrics it is scarce. Outcome results are also variable. Whereas in one retrospective study, parenteral nutrition was associated with better outcome, in the other three prospective studies no survival advantage was demonstrated.[31] In a prospective trial assessing calorie and protein needs of critically ill patients with anuria requiring CRRT, nitrogen balance was positively related to protein intake (better with >2 g/kg/day). Negative nitrogen balance has been associated with worse ICU and hospital outcomes in AKI patients receiving mixed nutritional support (enteral plus parenteral), though the use of the enteral route had a statistically significant better outcome. Enteral nutrition was also associated with a positive outcome in a large observational cohort of critically ill AKI patients. Physiologically, it has been seen that intravenously or enterally administered amino acids increases renal plasma flow and glomerular filtration rate in animals and in normal subjects, and glomerular filtration rate (GFR) can improve moderately but currently this amounts to only indirect evidence.

CONCLUSION

Patients with AKI are at high-risk of malnutrition, and the presence of malnutrition in the context of AKI has been linked to increased morbidity and mortality. The goals of nutrition support in AKI include prevention of protein energy wasting, preservation of lean body mass and nutritional status, avoidance of metabolic derangements and complications, improvement of wound healing, and support of immune function. The nutritional needs of critically ill children with AKI are not covered by nutrition support practices currently followed in most of the centers, moreover adequate nutrition support does not occur until 4–5 days after PICU admission, subjecting critically ill children to an extra burden of starvation and underfeeding. In absence of measured energy expenditure in children with AKI, estimation of energy needs should be based on predicted BMR. Efforts should be made to develop better nutritional assessment, to provide adequate nutrition in critically ill patients with AKI, and to prospectively evaluate risk and outcomes of nutrition management during AKI.

KEY LEARNING POINTS

- Patients with AKI are at high-risk of malnutrition which leads to increased morbidity and mortality.
- Most PICUs are not delivering optimum nutrition to children with AKI.
- Protein deficiency seems to be more prevalent than energy deficiency.
- Appropriate anthropometric and biochemical parameters are required to correctly reflect the nutrition status in the presence of fluid retention.
- Nutritional support by the enteral and/or parenteral route seems to be clinically helpful by rationally calculating the requirements of different nutrients.

REFERENCES

1. Metnitz PG, Krenn CG, Steltzer H, et al. Effect of acute renal failure requiring renal replacement therapy on outcome in critically ill patients. *Crit Care Med* 2002;30: 2051-2058.
2. Cano N, Fiaccadori E, Tesinski P, et al. ESPEN Guidelines on enteral nutrition: adult renal failure. *Clin Nutr* 2006;25:295-310.
3. Druml W. Nutritional management of acute renal failure. *Am J Kidney Dis* 2001; 37(Suppl. 1): 589-594.
4. Valencia E, Marin A, Hardy G. Nutritional therapy for acute renal failure. *Curr Opin Clin Metab Care* 2009;12:241-244.
5. Casaer MP, Mesotten D, Schetz MRC. Bench-to bedside review: metabolism and nutrition. *Crit Care* 2008; 12: 222-232.
6. Sethi SK, Maxvold N, Bunchman T, Jha P, Kher V. Nutritional management in the critically ill child with acute kidney injury: a review. *Pediatr Nephrol* 2017;32: 589-601.
7. Druml W, Fischer M, Sertl S, et al. Fat elimination in acute renal failure: long chain versus medium-chain trygliceride. *Am J Clin Nutr* 1992;5:468-472.
8. Zappitelli M, Goldstein SL, Symons JM, *et al*. Protein and calorie prescription for children and young adults receiving continuous renal replacement therapy: a report from the Prospective Pediatric Continuous Renal replacement Therapy Registry Group. *Crit Care Med* 2008;28:3239-3245.
9. Fiaccadori E, Lombardi M, Leonardi S, Rotelli CF, Tortorella G. Prevalence and clinical outcome associated with pre-existing malnutrition in acute renal failure: a prospective cohort study. *J Am Soc Nephrol* 1999;10:581-593.
10. Bellomo R, Ronco C, Kellum JA, Mehta RL, Palevsky P. Acute renal failure – definition, outcome measures, animal models, fluid therapy and information technology needs: the Second International Consensus Conference of the Acute Dialysis Quality Initiative (ADQI) Group. *Crit Care* 2004;8:204-212.
11. Kyle G, Arikan AA, Orellana RA, Jorge A. Nutrition Support among Critically Ill Children with AKI. *Clin J Am Soc Nephrol* 2013;8:568-574.
12. Fouque D, Kalantar AK, Kopple J, Chauveau P, Cuppari L. A proposed nomenclature and diagnostic criteria for protein-energy wasting in acute and chronic kidney disease. *Kidney Int* 2008;73:391-398.
13. Druml W, Metnitz B, Schaden E, Bauer P. Impact of body mass on incidence and prognosis of acute kidney injury requiring renal replacement therapy. *Intensive Care Med* 2010;36:1221-1228.
14. Mehta NM, Bechard LJ, Dolan M, Ariagno K, Jiang H. Energy imbalance and the risk of overfeeding in critically ill children. *Pediatr Crit Care Med* 2011;12: 398-405.
15. Druml W. Nutritional support in acute renal failure. In: Mitch W, Klahr S (Eds):. *Handbook of Nutrition and the Kidney*. 5th edn. Philadelphia: Lippincott Williams & Wilkins 2005. 95-114.
16. Gervasio JM, Cotton AB. Nutrition support therapy in acute kidney injury: distinguishing dogma from good practice. *Curr Gastroenterol Rep* 2009; 11: 325-331.
17. Gordon BR, Parker TS, Levine DM, Saal SD, Wang JC. Low lipid concentrations in critical illness implications for preventing and treating endotoxemia. *Crit Care Med* 1996;24:584-589.
18. Perez JR, Bes-Rastrollo M, Monedero P, Irala J, Lavilla FJ. Impact of prealbumin levels on mortality in patients with acute kidney injury: an observational cohort study. *J Ren Nutr* 2008;18:262-268.

19. Guimaraes SM, Lima EQ, Cipullo JP, Lobo SM, Burdmann EA. Low insulin growth factor-1 and hypocholesterolemia as mortality predictors in acute kidney injury in the intensive care unit. *Crit Care Med* 2008;36:3165-3170.
20. Scheinkestel CD, Kar L, Marshall Ket, al. Prospective randomized trial to assess caloric and protein needs of critically ill, anuric, ventilated patients requiring continuous renal replacement therapy. *Nutrition* 2003;19:909-916.
21. Cano N, Aparicio M, Brunori G, et al. ESPEN Guidelines on Parenteral Nutrition. Parenteral nutrition in adult renal failure. *Clin Nutr* 2009;28:401-414.
22. Btaiche IF, Mohammad RA, Alaniz C, et al. Amino acid requirements in critically ill patients with acute kidney injury treated with continuous renal replacement therapy. *Pharmacotherapy* 2008;28:600-613.
23. Fiaccadori E, Maggiore U, Rotelli C, et al. Effects of different energy intakes on nitrogen balance in patients with acute renal failure: a pilot study. *Nephrol Dial Transplant* 2005;20:1976–1980.
24. Fiaccadori E, Parenti E, Maggiore U. Nutritional support in acute kidney injury. *J Nephrol* 2008;21:645-656.
25. Berbel MN, Pinto MPR, Ponce D, Balbi AL. Nutritional aspects in acute kidney injury. *Rev Assoc Med Bras* 2011;57:587-592.
26. Singer P, Berger MM, VanderBerghe G, Biolo G, Calder P. ESPEN Guidelines on Parenteral Nutrition: intensive care. *Clin Nutr* 2009;28:387-400.
27. Chiolero R, Berger MM. Nutritional Support during renal replacement therapy. In: Ronco C, Bellomo R, Kellum JA (Eds): *Acute Kidney Injury*. Basel: Karger; 2007: 267-74.
28. Lipkin AC, Lenssen P. Hypervitaminosis A. Pediatric hematopoietic stem cell patients requiring renal replacement therapy. *Nutr Clin Prac* 2008;23:621–629.
29. Nakamura AT, Btaiche IF, Pasko DA, et al. In vitro clearance of trace elements via continuous venovenous hemofiltration. *J Ren Nutr* 2004;14:214–219.
30. Klein CJ, Moser-Veillon PB, Schweitzer A, et al. Magnesium, calcium, zinc, and nitrogen loss in trauma patients during continuous renal replacement therapy. *J Parenter Enteral Nutr* 2002;26:77–92.
31. Fiaccadori E, Regolisti G, Cabassi A. Specific nutritional problems in acute kidney injury, treated with non-dialysis and dialytic modalities. *NDT Plus* 2010;3:1–7.

PART 8: MISCELLANEOUS

32 Food Intolerance and Allergy

Edwin Dias

ABSTRACT

Food allergy is triggered by an immune reaction which is formed against food proteins, whereas food intolerances can be facilitated by any food constituent and do not include immunological mechanisms. The treatment of food allergies involves strict elimination from the diet of the offending food antigen, either by utilizing of a hypoallergenic infant formula or a detailed elimination diet. In patients with food intolerances small quantities of the allergenic food items are generally tolerated (dose-response relationship). Infants and young children with gastrointestinal food allergies, if presenting with recurrent vomiting or diarrhea, are at high-risk of failure to thrive, predominantly if there are associated feeding difficulties. Proper identification of food allergies and intolerances in infancy and childhood is essential in order to prevent growth impairment and nutritional deficiency states. Close monitoring of dietary intake and growth parameters, standard re-assessment of persistent allergies and dietary introduction of tolerated food proteins are vital steps in the nutritional management of children with food allergies.

Keyword: Diarrhea, Elimination diet, Faliure to thrive, Gastrointestinal food allergy, Food allergy, Food intolerance, Offending for antigens, Recurrent vomiting.

INTRODUCTION

Food allergy represent the failure to achieve or sustain immune tolerance to one or several food proteins.[1] There has been a recent remarkable increase in the incidence of food allergies in several developed countries (6% in children, 2% in adults).[2] Although, this rise in food allergies has been ascribed to low rates of early childhood infection or introduction to endotoxin (hygiene hypothesis), the exact basis for allergies increase remain unclear. Cow's milk, egg, peanut, tree nuts, fish, soybean and wheat causes about 95% of food allergies.[2,3] These allergies may present clinically with a range of systemic reactions (urticaria, angioedema, anaphylaxis), or involve the skin, gut and respiratory tract.[2,3] Multiple food allergies are frequent occur primarily in early childhood.

Food intolerance is characterized by an unfavorable reaction to any (nonprotein) food constituent without interacting with the immune system.[1] Examples are malabsorption of fat or carbohydrates which can present with abdominal bloating, pain or diarrhea.[4] Food intolerances may be a sign of underlying gastrointestinal conditions (e.g. celiac disease, intestinal lymphangiectasia) or metabolic disorders (e.g. hereditary fructose intolerance). Adverse food reactions is described in Box 1. In order to distinguish whether there is an adverse food reaction, many conditions have to be ruled out. The differential diagnosis of adverse food reactions has been listed in Box 2.

In order to make an appropriate diagnosis, the natural history and the cross reactivity between different food allergies is a must (Table 1). The clinical features and implications of IgE-mediated food allergy is elucidated in Table 2.

The treatment of food allergies is based on the exclusion of specific food proteins until tolerance has been established.[3-5] The treatment of food intolerance follows similar principles but may fluctuate according to the

Box 1: Adverse food reactions.

Food intolerance
Host Factors
Enzyme deficiencies—lactase (primary or secondary), fructase (maturational delay)
Gastrointestinal disorders—inflammatory bowel disease, irritable bowel syndrome
Idiosyncratic reactions—caffeine in soft drinks ("hyperactivity")
Psychologic—food phobias
Migraines (rare)
Food Factors
Infectious organisms—*Escherichia coli, Staphylococcus aureus, Clostridium*
Toxins—histamine (scombroid poisoning), saxitoxin (shellfish)
Pharmacologic agents—caffeine, theobromine (chocolate, tea), tryptamine (tomatoes), tyramine (cheese)
Contaminants—heavy metals, pesticides, antibiotics
Food hypersensitivities
IgE-Mediated
Cutaneous—urticaria, angioedema, morbilliform rashes, flushing, contact urticaria
Gastrointestinal—oral allergy syndrome, gastrointestinal anaphylaxis
Respiratory—acute rhinoconjunctivitis, bronchospasm
Generalized—anaphylactic shock, exercise-induced anaphylaxis
Mixed IgE- and Cell-Mediated
Cutaneous—atopic dermatitis, contact dermatitis
Gastrointestinal—allergic eosinophilic esophagitis and gastroenteritis
Respiratory—asthma
Cell—Mediated
Cutaneous—contact dermatitis, dermatitis herpetiformis
Gastrointestinal—food protein-induced enterocolitis, proctocolitis, and enteropathy syndromes, celiac disease
Respiratory—food-induced pulmonary hemosiderosis (Heiner syndrome)
Unclassified
Cow's milk–induced anemia
Immunoglobulin E (IgE)

Box 2: Differential diagnosis of adverse food reactions.

Gastrointestinal disorders (with vomiting ond/or diarrhea)
Structural abnormalities (pyloric stenosis, Hirschsprung disease)
Enzyme deficiencies (primary or secondary):
Disaccharidase deficiency—lactase, fructase, sucrase-isomaltase
Galactosemia
Malignancy with obstruction
Other: Pancreatic insufficiency (cystic fibrosis), peptic disease
Contaminants and additives
Flavorings and preservatives—rarely cause symptoms:
Sodium metabisulfite, monosodium glutamate, nitrites
Dyes and colorings—very rarely cause symptoms (urticaria, eczema):
Tartrazine
Toxins:
Bacterial, fungal (aflatoxin), fish-related (scombroid, ciguatera)
Infectious organisms:
Bacteria *(Salmonella, Escherichia coli, Shigella)*
Virus (rotavirus, enterovirus)
Parasites [*Giardia, Akis simplex* (in fish)]
Accidental contaminants:
Heavy metals, pesticides
Pharmacologic agents:
Caffeine, glycosidal alkaloid solanine (potato spuds), histamine (fish), serotonin (banana, tomato), tryptamine (tomato), tyramine (cheese)
Psychologic Reactions
Food phobias

underlying condition. The general scheme which can be followed to assess and manage a food allergy in a child is given as a Flowchart 1).

Gastrointestinal food allergies presenting with excessive vomiting, diarrhea or reduced protein/energy intake may be the basis for failure to thrive.[4,5] The exact and early diagnosis of food allergies is therefore primary in order to avoid nutritional deficiency states and growth impairment.[5]

PATHOPHYSIOLOGY

Two main types of food allergy can be illustrated based on the timing of the clinical reaction in relation to the food ingestion.[1-3] Sudden onset reactions take place within minutes after ingestion of a food box. In these patients the allergy is mediated by food-specific immunoglobulin E (IgE) antibodies.[2] Delayed onset reactions take place within several hours to days after ingestion and may include gut, skin or respiratory tract. These reactions are cell-mediated (lymphocytes, eosinophils) and typically lack confirmation of systemic IgE sensitization (skin prick tests and food-specific serum IgE antibodies negative).[2,3,6]

A mounting number of food allergens have been categorized, e.g. β-lactoglobulin in milk, ovomucin in hen's egg or ara c1 in peanut.[2] On each of these proteins, epitope regions have been mapped which interrelate with either IgE antibody or T-cell receptor. Conformational epitopes (with a

Table 1: Natural history of food allergy and cross-reactivity between common food allergies.

Food	Usual age at onset of allergy	Cross reactivity	Usual age at resolution
Hen's egg white	6–24 months	Other avian eggs	7 years (75% of cases resolve)
Cow's milk	6–12 months	Goat's milk, sheep's milk, buffalo milk	5 years (76% of cases resolve)
Peanuts	6–24 months	Other legumes, peas, lentils; coreactivity with tree nuts	Persistent (20% of cases resolve by 5 years)
Tree nuts	1–2 years; in adults, onset occurs after cross reactivity to birch pollen	Other tree nuts; coreactivity with peanuts	Persistent (20% of cases resolve by 7 years)
Fish	Late childhood and adulthood	Other fish (low cross reactivity with tuna and swordfish)	Persistent
Shellfish	Adulthood (in 60% of patients with this allergy)	Other shellfish	Persistent
Wheat	6–24 months	Other grains containing gluten	5 year (80% of cases resolve)
Soybeans	6–24 months	Other legumes	2 year (67% of cases resolve)
Kiwi	Any age	Banana, avocado, latex	Unknown
Apples, carrots, and peaches	Late childhood and adulthood	Birch pollen, other fruits, nuts	Unknown

Table 2: Clinical implications of cross-reactive proteins in immunoglobulin E-mediated allergy.

Food family	Risk of allergy to ≥1 member (%; approximate)	Feature(s)
Legumes	5	Main causes of reactions are peanut, soya, lentil, lupine, and garbanzo
Tree nuts (e.g. hazel, walnut, brazil)	35	Reactions are often severe
Fish	50	Reactions can be severe
Shellfish	75	Reactions can be severe
Grains	20	
Mammalian milks	90	Cow's milk is highly cross-reactive with goat's or sheep's milk (92%) but not with mare's milk (4%)
Rosaceae (rock) fruits	55	Risk of reactions to more than three related foods is very low (<10%)
Latex-food	35	For individuals allergic to latex, banana, kiwi, and avocado are the main causes of reactions

Source: Sicherer SH. Food allergy. *Lancet* 2002;360:701-710.

Flowchart 1: The general scheme to assess and manage a food allergy in a child.

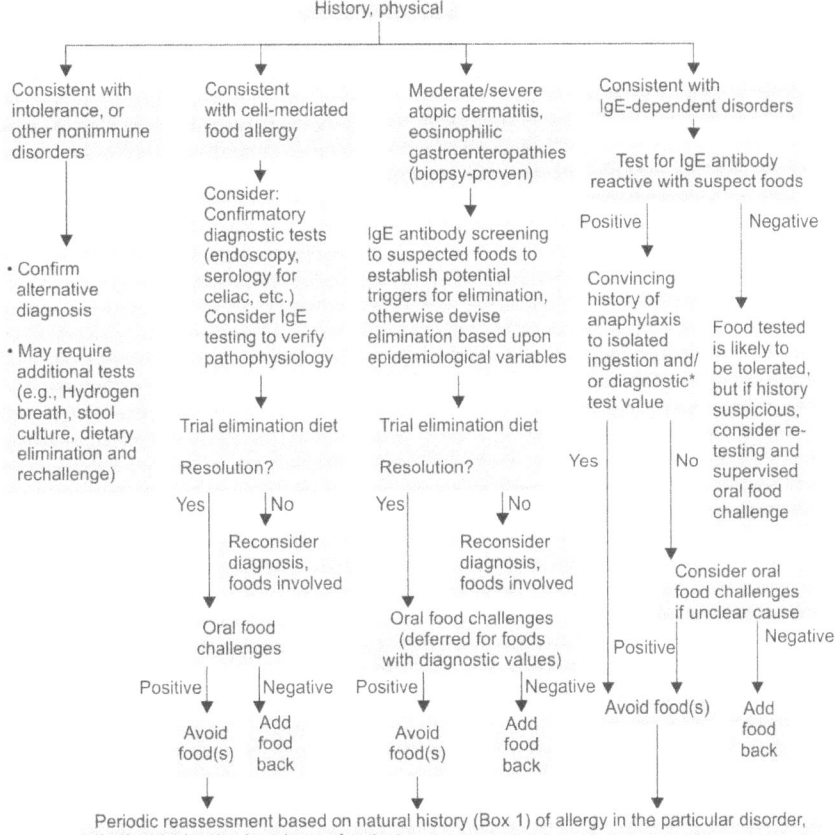

3-dimensional structure) may get inactivated by heating or acidification. For example, egg allergic patients may tolerate baked egg while uncooked egg causes unfavorable reactions.

CLINICAL MANIFESTATIONS OF FOOD ALLERGY

Food allergy may possibly present with a varied range of clinical manifestations.[3] Immediate reactions typically comprise of urticaria, angioedema, oral tingling or itching, vomiting or diarrhea. Anaphylaxis is a severe immediate type reaction with respiratory compromise (wheeze, stridor and cough) and/or hypotonia or collapse.[7] Anaphylaxis may be triggered in response to small doses of allergen and can be grave mainly in adolescents and young adults with concomitant unstable asthma.[7]

Delayed reactions consist chiefly of gastrointestinal or cutaneous reactions.[3,4,8] The contribution of food allergy in respiratory disorders, such as asthma, is not well elucidated. Atopic dermatitis with starting within the first months of life is to a large extent related to food allergy.[3] The gastrointestinal reactions can be divided into food protein-induced enterocolitis syndrome (FPIES) and proctocolitis.[4,8] Enteropathy and proctocolitis may come about in exclusively breastfed infants,[9] whereas FPLES seems to be caused by direct ingestion of the allergen by the infant.[10] Recently, eosinophilic esophagitis has been documented as a complication related to food allergy that often responds to dietary elimination.[11]

LACTOSE INTOLERANCE

Lactose is a disaccharide that is digested into glucose and galactose by a tiny intestinal brush border enzyme, lactase. Failure to absorb lactose will conclude in bacterial fermentation of the sugar, present as flatulence, diarrhea, acidic stools and perianal skin excoriation. Lactose malabsorption should not be puzzled with cow's milk allergy.[3,4] Dietary lactose restriction is usually adequate to control gastrointestinal symptoms. Secondary forms of lactose intolerance may be short-lived and resolve after the underlying gastrointestinal condition has remitted, e.g. viral gastroenteritis or celiac disease.

INVESTIGATION

The investigation of food allergy depends on three pillars: Coverage of food-specific serum IgE antibodies (by Radio-allergo-sorbent test (RAST) or CAP-FETA),[2] skin prick testing[6] and food challenge. In recent times, atopy patch testing has been recommended as a latest test for delayed food allergy, but its exact role has remained an area of current research.[12] Patients with confirmed food allergy must be reassessed on a regular basis in order to notice the development of tolerance to the offending food. This will often need open food challenges in order to demonstrate tolerance or ongoing allergies. Due to the risk of anaphylaxis these challenges should be taken care by a skilled allergist with access to resuscitation equipment.[7]

DIETARY MANAGEMENT OF FOOD ALLERGY

In children with specific IgE-mediated food allergy, e.g. cow's milk, egg or peanut, all food having the offending antigen needs to be kept away from its complications. As allergens are frequently masked in manufactured food products, this involves careful reading of ingredient labels.[5] In infants, allergies to multiple foods are common. For example, in infants with cow's milk allergy, concomitant, allergy to egg, soya or wheat may be present.[3]

Several hypoallergenic formulas are available for the treatment of infants with cow's milk and soy allergy. These hypoallergenic formulas are adjusted by at least 90% of infants with cow's milk allergy.[13] Cross-reactivity between cow's milk and soy is comparatively frequent in infants. Soy formula is no longer considered as a first-line cow's milk alternative mainly in infants under 6 months.[14] In breastfed infants, a maternal elimination diet may be valuable as intact food antigens in breast milk can elicit allergic manifestations in the infant.[9] However, the clinical benefit of maternal elimination diets is of importance. An adequate maternal intake of protein and micronutrients (recommended maternal calcium intake 1.2 g/day provided as separate portions distributed throughout the day) requirements has to be maintained.

There are two major types of hydrolyzed cow's milk formula, partially hydrolyzed and extensively hydrolyzed formula.[13,15] Partially hydrolyzed formula may play a role in allergic anticipation but it is not suitable for infants with well-known clinical signs of cow's milk allergy.[16] These infants have need of an extensively hydrolyzed formula or, if not tolerated, an amino acid-based formula.[15] In infants older than 6 months soy may also be a suitable substitute.[14] A dietician is usually mandatory to monitor broad-based elimination diets for nutritional adequacy.[5]

CONCLUSION

Hypoallergenic formulas (extensively hydrolyzed formula or amino acid-based formula) are part of the treatment of cow's milk allergy in formula fed infants. Soy formula may be appropriate in older infants, but cross-reactivity between cow's milk and soy protein are quite common.

- In breastfed infants with food allergic manifestations (e.g. early-onset atopic dermatitis, food protein-induced proctocolitis), a maternal elimination diet may control symptoms in the infant. Prolonged maternal elimination diets should be overseen by a dietician.
- Lactose intolerance is the most familiar food intolerance and is treated with a low-lactose diet. Causes of secondary lactose intolerance, such as celiac disease, should be considered in the differential diagnosis.

REFERENCES

1. Johansson SG, Bieber T, Dahl R, et al. Revised nomenclature for allergy for global use: Report of the nomenclature review committee of the world allergy organisation October 2003. *J Allergy Clin mmunol* 2004; 113:832-836.
2. Sampson HA. Update on food allergy. *J Allergy Clin Immunol* 2004; 113:805-819.
3. Hill DJ, Hosking CS, Heine RG. Clinical spectrum of food allergy in children in Australia and South East Asia: Identification and tatgets for treatment. *Ann Med* 1999;31:272-281.
4. Heine RG. Pathpphysiology, diagnosis and treatment of food protein induced gastrointestinal disease. *Curr Opin Allergy Clin Immunol* 2004; 2:221-29.
5. Mofidi S. Nutritional management of pediatric food hypersensitivity. *Pediatrics* 2003; 111:1645-1653.
6. Hill DJ, Heine RG, Hosking CS. The diagnostic value of skin prick testing in children with food allergy. *Pediatr Allergy Immunol* 2004; 15:435-441.
7. Sampson HA, Murioz-Furlong A, Campbell RL, et al. Second symposium on the definition and management of anaphylaxis: summary report-second national institute of allergy and infectious disease/food allergy and anaphylaxis network symposium. *J Allergy Clin Immunol* 2006; 117:391-397.

8. Sicherer SH. Clinical aspects of gastro intestinal food allergy in childhood. *Pediatrics* 2003; 111:1609-1616.
9. Jarvinen KM, Makinen-Kiljunen S, Suomalainen H. Cow's milk challenge through human milk evokes immune responses in infants with cow's milk allergy. *Allergy J Pediatr* 1999; 135:506-512.
10. Nowak-Wegryn A, Sampson HA, Wood RA, Sicherer SH. Food protein induced enterocolitis syndrome caused by solid food proteins. *Pediatrics* 2003; 111:829-835.
11. Furuta GT, Straumann A. The pathogenesis and management of eosinophilicoesophagitis. *Aliment Pharmacol Ther* 2006; 24:173-182.
12. Roher CC, Reibel S, Ziegert M, et al. Atopy patch tests together with determination of specific IgE levels reduce the need dor oral food challenges in children with atopic dermatitis. *J Allergy Clin Immunol* 2001; 107:548-553.
13. American Academy of Pediatrics: Committee on nutrition hypoallergenic infant formulas. *Pediatrics* 2000; 106:346-349.
14. Agostoni C, Axelsson I, Goulet O, et al. Soy protein infant formulae and follow on formulae: A commentary by the ESPHAN Committee on Nutrition. *J Pediatr Gastroenterol Nutr* 2006;42: 352-361.
15. De Boissieu D, Matarazzo P, Dupont C. Allergy to extensively hydrolyzed cow milk proteins in infants: identification and treatment with an amino acid-based formula. *J Pediatr* 1997; 131:744-747.
16. von Berg A, Koletzko S, Grubl A, et al. The effect of hydrolyzed cow's milk formula for allergy prevention in the first year of life: The German Infant Nutritional Intervention Study, a randomized double-blind trial. *J Allergy Clin Immunol* 2003; 111:533-540.

33 Drug-Nutrient Interaction

Uday Bodhankar, Sandeep Dhingra, Sheikh Minhaj Ahmed

ABSTRACT

Drug-nutrient interaction, defined as an alteration of the kinetics or dynamics of a drug or nutrient or the impairment of the nutritional status caused by physical, chemical, physiologic, or pathophysiologic relationship between a drug and nutrient, is a common occurrence in medical practice. However, it rarely leads to significant clinical consequences. Most drug-nutrient interactions require minor modification of the dosage or timing of administration of the drug or nutrient. There is a felt need that clinicians must have detailed knowledge of such interactions, and should anticipate, identify and address drug-nutrient interactions.

On identification of an interaction after a thorough clnical workup, a team-based approach involving dietician, nurse, pharmacist and a clinician is required for management of patients with interactions. In order to build on the knowledge of probable drug-nutrient interactions, continued encouragement for investigating and reporting interactions by the childcare providers is mandatory. Severity and the clinical significance of drug-nutrient interactions can vary. Hence, a rudimentary scoring system has been suggested which though, subjective, is a step in the right direction. Keeping optimal drug and nutrient management as the goal, high standard of clinical judgment goes a long way in understanding and preventing drug-nutrient interactions.

Keywords: Clinical judgment, Drug-nutrient interactions, Drug regimens, Enteral nutrition, Food drug interactions, Intestinal transporters, Nutritional status, Scoring system.

INTRODUCTION

There are plenty of drugs and nutritional products available with increasingly many people are taking pharmacologically active agent on a regular basis. Nutrient consumption on the other hand varies with availability, affordability, acceptability, palatability, cultural traditions and geography.

The number of potential interactions between medication and nutrition is overwhelming. However, the proportion of clinically significant interactions seems to be unknown. Significant interactions between drugs and nutrients are those which alter pharmacotherapeutic response or compromise the nutritional status in an individual. Traditionally, these interactions have been considered less significant than drug-drug interactions.

Classic examples of drug-nutrient interactions are seen with isoniazid on vitamin B_6 metabolism, iron on tetracycline absorption, and vitamin C deficiency on barbiturate action to name a few. Translation and integration of knowledge of drug nutrient interaction is still limited amongst clinicians, scientists, and regulators who in turn have the ability to make meaningful contributions to the subject.

DEFINITION: WHAT IS IT?

A drug-nutrient interaction is defined as an alteration of the kinetics or dynamics of a drug or nutrient or the impairment of the nutritional status caused by physical, chemical, physiologic, or pathophysiologic relationship between a drug and nutrient.[1, 2] A drug-nutrient interaction should ideally focus on the effect of a specific nutrient on a specific drug rather than what is covered under the umbrella term drug-food interaction.

Alteration in the *disposition* and *effect* of the drug or nutrient guide the clinical consequences of a drug-nutrient interaction. The term *disposition* refers to the physical and biochemical properties of absorption, distribution, and elimination of a drug or nutrient and the term *effect* to the action of a drug or nutrient at cellular or subcellular level.

A **precipitant agent** is the drug or nutrient that causes the interaction. An interaction can be caused by either addition of a drug or nutrient or removal of a drug or nutrient from an established regimen, and changing the dose of a drug or nutrient that is being administered at a stable dose for a long time. An **object agent** refers to the drug or nutrient that is the object of effect by the interaction after the introduction of the precipitant agent.[1]

Consensus on what makes a drug-nutrient interaction clinically significant based on objective terms is still lacking. A change by 20% of a pharmacokinetic or pharmacodynamic parameter from baseline in describing a drug-nutrient interaction as significant has been suggested by some authors.[3] This reference threshold of 20% is consistent with the Food and Drug Administration in determining therapeutic equivalence of drugs. [4]

CLASSIFICATION

To approach the drug-nutrient interactions in a systematic manner and to allow the clinicians to recognize, identify, manage and prevent the interactions, various authors have classified interactions based on mechanism of interaction (Table 1) and physiochemical or physiologic interactions (Table 2).

Classification system based on the physiologic sequence of administration and the mechanisms of the interactions as proposed by Chang[1] categorizes

Table 1: Examples of drug-nutrient interactions according to the mechanism-based classification system.[1]

Interaction type	Precipitant agent	Object agents	Proposed mechanism	Clinical outcome
Type I	Continuous enteral nutrition	Levothyroxine	Poor dissolution of levothyroxine tablets; possible adsorption to tubings	Risk of developing subclinical to overt hypothyroidism over-time
Type IIA	Grapefruit juice	Cyclosporine	Inhibition of intestinal CYP3A4 enzyme by grapefruit juice leading to an increased oral bioavailability of cyclosporine	Elevation of blood cyclosporine concentration that may lead to symptomatic toxicity
Type IIB	Valproic acid	L-carnitine	Competitive inhibition of intestinal SLC22A transport protein leading to malabsorption of dietary carnitine	Symptomatic carnitine deficiency (Hyperammonemia and acute altered mental status without evidence of hepatic injury) in susceptible patients
Type IIC	Oral calcium supplements	Ciprofloxacin (oral)	Chelation and complexation of ciprofloxacin by calcium ions	Significantly reduced oral bioavailability of ciprofloxacin; possible treatment failure
Type III	Tyramine (large amount)	Rasagiline	Rasagiline is a type B monoamine oxidase inhibitor (MAOI-B). Although the interaction potential with tyramine is lower than that of MAOI-A, ingestion of a large amount of tyramine may still lead to the "cheese reaction"	Hypertensive crisis secondary to the presence of a large amount of epinephrine in the systemic circulation
Type IV	Dietary sodium restriction	Lithium	Sodium restriction can enhance the renal tubular reabsorption of drugs such as lithium	Lithium toxicity

Table 2: Location and mechanisms of drug-nutrient interactions.[5]

Site of interaction	Consequence	Mechanism of interaction
In drug (or nutrient) delivery device or gastrointestinal lumen	Reduced bioavailability	Physicochemical reaction and inactivation
Gastrointestinal mucosa	Altered bioavailability	Altered transporter and/or enzyme function
Systemic circulation or tissues	Altered distribution / effect	Altered transporter, enzyme, or other physiologic function
Organs of excretion	Altered clearance	Antagonism, impairment, or modulation of elimination

the drug-nutrient interactions into 4 main types. These are described as under:

Type I: Ex Vivo Bioinactivations

Interactions involving chemical and physical reactions that take place before the drug and nutrient involved have entered the body are classified as ex vivo bioinactivation. This mechanism occurs during direct physical contact of drug and nutrient and is commonly seen in relation to the preparation and infusion of a drug and nutrient formulation in patients receiving enteral nutrition or parenteral nutrition. Mixing certain drugs with food may also lead to this type of interaction. Type I interactions can be avoided by separating implicating drugs and nutrients in the absence of data confirming a lack of interaction.

Type II: Absorption Phase-associated Interactions

Type II interactions are the most commonly encountered interactions and are limited to drugs and nutrients delivered orally or enterally. In this type of interaction function of an enzyme (type A interaction) or a transport protein involved in transport of the object into systemic circulation (type B interaction) is modified by the precipitant agent. Type C interaction involves complexation, binding, and/or other deactivating processes that occur in the gastrointestinal tract. It is possible to predict the likelihood of drug-nutrient interactions mediated by the same mechanism. Type II interactions can be minimized by modifying the administration schedule of the precipitant or object agent.

Type III: Physiologic Action-associated Interactions

Interactions which occur after the absorption phase between the precipitant agent and the object agent are termed as physiologic action-associated interactions (type III). The mechanisms involve changing the cellular or tissue distribution, systemic metabolism or transport, or penetration to specific organs or tissues of the object compound. In some cases, these interactions take place at the receptors of the target cells or tissues. Separating administration time does not resolve the interaction and requires dose adjustment for optimization of therapy or to avoid adverse events.

Type IV: Elimination Phase-associated Interactions
Interactions which may involve the modulation, antagonism, or impairment of renal or enterohepatic elimination are termed as type IV. Competition for certain tissue-specific transport proteins for elimination may be the reason for such type of interactions.

FACTORS AFFECTING DRUG AND NUTRIENT DISPOSITION

Mechanism of how a drug and nutrient interact depends on the physiologic sequence of events after a drug or nutrient is ingested. The physiologic effects may be a change in pH which may affect the dissolution and binding of drugs and nutrients, presence of compound-specific transport proteins, receptors, and enzymes in different tissues which might alter the location where drugs and nutrients interact and other characteristics.

Nutritional Status
Malnutrition influences the pharmacokinetics of the drugs by modifying the distribution and clearance which may lead to alteration of therapeutic effectiveness and risk for toxicity. Nutritional status may also modify the susceptibility to other chemical exposures as well.[6] Role of antimicrobials in obesity has been much researched in view of the clinical effects of not accounting for altered drug distribution or clearance.[7] This has also been suggested in the case of antibiotics used in undernourished children.[8]

Food Effect
Food effect in general: Drug absorption may be altered whenever food intake along with drugs modifies the physicochemical conditions within the gastrointestinal tract. Bioavailability of drugs also depends upon the constituents of food (amount of protein, fat or carbohydrate) which may lead to either increase or decrease in drug bioavailability. In a classical example bioavailability of deferasirox is increased when taken with food and especially in presence of higher fat content of the meal. Hence, the recommendation is to administer deferasirox 30 minutes before meals.[9]

Specific foods or food components may also have a unique influence on drug disposition. Dietary products are known to chelate the fluoroquinolone antibiotics and reduce their bioavailability. Xanthine oxidase content in cow's milk may reduce drug bioavailability of mercaptopurine and lead to its transformation to the inactive 6-thiouric acid by the enzyme.[10] Soy protein isolates reduce the expression and activity of the cytochrome P450 (CYP)-metabolizing isoenzyme CYP1A1. Fruit juices can have an influence on drug disposition based on furanocoumarin and flavonoid content. Juices from pureed vegetables can have an influence on drug transporters and metabolizing enzymes.

Other food constituents: Enteral nutrition alters the bioavailability of variety of drugs by multiple mechanisms.[11,12] Parenteral nutrition although considered a prescription medication and is administered directly into the circulation has the ability to interact with medications. Parenteral nutrient admixtures and other individual nutrients (e.g. potassium chloride, magnesium sulfate, multivitamins) can interact at many levels.

Effect of Specific Nutrients or Other Dietary Supplement Ingredients on Drug Disposition

The effect of a nutrient on drug disposition may lead be positive outcome (example being use of pyridoxine in the prevention of isoniazid toxicity).[13] Polyphenolic compounds like flavonoids, terpenes, and vanilloids which are contained in culinary herbs and spices may carry health benefits but may also influence drug disposition as they are substrates for drug-metabolizing enzymes and transporters.[14]

INFLUENCE OF DRUGS ON OVERALL NUTRITIONAL STATUS

Food intake and absorption: Medication can alter the nutritional status by a variety of mechanisms which include food intake, digestion, and absorption. Food intake may be altered by a drug by direct effect on the gastrointestinal tract or through the gut–brain axis. Common adverse effects of drugs like nausea, vomiting, diarrhea and others like stomatitis, dysgeusia can also lead to adverse effect to nutritional status.

Metabolism: Many drugs may lead to metabolic adverse effects (e.g. weight gain, hyperglycemia, dyslipidemia, osteoporosis). Change in the overall nutritional status like weight gain is a well-known adverse effect caused by steroids and antipsychotics.

Influence of medication on the status of specific nutrients: Nutrient absorption, distribution, metabolism, and excretion may be altered by specific medications and their deficiencies may be associated with clinical manifestations. Such nutrient deficits may be dose-related, duration-related, or idiosyncratic in nature. Clinically, significant examples of such type of interactions are seen with carbamazepine which alters biotin status by decreasing absorption and increasing clearance.[15-17] Sodium valproate can lead to carnitine deficiency and subsequent tissue depletion which may in part be due to an inhibition of tissue uptake.[18] Changes in acylcarnitine subspecies with sodium valproate treatment reflect impaired intermediary metabolism and is the likely cause for drug-induced hepatotoxicity[19] including hyperammonemia.

Improvements in nutrient status may be seen with some drug treatment regimens especially during highly active antiretroviral therapy in management of HIV infection which leads to improved concentrations of α-carotene, β-carotene, α-tocopherol, vitamin B_{12}, and folate.[20] Vitamin D status may be improved with the use of HMG-CoA reductase inhibitors and lead to the drug's therapeutic benefit beyond cholesterol concentration modification.[21]

POPULATION AT RISK

Patients with chronic disease who use multiple medications, especially using drugs with a narrow therapeutic index are susceptible to drug-nutrient interaction. Other risk factors include extremes of ages, poor nutritional status, impaired organ function, and genetic variation in drug transporters, enzymes, or receptors.

CLINICAL APPROACH

Identification

To identify drug-nutrient interaction it becomes necessary to systematically assess the drug regimen and nutrient intake. To achieve this, a thorough nutritionally focused history, and physical examination to allow identification of potential nutrient deficits needs to be undertaken. Checklists for identifying patients with a potential drug-nutrient interaction and procedures regarding responsibilities and documentation of each intervention would be critical.

Management

Patient management will be based on the severity of the presenting drug-nutrient interaction or the risk potential for an interaction. Most clinically relevant interactions require only close monitoring or minor modification of the dosing schedules, while interactions which require either the drug or nutrient to be discontinued are rare. If the therapeutic efficacy of a drug regimen is different than expected, the clinician could evaluate whether this outcome is related to the patient's nutritional status, dietary habits, or specific nutrient or other dietary supplement intake. The drug Interaction Probability Scoring System and Scale[22] may be used to make an association between drug-nutrient pairs.

Prevention

Prevention can begin with increased awareness and attention paid by clinicians towards patient's nutritional status and dietary habits before and during drug therapy. Particular attention could also be paid to medication used in the elderly, critically ill, or those receiving enteral or parenteral nutrition therapy. A multidisciplinary approach to suspected drug-nutrient interaction involving the dietician, nurse, pharmacist and clinician will help in review of the policy, procedure, and interventions by the pharmacy and therapeutics committee. However, drug-nutrient interactions are difficult to predict and can still recur in view of intraindividual variability of therapeutic or toxic responses.

DRUGS AND THEIR INTERACTIONS

The interaction of natural products and drugs is a common hidden problem but not always leads to clinically significant interaction. The common interactions leading to clinically significant effects are listed (Table 3) and should be kept

Table 3: Summary of some significant drug-food interactions.

Drugs	Food	Dugs-food interaction
Warfarin	• High-protein diet • Vegetables containing vitamin k • Charbroiled • Cooked onions • Cranberry juice • Leafy green vegetables	• Raise serum albumin levels, decrease in international normalized ratio (INR) • Interferes with the effectiveness and safety of warfarin therapy • Decrease warfarin activity • Increase warfarin activity • Elevated INR without bleeding in elderly • Thromboembolic complications may develop
Monoamnine oxidases	Tyramine-containing food	Hypertensive crisis
Propranalol	Rich protein food	Serum level may be increased
ACE inhibitors	Empty stomach	Absorption is increased
Ca channel blockers	Grapefruit juice	Increases the bioavailability
Antibiotics	With milk products	Complex with some antibiotics and prevent their absorption, reduced bioavailability
Acetaminophen	Pectin	Delays its absorption and onset
NSAIDs	Alcohol Beverages	Can increase risk of liver damage or stomach bleeding The Cmax and $AUC0\text{-}\alpha$ significantly increased
Theophyline	High-fat meal and grapefruit juice Caffeine	Increase the bioavailability Increases the risk of drug toxicity
Esomeprazole	High-fat meal	Bioavailability was reduced
Isoniazid	Plants, medicinal herbs, oleanolic acid	Exerts synergistic effect
Glimepiride	With breakfast	Absolute bioavailability
Mercaptopurine	Cow's milk	Reduce bioavailability
Tamoxifen	Sesame seeds	Negatively interferes with tamoxifen in inducing regression of established MCF-7 tumor size but beneficially interacts with tamoxifen on bone in ovariectomized athymic mice
Levothyroxine	Grapefruit juice	Delay the absorption

in mind whenever prescribing these medication.[23] The interactions between natural products and drugs are based on the same pharmacokinetic and pharmacodynamic principles as drug-drug interactions. Several fruits and berries contain agents that affect drug-metabolizing enzymes.[24] Grapefruit is the most well-known example which can inhibit cytochrome P4503A4 (CYP3A4) which is involved in metabolism of almost all drugs metabolized in liver.[25]

FUTURE RESEARCH

Pharmacokinetic and pharmacodynamic properties of various drugs and knowledge of cellular signaling pathways, transporters and enzymes involved in nutrient metabolism are areas where research can lead to better understanding of the drug-nutrient interactions. Drug-nutrient interaction models need to be developed to evaluate single and multiple enzymatic and transporter pathways and which might help in predicting clinically relevant drug-nutrient interactions.

Another area of research includes the pharmacogenomic aspects of select drug-nutrient interactions and its effect on absorption, distribution, metabolism and excretion. Standardized experimental design used in research of drug development could also be extended to nutrition research and physiologically based modeling can be used to predict parameters of interest.

Research on the drugs which are already in the marketplace is the need of the hour and should first focus on drugs having a narrow therapeutic index with well-characterized transport and metabolic pathways. Depletion of micronutrients secondary to drugs (e.g. pyridoxine with isoniazid or folic acid with phenytoin) and the effect of supplementation of these micronutrients could be studied prospectively.

CONCLUSION

Nutrition-drug interactions, a common occurrence, require minor modification of the dosage or timing of administration of the drug or nutrient. However, clinicians must have detailed knowledge of such interactions, and should anticipate, identify and address drug-nutrient interactions. A thorough history focusing on nutrition, examination to identify risk factors, and vigilance for development of interactions is important to allow for identification of potential adverse interactions especially in high-risk groups. On identification of an interaction a team-based approach involving dietician, nurse, pharmacist and clinician are required for management of patients with interactions. A rudimentary scoring system is a step in the right direction. High standard of clinical judgment is warranted safeguarding from drug-nutrient interactions.

> **KEY LEARNING POINTS**
>
> - A drug-nutrient interaction is defined as an alteration of the kinetics or dynamics of a drug or nutrient.
> - Drug-nutrient interactions are classified into 4 main types. They are ex vivo bio-inactivations, absorption phase-associated interactions, physiologic action-associated interactions and elimination phase-associated interactions.
> - Factors affecting drug and nutrient disposition include nutritional status, food effects, influence of drugs on overall nutritional status and influence of medication on the status of specific nutrients.
> - For identification of drug-nutrient interaction it is necessary to systematically assess the drug regimen and nutrient intake.
> - Clinically relevant interactions require close monitoring or minor modification of the dosing schedules, while interactions which require either the drug or nutrient to be discontinued are rare.
> - Prevention is important and can begin with increased awareness and attention paid by clinicians towards patient's nutritional status and dietary habits before and during drug therapy.

REFERENCES

1. Chan LN. Drug-nutrient interactions. In: Shils ME, Shike M, Olson JA (Eds). *Modern Nutrition in Health and Disease*. 10th edn. Philadelphia, PA: Lippincott Williams and Wilkins 2006:1539-1553.
2. Santos CA, Boullata JI. An approach to evaluating drug–nutrient interactions. *Pharmacotherapy* 2005;25:1789-1800.
3. Chan LN. Drug-Nutrient interactions. *J Parenter Enter Nutr* 2013;37:450-459.
4. US Food and Drug Administration (FDA). *Guidance for Industry: Food-effect Bioavailability and Fed Equivalence Studies*. Rockville MD: FDA 2002. Available at: http://www.fda.gov/downloads/Drugs/GuidanceComplianceRegulatoryInformation/Guidances/ucm070241.pdf Accessed on:18 January 2018.
5. Chan LN. Drug–nutrient interaction in clinical nutrition. *Curr Opin Clin Nutr Metab Care* 2002;5:327-332.
6. Kordas K, Lonnerdal B, Stoltzfus RJ. Interactions between nutrition and environmental exposures: effects on health outcomes in women and children. *J Nutr* 2007;137:2794-2797.
7. Pai MP, Bearden DT. Antimicrobial dosing considerations in obese adult patients. *Pharmacotherapy* 2007;27:1081-1091.
8. Maitland K, Berkley JA, Shebbe M, et al. Children with severe malnutrition: can those at highest risk of death be identified with the WHO protocol? *PLoS Med* 2006;3:2431-2439.
9. Novartis Pharmaceuticals Corp. Exjade (deferasirox) Tablets for Oral Suspension prescribing information. East Hanover, NJ; 2007. Available at: http://www.fda.gov/cder/foi/label/2007/021882s003lbl.pdf. Accessed on: 18 January 2018.
10. DeLemos ML, Hamata L, Jennings S, Leduc T. Interaction between mercaptopurine and milk. *J Oncol Pharm Pract* 2007;13:237-240.
11. Dickerson RN. Medication administration considerations for patients receiving enteral tube feedings. *Hosp Pharm* 2004;39:84-89, 96.

12. Rollins C, Thomson C, Crane T. Pharmacotherapeutic issues. In: Rolandelli RH, Bankhead R, Boullata JI, Compher CW (Eds): *Clinical Nutrition: Enteral and Tube Feeding*, 4th edn. Philadelphia: Elsevier/Saunders 2005:291-305.
13. Morrow LE, Wear RE, Schuller D, Malesker M. Acute isoniazid toxicity and the need for adequate pyridoxine supplies. *Pharmacotherapy* 2006;26:1529-1532.
14. Kaefer CM, Milner JA. The role of herbs and spices in cancer prevention. *J NutrBiochem* 2008;19:347-361.
15. Said HM, Redha R, Nylander W. Biotin transport in the human intestine: inhibition by anticonvulsant drugs. *Am J Clin Nutr* 1989;49:127-131.
16. Mock DM, Dyken ME. Biotin catabolism is accelerated in adults receiving long-term therapy with anticonvulsants. *Neurology* 1997;49:1444-1447.
17. Rathman SC, Eisenschenk S, McMahon RJ. The abundance and function of biotin-dependent enzymes are reduced in rats chronically administered Carbamazepine. *J Nutr* 2002;132:3405-3410.
18. Tein I, DimAuro S, Xie ZW, et al. Valproic acid impairs carnitine uptake in cultured human skin fibroblasts: an in vitro model for pathogenesis of Valproic acid-associated carnitine deficiency. *Pediatr Res* 1993;34:281-287.
19. Werner T, Treiss I, Kohlmueller D, et al. Effects of Valproate on acylcarnitines in children with epilepsy using ESI-MS/MS. *Epilepsia* 2007;48:72-76.
20. Drain PK, Kupka R, Mugusi F, Fawzi WW. Micronutrients in HIV-positive persons receiving highly active antiretroviral therapy. *Am J Clin Nutr* 2007;85:333-345.
21. Pe´rez-Castrill ´on J, Vega G, Abad L, et al. Effects of atorvastatin on vitamin D levels in patients with acute ischemic heart disease. *Am J Cardiol* 2007;99:903-905.
22. Horn JR, Hansten PD, Chan L-N. Proposal for a new tool to evaluate drug interaction cases. *Ann Pharmacother* 2007;41:674-680.
23. Bushra R, Aslam N, Khan AY. Food-Drug Interactions. Oman Med J 2011; 26:77-83.
24. Molden E, Spigset O. Fruit and berries–interactions with drugs. *Tidsskr Nor Laegeforen* 2007;127:3218-3220.
25. Kirby BJ, Unadkat JD. Grapefruit juice, a glass full of drug interactions? *Clin Pharmacol Ther* 2007;81:631-633.

34
Sports Nutrition

VN Tripathi, Rakhi Jain, Piyush Upadhyay

ABSTRACT

Healthy nutrition, besides its role in growth and development is crucial for optimal performance by sportspersons and athletes, both children and adolescents. Macronutrients, micronutrients and fluids in the proper amounts are essential to provide energy for growth and activity. Sports drink containing sodium chloride and potassium chloride are recommended. Athlete should consume 1.5–3 L of water beyond normal intake, the day before event, 0.5–1 L 2 hour prior to event, empty bladder for 15 minutes prior to event and sip 0.25–0.3 L every 15–20 minutes during the event. The sportspersons must be educated about what and when to eat and drink not only during the event but also before and after activity. Pre-event meal should stress on high carbohydrate intake to enrich glycogen stores. For a morning event, night meal should be highly rich in carbohydrates and breakfast should be light. Use of performance-enhancing drugs is not permitted in view of their adverse effects.

Keywords: Adolescents, Athletes, Macronutrients, Micronutrients, Nutrition, Performance enhancing drugs, Sports, Sports event.

INTRODUCTION

By definition, the term *nutrition* is the study of food and nutrients and their effect on health, growth and development. Its importance in sustaining a healthy life is immense. Sports nutrition deals with an application of principles of nutrition to the field of sports, athletics and games so that the performance can be enhanced to the maximum potential. It enhances performance by decreasing fatigue and helps to protect against injury and aids quicker recovery.[1] Genes, training and nutrition are the main factors that play key roles to excel in sports. Since genetic makeup of an individual is a constant factor, training in sports achieves a significant role and good training can never be attained without appropriate nutrition. Athletes should know what and when to eat before, during and after the training session or the main event.

Energy requirement varies with age, weight, gender of the sportsperson and it also depends on the nature of sport or physical activity involved. Decreased energy intake may lead to delayed puberty, short stature, menstrual dysfunction, loss of muscle mass and increased susceptibility for fatigue, injury or illness.[2,3]

MACRONUTRIENTS

Carbohydrates form the major fuel for sports activity, one gram releasing four kilocalories of energy. Glucose is stored as glycogen in muscle and liver which is most readily available for working muscle. Carbohydrates should form 45 to 65% of total intake 4-18-year-old children.[4] Focus should be on inclusion of wholesome unrefined complex carbohydrates like whole grains or products with whole grain as first ingredient in the menu for athletes as they are rich in fiber, vitamins, minerals, phytochemicals, antioxidants and have essential fatty acids. Carbohydrate rich diet is bulky hence, many athletes may need to change their food habits from three major meals to more frequent smaller meals and to take 30-50% of total daily energy intake as intermediate snacks.

Proteins build and repair muscle, hair, nails and skin. For exercise of short duration or mild in intensity proteins do not act as a primary source of energy. As exercise duration increases, proteins help to maintain blood glucose through liver gluconeogenesis.[2] One gram of protein provides four kilocalories of energy. Protein should comprise approximately 10-30% of total energy intake for 4- 18-year-old.[4] Recommended daily allowance for protein for most people is 0.8 g per kg body weight. It may vary with the kind of sport. Protein needs are easily met by normal diet hence protein supplements are not indicated. Excess intake of protein may adversely affect the performance.

Fats provide essential fatty acids, help to absorb fat-soluble vitamins (A, D, E, K) and provide insulation. One gram provides nine kilocalories hence is energy dense. It should be 25-35% of total energy intake for 4- 18 year-old.[4] Saturated fats should comprise around 10% of energy.[1,3]

MICRONUTRIENTS

Vitamins and minerals are important for good health. Athletes should pay special attention to consume adequate amounts of iron, calcium and vitamin D and iron. Calcium is important for healthy bones, normal enzyme activity and muscle contraction. The daily recommended intake of calcium is 1,000 mg/day for children 4-8-years of age and 1300 mg/day for 9-18 year-old.[4,5]

Vitamin D is necessary for regulation of calcium absorption and regulation and maintains bone health. Requirement of vitamin D varies depending on geographical condition and race. Athletes living in northern latitudes or who train indoors (e.g. figure skaters, gymnasts, dancers) are more likely to be vitamin D deficient.[2]

Iron is an important mineral for oxygen transport and several reactions at cellular level. During adolescence, more iron is required to support growth as well as increases in blood volume and lean muscle mass as it is important for oxygen delivery to body tissues.[1] Iron depletion is common in athletes because of diets poor in meat, fish and poultry, or increased iron losses in urine, feces, sweat or menstrual blood.[2] Therefore, athletes particularly female athletes, vegetarians and distance runners should be screened periodically for iron status.[2]

FLUIDS

Fluids, particularly water, form an important component of nutrition for athletes. Athletic performance can be affected by the amount of fluid consumed by athletes. Fluids help to regulate body temperature and replace sweat losses during exercise.[5,6] Fluid loss in sweat and fluid intake required by an athlete is affected by environmental temperature and humidity.[1,6,7] Increased temperature and higher humidity result in increased fluid requirement needed to maintain hydration. Dehydration can decrease performance and increase the risk of heat stroke.[1,6,7] The amount of fluid required depends on many factors including age and body size.[6,7] Fluid balance is critical. There are huge fluid losses both in training and in events. Athlete should consume 1.5 to 3 L of fluid beyond normal intake the day before event, 16-32 ounces (400-600 mL) 2 hour prior to event, empty bladder 15 minutes prior to event and sip 8-10 ounces (or 150 to 300 mL) every 15-20 minutes during the event.[1,6,7] Along with sweat electrolytes are also lost. Hence sports drink containing sodium chloride and potassium chloride are preferred (some recommend drinks containing carbohydrates 6%).[3,6,8] Following activity, athletes should drink enough fluid to replace sweat losses. This usually requires consuming approximately 1.5 L of fluid/kg of body weight lost.[1,7] Routine ingestion of carbohydrate containing sports drinks in nonathletes should be avoided as it can result in excessive calories, increasing the risks of overweight and obesity as well as dental caries.[8]

RECOVERY FOODS

Recovery foods should be consumed initially within 30 minutes of exercise, and then again within 1-2 hours of exercise, to help replenish muscles with glycogen and allow for proper recovery. These foods should include protein and carbohydrates.[2,9] Examples include graham crackers with peanut butter and juice, yogurt with fruit, or a sports drink with fruit and cheese.

PERFORMANCE ENHANCING SUBSTANCES

Performance enhancement substances are ergogenic substances or drugs like anabolic steroids, stimulants and narcotics are commonly known as 'doping' are strictly prohibited as they are injurious to health and are banned by International Olympic Committee and other sports organization.[10]

Table 1 presents the classification of sports and games according to energy expenditure.

Table 2 presents the average body weight and energy expenditure levels assumed and allowances suggested.

Table 3 presents the key points for workout.

CONCLUSION

Table 1: Classification of sports and games according to energy expenditure.

Category	Event
Group i	Power event of higher weight category (80 kg and above): Weight lifting, wrestling, boxing, judo, throwing events
Group ii	Endurance events: Marathon, long distance running, cycling, rowing middle and long distance swimming
Group iii	Team events, athletics and power events of middle weight category (65 kg), hockey, football, volleyball, basketball, tennis, sprints, jumpers, boxing, wrestling, weight lifting, judo and swimming
Group iv	Events of light weight category: Gymnastics, table tennis, yatching, boxing wrestling, weight lifting, judo
Group v	Skill games shooting, archery and equestrain

Source: National Institute of Nutrition

Table 2: Average body weight and energy expenditure levels assumed and allowance suggested.

Event Category	Body weight (kg)	Energy allowances		Calories ratio
		Kcal/kg/day	Kcal/day	Cho:Prot:Fat
Group i	85	70	6000	55 : 15 :30
Group ii	65	80	5200	60 : 15 :25
Group iii	65	70	4500	60 : 15 :25
Group iv	60	60	3600	65 : 15 :20
Group v	60	50	3000	55 : 15 :30

(CHO: carbohydrate; Pro: protein)

Table 3: Key points for workout.

Pre-exercise
Start exercise well hydrated
- Start exercise glycogen loaded in both muscles and liver
- Supper: Pre-event meal high in carbohydrate. If planning to exercise for more than 4 hours, or 2 hours in high heat and humidity add salt to foods
- Breakfast: Cyclist aim for at least 1,000 calories. Runners may not be able to eat as much – perhaps only a few hundred calories. Walkers and triathletes will be in between
- Preworkout calories benefit both endurance and strength in athletes, both aerobic and anaerobic work
- Start prolonged exercise in the heat salt-loaded
- Be prepared for start delays. At the event have easily digestible fluids and calories available in case of start delay

Contd...

Contd...

During Exercise
- Hydrate
  - Aim for 8 ounces (250 mL) of fluids, every 15 to 30 minutes depending upon the heat
  - Have carbohydrate-in-water solutions (for example maltodextrin).
  - Cyclist: Carry two waterbottles or use a hydration systems (e.g. camelbak) while runners carry bottles.
- Calories
  - For events longer than 1 hour, consume at least 300 calories per hour of exercise.
- Salt
  - For multi-hour event in conditions of heat and humidity, consume salty food, sodium-rich solutions and gels.

Postexercise
- Refueling after exercise is a key recovery strategy
- The sooner the better. Refueling during exercise is the best
- Prompt refueling benefits both endurance and strength athletes
- Prompt refueling benefits aerobic and anaerobic work
- Aim to ingest at least 50 g of carbohydrate (200 calories) within the first 30 minutes after exercise and again every hour for the next 3 hours, up to caloric deficit
- Some fat and some protein with the carbohydrate is no problem
- Real food is better than the "specialty sports products".

Good, balanced nutrition in sports is the fulcrum on which physical training and efficiency of the sportsperson during the sports event depends. Proper meal planning in accordance with the sports category and phase of training or sports event goes a long way in enhancing performance and overcome muscle injury. A balance diet providing all the nutrients in apt quantity eliminates the need of sports supplements. Performance enhancing substances are strictly prohibited as they are injurious to health and are banned.

KEY LEARNING POINTS

- Importance of nutrition in sports performance should be emphasized and facilities provided to ensure good quality and quantity of nutrition to the athlete.
- Dietary history, medical checkups of athletes to monitor body weight changes, micronutrient balance, lipid profile in response to diet planned should be done periodically.
- Energy need varies from 3,000 calories for skill games to 7,000 calories for power events of super heavy category.
- Nutritional needs of junior athlete varies from that of adults. They need more proteins (2 g/kg body weight) so that their muscle mass development, muscle regeneration and additional requirement of activity can be taken care of. They should start the day with breakfast, have snacks in morning and evening apart from lunch and dinner. Intake of plenty of oral fluids is a must.
- Diet plan varies according to the phase of training. Need of nutrients is less in the transition phase than the precompetitive phase while competitive phase requires more nutrients than the precompetitive phase.

Contd...

Contd...

- ¤ The diet should be balanced in terms of both micro-and macronutrients. This eliminates the need of nutritional supplements. Supplements are required for those who are deficient in nutrients.
- ¤ Pre-event meal should stress on high carbohydrate intake to enrich glycogen stores. For example, for a morning event, night meal should be highly rich in carbohydrates and breakfast should be light.
- ¤ Fluid balance is critical. There are huge fluid losses both in training and in events. Along with sweat electrolytes are also lost. Hence sports drink containing sodium chloride and potassium chloride are preferred. Athlete should consume 50-100 ounces of water beyond normal intake, the day before event, 16–32 ounces 2 hour prior to event, empty bladder 15 minutes prior to event and sip 8–10 ounces every 15–20 minutes during the event.
- ¤ Performance enhancing substances are strictly prohibited as they are injurious to health and are banned by International Olympic Committee and other sports organization.

REFERENCES

1. Hoch AZ, Goossen K, Kretschmer T. Nutritional requirements of the child and teenage athlete. *Phys Med Rehabil Clin N Am* 2008;19:373-398.
2. Dietitians of Canada, the American Dietetic Association, and the American College of Sports Medicine. Joint position statement: Nutrition and athletic performance. *Can J Diet Pract Res* 2000;61:176-192.
3. Meyer F, O'Connor H, Shirreffs SM. International Association of Athletics Federations Nutrition for the young athlete. *J Sports Sci* 2007;25(Suppl 1):S73-S82.
4. Otten JJ, Hellwig JP, Meyers LD. *Dietary Reference Intakes: The essential Guide to Nutrient Requirements.* National Academies Press 2006.
5. Institute of Medicine. Dietary reference intakes for calcium and vitamin D. Consensus Report, November 30, 2010. Available at: www.iom.edu/Reports/2010/Dietary-Reference-Intakes-for-Calcium-and-Vitamin-D.aspx Accessed on: 12 March 2018.
6. Rowland T. Fluid replacement requirements for child athletes. *Sports Med* 2011; 41:279–288.
7. American College of Sports Medicine. Position stand: Exercise and fluid replacement. *Med Sci Sports Exerc* 2007;39:377-390.
8. American Academy of Pediatrics, Committee on Nutrition and the Council on Sports Medicine and Fitness. Sports drinks and energy drinks for children and adolescents: Are they appropriate? *Pediatrics.* 2011;127:1182-1189.
9. Laura K Purcell and Canadian Paediatric Society, Paediatric Sports and Exercise Medicine Section: Sport nutrition for young athletes. *Pediatr Child Health* 2013;18: 200-202.
10. International Life Science Institute, National Institute of Nutrition and Sports Authprity of India. *Nutrition and Hydration Guidelines for Excellence in Sports Performance.* Available at: http://www.ilsi-india.org/PDF/Conf.%20recommendations/Nutrition/Nutrition%20&%20Hyd.%20Guidelines%20for%20Athletes%20Final%20report.pdf. Accessed on: 12 March 2018.

35. Nutritional Supplements

VN Tripathi, Piyush Upadhyay, Rakhi Jain

ABSTRACT

Increased awareness about health has led to increased intake of nutritional supplements although routine use of such supplements in a healthy individual is not recommended. This has undermined the importance of the fact that a healthy diet including a variety of nutrients is the best method to achieve dietary nutrients. People need to be educated about the importance of natural sources of nutrients. Only those that are deficient in the intake of recommended amounts need to be supplemented after discussion with a pediatrician. This alone can help to curb the indiscriminate use of commercially available dietary supplements.

Keywords: Indiscriminate use, Nutrients, Nutrition, Nutritional supplements.

INTRODUCTION

Nutrition has a central role in growth and development of children. The use of dietary supplements is in vogue in this era of increased awareness about health and diet. Often, the information gained through media and internet is incomplete or incorrect. Nutritional supplements are very often considered as a replacement of a balanced diet. Primary reason for using dietary supplements in children is to improve or maintain health.[1] The use of supplements to treat or prevent specific health conditions was very low. Only about one-quarter of children used dietary supplements to enhance nutrient intake from food. Multivitamins/mineral (MVM) are commonly used by children. Vitamin C, calcium, and botanicals/herbals as stand-alone products or as ingredients of or multivitamin products are also used. Factors associated with greater use among children included younger age, more healthful diets, greater food security, greater physical activity, and better access to health care.[2]

DEFINITION

Nutrient supplements are regulated by the Food and Drug Administration (FDAs) Center for Food Safety and Applied Nutrition. The Dietary Supplement Health and Education Act (DSHEA) of 1994 sets safety and labeling requirements for dietary supplements.[3] The DSHEA defines a dietary supplement, in part, as a product intended to supplement the diet that contains any of the following dietary ingredients: Vitamin; mineral; an herb or other botanical; amino acid; a dietary substance for use by humans to supplement the diet by increasing the total dietary intake;or a concentrate, metabolite, a constituent, extract, or combination of any ingredient mentioned above.[3,4] Dietary supplements are intended to be taken by mouth and can be in many forms, including pills, capsules, tablets, liquids, powders, or other forms as long as they are not represented for use as a conventional food or as a sole item of a meal or diet.[3,4] They must also be identified on the label as a dietary supplement.

OPTIMAL INTAKES

Food Based Recommendation

Wise selection of a variety of nutrient-rich foods is generally the best strategy for meeting nutrient needs. Plant foods, such as fruits, vegetables, whole grains, beans, nuts, seeds, and tea provide an array of other health-promoting substances beyond vitamins and minerals including carotenoids and polyphenols, such as flavonoids. Data suggest that positive health outcomes are related more to dietary patterns, the types and amounts of foods consumed, than to intakes of individual nutrients.[5]

Nutrient Based Recommendations

Optimal nutrient intakes are those that promote health and reduce risk for chronic disease while minimizing risk of excess. The Institute of Medicine's (IOM's) Dietary Reference Intakes (DRIs) are the best available evidence-based nutrient standards for estimating optimal intakes. They include the recommended dietary allowances (RDAs), adequate intakes (AIs), estimated average requirements (EARs), and tolerable upper intake levels (ULs).[6] The RDAs and AIs (when data was not sufficient to determine an EAR and thus an RDA) serve as intake goals for healthy individuals but may not be sufficient for those who are malnourished.[6]

NUTRIENT SUPPLEMENTS IN PRACTICE

The optimal means of obtaining nutrients and vitamins for individuals of all ages, especially children, is through a balanced and nutritious diet, many parents offer their child a variety of nutritional supplements commercially available for children to ensure that their nutritional targets are met. These supplements may be in the form of flavored chewables, gummies, gumballs, and liquid formulations. Special MVM formulations targeting specific age group of pediatric population are available to meet their nutritional needs. Some supplement formulations even claim to promote immune health, bone health, and provide energy and brain support. Liquid nutritional supplements (commercially available powders or energy drinks provide children with protein, fat, fiber, and a combination of vitamins and minerals to aid in growth and promote weight gain. MVM supplements for children may include omega-3 fatty acids for healthy brain development, extra vitamin C to promote immune support, as well as iron, calcium, zinc, vitamin D, vitamin B, and vitamin E but should be consumed by children only after evaluating the actual need of the child.[7] Certain forms of nutrients provide better nutrient adequacy based on their molecular structure and chemical formula. For example, folic acid from supplements and fortified foods is more bioavailable than folate from foods due to the ease of absorption of the unconjugated form.[8]

When to Consider Supplementation

Currently, the American Academy of Pediatrics (AAP) and the American Dietetic Association emphasize that eating a balanced, nutritious diet is the best possible method for children to obtain essential nutrients (Box 1).[9-11] AAP does not recommend nutritional supplementation in healthy children over the age of 1 year. MVM supplement should not be given without discussing the necessity of such supplement with treating pediatrician.

AAP recommends the following groups of healthy infants and children to receive 400 IU daily of supplemental vitamin D: All infants who are exclusively or partly breastfed (beginning the first few days of life and continued unless infant is weaned to at least 1 qt/day vitamin D–fortified formula or, if older than 12 months, whole milk or low-fat milk when appropriate); all non-breastfed infants and older children who consume less than 1qt/day vitamin D–fortified formula or milk; and adolescents with dietary intakes <400 IU/day.[12] Children at an increased risk for vitamin D deficiency, such as those with fat malabsorption and those taking seizure medications may need higher amounts to achieve normal vitamin D status as determined by laboratory results.[12]

Box 1: Daily MVM supplement may be needed for the following groups of children.[9-11]

- Children who do not eat a regular, balanced diet that includes foods from a variety of food groups
- Children with a poor appetite or picky food habits
- Children who have a restrictive diet, such as a vegetarian or dairy-free diet
- Children with chronic medical conditions
- Children who are underweight
- Children with diagnosed deficiency disease of one or more micronutrients
- Children on medications that may cause specific nutrient deficiency like corticosteroids and antiepileptic drugs among others

Tips Regarding Safe Use of Multivitamin/Mineral Supplements

- As with all medications, MVM supplements should always be kept out of reach of children to prevent accidental overdose, especially because many of these supplements can easily be mistaken for candy.
- Excessive doses of MVM supplements, especially fat-soluble vitamins, can cause toxicities.
- Always remember to give children only the MVM formulations that are marketed for use in children and to administer only the recommended dose.
- Always read the label before giving your child any medication or supplement including MVM supplements, and check for expiration dates.
- Store MVM supplements in a cool, dry place.
- Remember that MVM supplements are intended for use as an adjunct to eating a well-balanced, nutritious diet; they are not intended as a substitute for eating a healthy variety of foods consisting of whole grains, fruits, and vegetables.
- MVM supplements are intended to prevent nutritional deficiencies and to maintain nutritional stores; they are not intended for the self-treatment of vitamin deficiencies. If your child is exhibiting signs of nutritional deficiencies, see your pediatrician immediately.
- If you are unsure whether your child requires supplementation, discuss the use of MVM supplements with your pediatrician to determine how best to meet your child's nutritional needs.
- Children on medications for treatment of diseases like asthma, allergies, and attention deficit hyperactivity disorder should be looked for possible interactions before recommending supplements.[13]

ROLE OF PEDIATRICIAN/DIETETICS PRACTITIONERS

A pediatrician must be updated on the safety and efficacy of the supplement formulations prescribed (Box 2).

Box 2: The roles and responsibilities of pediatrician/physician.[4]

- Assessing nutritional status of children to determine inadequate or excessive intake of vitamins and minerals and find the actual need of a supplement.
- Evaluating the therapeutic benefit or harm of nutrient supplementation as per the child's age and nutritional status.
- Evaluating the safety of a nutrient supplement in terms of dose and its interaction with food, other dietary supplements and prescribed medications.
- Educating parents regarding the benefits of a balanced diet and nutrition achieved through conventional and fortified foods.
- Recommending supplementation when food intake is inadequate to meet particular nutrient requirements.

Some characteristics of a healthy plate are given in Box 3.

> **Box 3:** Some characteristics of a healthy plate.[14]
>
> **Milk**
> - Children who consume dairy products, such as milk, milk substitutes, yogurt, and cheese get many important nutrients. Children >2 years of age should consume fat-free and low-fat milk (1% fat) during the day in order to.
>   - Provide them nutrients, such as protein, calcium, vitamin D, and potassium.
>   - Help build strong bones, teeth, and muscles in growing children.
>   - Increase the tendency of the child to continue milk intake when they are older.
>
> **Sugar**
> - Provide food and beverages with fewer added sugars by providing fresh fruits and resins as:
>   - Increased sugar can lead to fullness and early satiety causing decreased nutrient intake from other food items.
>   - Extra calories added to diet without nutrients.
>   - Increase risk of dental caries.
>
> **Salt**
> - Provide food with decreased salt or sodium content as:
>   - Children tasting salty food regularly makes them used to salty food. Increased intake of salt or sodium increases chances of hypertension.

CONCLUSION

Consuming wide variety of nutritious foods is the best way to maintain health and promote growth. It is an important responsibility of dietician or pediatrician to educate the public on healthful dietary patterns and utility of a balanced diet to their child. The frivolous and routine use of supplements should be discouraged. A safe and appropriate nutrient supplement should be used if needed depending on the nutritional assessment of the child to meet their nutrient needs.

> **KEY LEARNING POINTS**
>
> - A balanced diet with a variety of nutrients is the best method to achieve nutrients.
> - Supplements should be given only after discussion with the pediatrician/physician.
> - Nutritional status of the child determines the requirement of nutritional supplements.
> - Caution needs to be exercised regarding safety and dosage while giving nutritional supplements as their overdose may lead to toxicity.

REFERENCES

1. Bailey RL, Gahche JJ, Thomas PR, Dwyer JT. Why US children use dietary supplements *Pediatr Res* 2013;74:737-741.
2. Shaikh U, Byrd RS, Auinger P. Vitamin and mineral supplement use by children and adolescents in the 1999-2004 National Health and Nutrition Examination Survey: Relationship with nutrition, food security, physical activity, and health care access. Arch *Pediatr Adolesc Med* 2009;163:150-157.

3. Dietary Supplement Health and EducationAct of 1994. Public L No. 103-417 (codified at42 USC 287C-11).
4. American Dietetic Association. Position of the American Dietetic Association: Nutrient Supplementation. *J Am Dietet Assoc* 2009;109:2073-2085.
5. Lichtenstein AH, Russell RM. Essential nutrients: Food or supplements: Where should the emphasis be? *JAMA*. 2005;294:351-358.
6. Institute of Medicine, Food and Nutrition. Board. *Dietary Reference Intakes: Applications in Dietary Assessment*. Washington, DC: National Academies Press 2000.
7. Peaslee K. Supplements: nutrition insurance for children. *Today's Dietitian*. Available at: www.todaysdietitian.com/newarchives/tdjan2008pg50.shtml. Accessed on: 3 April 2018.
8. Institute of Medicine, Food and Nutrition Board. *Dietary Reference Intakes for Thiamin, Riboflavin, Niacin, Vitamin B6, Folate, Vitamin B12, Pantothenic Acid, Biotin, and Choline*. Washington, DC: National Academies Press 1998.
9. Moreno M. Advice for patients: vitamin and mineral supplementation in children. *Arch Pediatr Adolesc Med* 2009;163:192.
10. Science Daily. Vitamin use is highest in kids who don't need them, study finds. Available at: http://www.sciencedaily.com/releases/2009/02/090202174657.html. Accessed on: 3 April 2018.
11. Ifat S, Byrd RS, Auinger P. Vitamin and mineral supplement use by children and adolescents in the 1999-2004 National Health and Nutrition Examination survey: Relationship with nutrition, food security, physical activity, and health care access. *Arch Pediatr Adolesc Med* 2009;163:150-157.
12. Wagner CL, Greer FR. Section on Breastfeeding and Committee on Nutrition. Prevention of rickets and vitamin D deficiency in infants, children, and adolescents. *Pediatrics* 2008;122:1142-1152.
13. Terrie YC. The ABCs of Pediatric Multivitamin/Multimineral Supplements. *Pharmacy Times*, 2013.
14. Build a Healthy Plate With Milk. Available at: http://www.teamnutrition.usda.gov/library.html. Accessed on: 4 April 2018.

Index

Page numbers followed by b refer to box, f refer to figure, fc refer to flowchart, and t refer to table

A

Abdomen 294
Abortion 98
Accidental contaminants 403
Accredited social health activists 216
Acetaminophen 416
Acetyl-CoA carboxylase 49
Acetylhydrolase 151
Achar's grading 209t
Achondroplasia 99
Acidosis
  metabolic 237
  renal tubular 88, 90
Aciduria, methylmalonic 52
Acquired immunodeficiency syndrome 180
Acrodermatitis enteropathica 9, 11, 99f, 100, 129
Acute respiratory distress syndrome 11, 25
Addison's disease 107
Adenosine triphosphate 223
Adiponectin 151
Adolescent 325
  dieters 180
  friendly health services 178
  growth and development 171
  nutrition 169
    interventions for 180b
  nutritional
    dwarfing 99
    status of 177
Adverse food reactions 402b
  differential diagnosis of 403b
Aflatoxin 403
  contamination hypothesis 190
Alanine aminotransferease 295
Albumin 12, 390
Alkaline phosphatase 75
Alkalosis, metabolic 237
Allopurinol 12
Alpha linoleic acid 272
Alzheimer disease 53
American Academy of Pediatrics 114, 150, 290, 310, 428
Amino acid 12, 38, 191, 380, 395
  aromatic 381
  branched chain 381
  levels, low 196
  nonessential 12
Ammonia genesis 382
Amnesia
  anterograde 237
  retrograde 237
Anaphylaxis, exercise-induced 402
Anasarca 207
Anemia 48, 50, 99, 101, 110t, 212, 213, 223, 237, 371, 381
  adverse effects of 176fc
  cow's milk-induced 402
  hemolytic 11, 61, 81
  maternal 138, 138b
  megaloblastic 51, 53
  microcytic-hypochromic 9
  nutritional 116
  pernicious 51
  refractory 9
  severe 217
Anganwadi worker 216, 230, 264
Angioedema 401, 402
Annaparasana 186
Anorexia 58, 99, 118, 129, 229, 237, 380
  nervosa 235, 239
Anthropometry 33, 281, 293, 390
Antibiotics 402, 416
  oral 60
Antibody 277
  levels 248
  vaccination responses 248
Anticonvulsants 292
  therapy 88
  tricyclic 292
Antiepileptic drugs 89
Antigens 194

Anti-inflammatory activities 375
Antimicrobial factors 244
Antioxidants 11, 16, 16f, 20, 21, 40
  dietary 141
  extracellular 12
  foods rich in 22
  intracellular 12
  nutritional 12
  potential hazards of 25
  role of 24, 25
  treatment, failure of 26
  types of 12
  vitamins, dietary sources of 23t
Antipsychotic agents 292
Antituberculous therapy 217
Appetite 211
  test 218
Arachidonic acid 7, 272, 381
Areflexic paralysis 222
Arginine 12, 13
  vasopressin 289
Arnold classification 200
Arrhythmia 237, 390
  cardiac 223
  paroxysmal atrial 237
  ventricular 237
Arsenic 105
Arthralgia 105
Arthritis, rheumatoid 11, 99
Arthropathies, weight related 300
Ascites 207
Ascorbic acid 1, 8, 11, 18, 23, 53, 143, 174
Aspartate aminotransferase 295
Assisted feeding, methods of 276f
Asthma 290, 292, 402
Ataxia 9, 237
Atresia 207
Atrophy
  infantile 207
  villous 195
Attention-deficit hyperactivity disorder 121
Auditory evoked brain stem response 121
Autoimmune disorder, chronic systemic 356
Auxiliary nurse midwife 216
Avidin 49
  biotin complex 49

B

Baby-friendly
  hospital initiative 162, 267
  techniques 155
Bacteria 403
Bangle method 34, 35
Bardet-Biedl syndromes 294
Bariatric surgery, criteria for 300b
Basal ganglia disorder 103
Basal metabolic rate 134, 192
Basal metabolism, maintenance of 4
Behavioral changes 118, 129
Behavioral modifications 313
Behavioral therapy, cognitive 331
Beriberi 41, 237
Beta-carotene 1, 12, 22, 141, 174
  supplements of 26
Bifidus factor 151
Bile salt lipase 151
Biliary obstruction 60
Bilirubin 12
Biochemical
  changes 207
  parameters 392
  tests, special 37
Bioelectrical impedance analysis 382, 391
Biotin 8, 41, 49, 272, 279, 397
  deficiency 50
Birth defects 129
Birth weight 229, 271, 291
  prematurity 80
Bitot spot 55, 65, 66, 66f, 263
Bleeding 213, 390
  diathesis, complication of 213f
  disorders 111
  increased risk of 382
Blepharitis 129
Blind loop syndrome 51
Blindness 129
Blood 247
  count, complete 229
  glucose 229, 324
    postprandial 320
  loss, chronic 99
  peripheral 194
  pressure 293
  sampling 111
  smear 229

sugar 207
   random 218
   thiamine level 43
   transfusion 233
   urea nitrogen 392
      final collection of 392
Blount disease 290
B-lymphocytes 248
Body
   fat, total 390
   image disorders 347
   mass index 34, 37, 286, 289, 295, 304, 318, 343, 370, 390, 391
   organ systems 126
   water, total 190
   weight 230
      loss 390
Bone
   disease, metabolic 88
   marrow 51f
   mineral density, reduced 373
   mineralization 103
Borderline malnutrition 37
Bow legs 83
Bowel disease, inflammatory 11, 13, 51, 129, 347, 369, 402
Bowel syndrome, pediatric irritable 330
Bradycardia 237
Bradykinesia 222, 258
Brain 126, 255
   and glial cell line-derived neutrophic factor 151
   development 136
   energy metabolism 117, 118
   iron rich area in 117b
Breast
   abscess 161
   engorged 160f
   engorgement 160
   milk 148, 267
      advantages of 148
      composition of 149
      expressed 273
      nutritive value of 149
      volume of 159
   problems 160
Breastfeeding 161, 180, 336
   role of 267
   technical aspects of 152

Breath
   holding
      episodes 118
      spells 120
   shortness of 292
Bronchopneumonia 206
Bronchospasm 402
Brunner's glands 344
Bulging staphyloma 67f
Burning feet syndrome 47, 48

C

Caffeine 402, 403
Caffey's disease 58
Calamine lotion 126
Calcium 9, 10, 17, 17f, 105, 139, 143, 150, 174, 176, 191, 272, 279, 358, 397
   channel blockers 416
   deficiency 307
      rickets 105
   D-pantothenate 48
   transport protein 56, 79
Calorie 4, 150, 174, 188
   daily requirement for 3t
   deficiency 189
   requirement 3, 4
   total 5
Calorimetry 391
Carbohydrates 1, 2, 5, 16f, 135, 192, 236, 272, 279, 320, 322, 324, 394, 395, 397, 421, 423
   less complex 2
   nutritional requirements of 18
Carbonic anhydrase 128
Carboxylation reactions needing biotin 49b
Carcinoma, hepatocellular 382
Cardiac arrest 237
Cardiac disease 295
Cardiac failure, congestive 43, 197, 213
Cardiomyopathy 103, 237
Cardiovascular disease 8
Cardiovascular system 228
Carotenes 23
Carotenoids 23
Casal necklace 46
Catabolic losses, enhanced 194
Catalase 12
Cataract 129

Catch-up growth 218
Catecholamines 289
Celiac disease 64, 70, 74, 347, 356, 357, 402
    management of 358t
Celiac subjects, nutritional status of 357
Cell
    death 255
    function 128
Cellular immune function 247
Center for Disease Control 290
Center for Food Safety and Applied Nutrition 427
Central nervous system 58, 105, 188
Cerebellar nuclei 117
Cerebrospinal fluid 42
Champagne glass appearance 87
Cheilosis 45, 45f
Chemokines 151
Chest, violin-shaped deformed 81
Child abuse and neglect 85
Chloride 272, 279
Cholecalciferol 8
Cholelithiasis 300
Cholera 106
Cholestasis 103
Cholesterol 5, 7, 16, 16f, 390
    total 388
Choline 136, 272, 279
Chromium 10, 191, 272, 396
Chronic obstructive pulmonary disease 25
Cinnamic acid 12
Ciprofloxacin 411
Cleft
    lip 53
    palate 53
Clubbing 206, 210
Cobalamin 272
Cobalt 101
Coenzymes 40
Colchicine 51
Colitis, ulcerative 369
Colostrum 149
Coma 222, 237
Community-based therapeutic care 219
Complement system 194
Comprehensive multidisciplinary intervention 298
Concave depression, saucer-like 86
Conjunctiva
    palpebral 97f
    pigmented 66f
    wrinkled bulbar 65f
    xerotic 69
Conjunctival impression cytology 69
Connective tissue defects 129
Constipation 58, 84, 237, 347
    resolution of 331
Continuous venovenous
    filtration 396
    hemodiafiltration 396
Contraceptive
    oral 292
    use of 48
Copper 9, 100, 137, 191, 194, 272, 279, 396
    deficiency 9
Cori cycle 236
Corneal scar 55, 66, 67
    bilateral 68f
Corticosteroid use, minimization of 376
Corticotropin-releasing hormone 289
Cortisol 196
Costochondral junction, enlargement of 308
Coumarin derivatives 12
Cranial nerve palsies 118, 121
C-reactive protein 246
Crohn's disease 369, 375
Cryptosporidium 243
Cushing's syndrome 288, 295
Cyanocobalamin 8, 50, 138
Cyclic adenosine monophosphate 106
Cyclosporine 411
Cystathioninuria 48
Cystic fibrosis 11, 64, 88, 342, 344, 347, 350-352, 403
    transmembrane conductance regulator gene 342
Cystinosis 90
Cysts, epidermal 89
Cytokine 151, 249
    production, reduced 194

D

Daily energy intake, low 390
Daytime sleepiness 292
Deep venous thrombosis 290
Deformities 84
Dehydration 58, 213, 218, 231
    severe 217
    treatment of 232

Dehydroepiandrosterone 295
Delirium 237
Dementia 46, 53
Dental caries 10
Deoxyribonucleic acid 50
Depigmentation 9
Depression 53, 237, 292
Dermatitis 381, 382
   acral 129
   atopic 402
   contact 402
   herpetiformis 402
Dermatosis 46
   classical 209
   mosaic 205f
   typical 211
Desferrioxamine 12
Diabetes 180, 290, 295, 317, 361
   maternal gestational 291
   mellitus 10, 286, 292, 300
Diaphragm
   impaired contractility of 222
   weakness 237
Diarrhea 10, 46, 99f, 106, 194, 195, 195b, 210, 211, 217, 237, 243, 335, 336, 340, 403
   acute 336
   chronic 70, 111, 339, 340
   nutritional management of 335
   osmotic 195
   persistent 10, 338
   protracted 99
   three dietary plans in 339t
   worldwide 335
Diarrheal disease, chronic 65, 101
Diarrheal disorder, acute 335
Diet 282, 287, 338, 339, 369, 379
   high-protein 416
   types of 339
Dietary sources 43, 46, 50, 58, 101
Dietary supplement
   Health and Education Act 427
   role of 24
Disability adjusted life year 216
Disaccharidase deficiency 195, 403
Diuretic therapy 106
Diverticulitis 6
Docosahexaenoic acid 7, 272, 381
Dopamine 119
Down syndrome 295
Drip drop technique 160

Drowsiness 217
Dry beriberi 41, 42
Dry skin 68
Dual nutrition burden 304
Dual-energy X-ray absorptiometry 291, 347
Dugdale index 34, 35
Duodenal enzymes 207
Dyguesia 382
Dyselectrolytemia 224
Dysgeusia 380
Dyslectrolytemia 213
Dyslipidemia 300
Dysmotility 347
Dysphagia 292
Dysplasia 11
   metaphyseal 85
Dyspnea 222
Dystrophy, renal 92

E

Eating disorders 347
Eczema 129, 202f, 211, 237, 403
Edema
   bilateral pitting 218
   chest 207
   grading of 34b
   pediatric 204f, 207, 210f
   periorbital 204f
   pulmonary 237
   refeeding 221
Eicosanoids 135
Eicosapentaenoic acid 7
Electrocardiogram 212
Electrocardiography 197
Electrolyte 190, 218, 237, 394
   abnormality 237
      correction of 239
   disturbances 207
   imbalance 231
   serum 218
Encephalitis like syndrome 222
Encephalopathy 103
   hepatic 382
   hypoxic-ischemic 11
Endemic tropical sprue 51, 88
   part of 51f
Endocrine 188, 288
   disorders 288
   dysfunction 380

problems 292
system 229
Energy 16f, 143, 174, 188, 192, 272, 279, 383, 394, 397
   balance 318
   expenditure, break-up of 2t
   intake 318
   requirement 1, 3
      break-up of 4b
Entamoeba histolytica 206
Enteral infectious disease 347
Enteral nutrition 369, 374
Enteritis 206
Enterocolitis, necrotizing 11, 273
Enteropathy syndromes 402
Enterovirus 403
Enzyme 151
   deficiencies 403
      primary 403
      secondary 403
   therapy 362
Eosinophils 403
Epinephrine 289
Epithelial barrier function 375
Epithelium 54
Erythrocyte
   sedimentation rate 37
   zinc protoporphyrin level 112
Erythropoietin 151
Escherichia coli 336, 402, 403
Esomeprazole 416
Esophageal web 111
Esophagitis, allergic eosinophilic 402
European Society for Clinical Nutrition and Metabolism 346, 383
European Society for Pediatric Gastro-enterology, Hepatology and Nutrition 338, 371
European Society of Clinical Nutrition and Metabolism Guideline 394
European Society of Pediatrics Gastro-enterology and Nutrition Guidelines 271
Extensive superficial infection 217
Extracellular superoxide dismutase and catalase 12
Extremities 82
Eye problems 129

F

Facial
   nucleus 117
   puffiness 207
Failure to thrive 99, 101
Fanconi's syndrome 88, 90
Fat 1, 2, 5, 6, 16, 16f, 135, 150, 174, 176, 279, 321, 383, 421
   larger quantity of 2
   malabsorption 380
   nutritional requirements of 18
   soluble vitamins 7, 41, 54, 64, 70, 344, 373
      deficiency of 381
   tissue 389
   wasting, subcutaneous 211
Fatigue 237
Fatty acid 12
   essential 7, 135, 351
   long chain polyunsaturated 277, 381
   monounsaturated 7, 321
   omega-3 polyunsaturated 7, 12, 13, 321
   polyunsaturated 7, 150, 249, 321, 370
   synthesis of 49, 106
Fatty liver 192
   disease, nonalcoholic 286, 290, 292, 295
Feeding 148, 164, 165, 232
   alternative methods of 384
   complementary 164
   guidelines 304, 310
   inadequacy 219
   intervals and modes 275
   method, initial 273
   position 153f
   reflexes 157
      maternal 158f
      neonatal 159
   route of 394
   skills, maturation of 273
Ferric carboxymaltose injection 113
Fetal defects 68
Fetus
   growth of 134f, 135
   visual development of 136
Fever 56, 229
Fiber 2, 6, 135, 322
   advantages 6
   containing foods 6

daily requirement 6
dietary 322
disadvantage 6
types 6
Flavanols 12
Flavin
  adenine dinucleotide 43
  mononucleotide 43
Flavones 12
Flavonoids 12
Flavoprotein coenzymes 43
Fluid 4, 272, 422
  adequate 135
  imbalance, correction of 239
  retention 237
Fluoride 9, 10, 103, 272
Fluorosis 10, 85
Flushing 402
Folacin 52
Folate 52, 174
Folic acid 8, 41, 52, 137, 272, 279, 381, 397
  deficiency, maternal 53*f*
  requirements 138
  sources of 52*f*
  therapy, periconceptional 53, 53*f*
Follicle stimulating hormone 295
Food
  allergy 401, 405
    clinical manifestations of 405
    dietary management of 406
    natural history of 404*t*
    types of 403
  and Drug Administration 427
  components 318, 320, 414
  effect 413
  guide pyramid 299*f*
  intake and absorption 414
  intolerance 402
    and allergy 401
  phobias 402, 403
  protein-induced enterocolitis syndrome 402, 406
Foot pain 292
Foremilk 149
Formula-fed infants 57, 79
Fractures 84, 88
Fragile X syndrome 295
Free radicals 11, 21
  characteristic features of 21
  Golden's hypothesis of 190
Fructase 2, 402, 403
  intolerance, hereditary 402

Fundal changes 129
Fundus ophthalmicus 67
Funnel-chest deformity 83*f*

G

Gait, painful 292
Galactosemia 162, 403
Gallbladder disease 292
Gallstones 290
Gamma aminobutyric acid 119
Gastroenteritis 106, 402
Gastroesophageal reflux 292
  disease 290, 300, 347
Gastrointestinal
  anaphylaxis 402
  bleed 111
    aggravation of 112
  changes 134
  disease 13, 357
    eosinophilic 347
  disorders 402, 403
    functional 330
  food allergies 403
  infection, superimposed 195
  intestines 188
  manifestations 99, 206, 209
  problems 292
  surgery 111
  system 228
  tract 48, 104, 312, 393
  upset 9
Gavage feeding 276*f*
Genitourinary system 229
Genu valgum 82, 83*f*, 104
Genu varum 83
Genu varus 84*f*
Gestational age 271, 273
Ghrelin 151
Giardiasis, chronic 65
Glaucoma 129
Glimepiride 416
Globus pallidus 117
Glomerular filtration rate 90, 398
Glossitis 45*f*, 50*f*, 111, 381
Glucagon 196
Glucocorticoids 289
Glucogenesis, boosting of 196
Glucose 2, 3, 12
  tolerance, impaired 10
Glutamate decarboxylase 119
Glutamine 12
  supplementation 13

Glutathione 11
  concentration 24
  peroxidase 11, 12, 18, 152
  analogue 11
  selenium compounds like 12
Gluten-free diet 358, 362, 364
  benefits of 359
Glycemic index 7, 320
Glycogen deficit 380
Glycogenesis 236
Glycosidal alkaloid solanine 403
Goiter 10, 97, 98, 101, 103, 295
Golden's hypothesis 190
Gomez classification 198
Gomez syndrome 184, 221
Gopalan's hypothesis 190
Green classification 265
Growth 1, 4
  and nutrition, monitoring of 281
  childhood 287
  disorders 129
  documentation of 304
  factor 151
    epidermal 151
    insulin-like 151, 229, 381, 391
    transforming 151
  failure 68, 173, 189, 211, 371
    pathogenesis of 371f
  hormone 196, 229
    deficiency 288
  monitoring 166, 372
  parameters 346
  retardation 70, 99, 118, 201f, 202f, 211, 224, 382
Gulf syndrome 56, 58

H

Hair
  changes 203, 209
  loss 47
  premature graying of 47
Hallucinations 237
Handgrip strength 382
Haptoglobin 12
Harrison's groove 308
Harrison's sulcus 81
Headache 48
Health and nutritional education 265
Hearing loss 53
  sensorineural 118

Hearing problem 121
Heart
  autonomic control of 106
  block 10
  disease
    congenital 81
    cyanotic 81
    reduces incidence of 136
  failure 97f, 229, 237
Heavy metals 402, 403
Height for age 33, 39, 199
Heiner syndrome 402
Hematological effects 111
Hemochromatosis 11, 97
Hemoglobin 37, 218
  normal 306
Hemolysis 222, 237
Hemorrhage, intraventricular 11
Hemorrhagic disease 61, 150
  very-late vitamin K deficiency-related 61
Hemosiderosis 9, 97
  food-induced pulmonary 402
Hepatosplenomegaly 99
Hindmilk 150
Hip pain 292
Hirschsprung disease 403
Histamine 402, 403
Holliday and Segar formula 4t
Homocystinuria 48
Hookworm 111, 206
Hormone 40, 128
  luteinizing 295
  melanocyte-stimulating 289
  metabolism regulating 151
  parathyroid 73, 75
Human growth hormone 352
Human immunodeficiency virus 180, 216, 219
Human leukocyte antigen 356
Human milk
  fortification of 270, 278
  fortifier 278
  oligosaccharides 151
Hydroxyanisole, butylated 12
Hydroxyproline assay kit 38
Hymenolepsis nana 206
Hyperbilirubinemia 61
Hypercalcemia
  idiopathic 105
  severe 58

Hypercholesterolemia 50
Hyperesthesia 50
Hyperglycemia 237
Hyperkeratosis 56, 129
　follicular 68
Hyperlipidemia 50, 290
Hypernatremia 58
Hyperoxaluria 48
Hyperparathyroidism, secondary 308
Hyperpigmentation 9
Hypertension 58, 290, 291, 295, 300
　benign intracranial 121
　idiopathic intracranial 290
Hypertrophy 68
Hypervitaminosis 56, 58
Hyperzincuria 99
Hypoalbuminemia 196
Hypocalcemia 237, 307
　clinical features of 74
Hypogeusia 99
Hypoglycemia 192, 213, 217, 218, 231, 380, 388
　treatment of 231
Hypogonadism 9, 99
Hypokalemia 191, 237
Hypomagnesemia 237
　acute severe 106
Hyponatremia 237
Hyponatremic state 107
Hypophosphatemia 222b, 235, 237, 307
Hypotension 222, 237
Hypothermia 213, 217, 218, 229, 231
　treatment of 231
Hypothesis
　adaptation 189
　dietary 189
Hypothyroidism 288, 295
　congenital 98
　neonatal 98
Hypoxia, anemic 120

I

Ileitis, regional 99
Immune deficiency disorders 13
Immune system 229
　dysfunction of 382
　innate 245
Immunity
　acquired 247
　cell mediated 192, 194
Immunoglobulin 194, 277, 402

E-mediated allergy 404t
India's National Goiter Control Program 98
Indian Academy of Pediatrics Classification 198
Indian Childhood Cirrhosis 10, 11, 101
Indian Council of Medical Research 14, 15
Infant feeding, components of 148
Infantile tremor syndrome 10, 51, 100
Infections 127, 218, 231, 300
　bacterial 248
　fulminant 217
　treatment of 232
Infertility 68
Infestations 180
Inositol 272
Insomnia 48
Insulin 196
Integrated Child Development Service
　Program 263
　Scheme 264
Intensive care unit 273
Interaction Probability Scoring System and Scale 415
Interleukins 277
International Society of Renal Nutrition and Metabolism 392
Intestinal barrier defect, correction of 363
Intestinal
　microbiota 375
　mucosa, barrier function of 244
　parasitosis, chronic 60
Intracranial pressure, raised 56
Intrauterine growth
　restricted babies, feeding in 276
　restriction 37, 134, 277
Iodine 9, 10, 97, 137, 141, 177, 272
　deficiency 258
　　disorder 97, 98b
　deficient drinking water 97
　utilization 101
Iron 1, 9-13, 17, 17f, 18, 24, 96, 109, 116, 123, 137, 150, 174, 176, 191, 194, 272, 279, 315, 371
　absorption 101
　deficiency 49, 111, 116, 119t, 120, 120b, 121-123, 129, 306
　　anemia 9, 40, 41, 81, 96, 97f, 109, 115, 116, 195, 307, 308fc
　　causes of 110

neurologic sequelae of 119
neurological manifestation of 118*t*
dextran complex 113
dietary 110
ferric gluconate 113
oral 113*b*
overload 11
recommended dietary allowance of 110*t*
sucrose 113
therapy, parental 112
Irritable bowel 330, 339, 402
Isoniazid 416
Isonicotinyl hydrazide 57, 79

J

Jejunostomy, percutaneous endoscopic 384
Jelliffe classification 190, 198
Joints, hypermobility of 129
Joulie's solution 91
Junk foods 180

K

Kahn syndrome 222, 258
Kanawati index 34, 37
Kangaroo mother care 158*f*, 231
Keratomalacia 55, 66
Kernicterus 61
Kidney 52
  disease 104
    acute 393
    chronic 90, 390
  function, complete loss of 389
  injury
    acute 386-387, 394
    chronic 107
Knock-knee 73, 83
  deformity 104
  physiological 85
Koilonychia 111
Korsakoff's dementia 381
Korsakoff's psychosis 237
Kreb's cycle 49, 236
Kwashiorkor 11, 32, 188, 190, 192, 196, 197, 200, 201*f*, 202*f*, 204*f*-205*f*, 207, 210, 211, 211*t*, 212, 235, 239, 243, 244, 247, 248
  grading of 202*t*, 207*b*

marasmic 197, 198, 210, 210*f*, 242, 243
tissue paper intestine of 244
Kynureninase deficiency 48

L

Lactase 403
  deficiency 339
  enzyme 339
  primary 402
  secondary 402
Lactation 143
Lactic acid dehydrogenase, serum 52
Lactic acidosis 237
Lactoferrin 151, 277
Lactose 150, 339
  diet, low 339
  free diet 339
  intolerance 406
Lamblia giardia 206
Laparoscopic adjustable silicone gastric banding 300
L-ascorbic acid 272
Laurence-Moon syndromes 288, 294
L-carnitine 279, 411
Lecithin 7
Legs
  bowing of 73
  physiological bowing of 85
Leptin 151
  hormone injections 300
Lethargy 217, 222, 361
Leucine, catabolism of 49
Leukocyte 151
  count, total 245
  dysfunction 222, 237
Leukotrienes 249
Levothyroxine 411, 416
Limbs 294
Linoleic acid 7, 135, 272
Linolenic acid 7, 135
Lipids 135, 192, 272, 394, 395, 397
Lipolysis 196, 236
  augmentation of 196
Lipoprotein
  antioxidant 12
  high-density 9, 388, 389
  low-density 388, 389
  very low density 388, 389
Lithium 411
Liver 52, 188, 212, 224

disease 70, 92, 104, 347, 350
   cholestatic 11
   chronic 57, 74, 79, 88, 379, 380*t*
   protein synthesis, promotion of 196
Low birth weight 10, 80, 96, 134, 185
   babies 158*f*, 161, 270, 280
   feeding of 270, 271
Low glycemic index food items, advantages of 8
Lowe syndrome 88, 90
Lung disease, restrictive 290
Lycopene 1, 11, 12, 18
Lymphangiectasia, intestinal 402
Lymphocytes 151, 247, 403
Lymphokine production 194
Lymphopenia 194
Lymphoreticular system 188
Lysozymes 151, 277

M

Maclaren classification 198
Macrominerals 2, 8, 95, 96, 105
Macronutrients 2, 135, 137, 421
   dietary 372
Macrophages 151
Magnesium 9, 10, 105, 140, 174, 191, 236, 237, 272, 279, 358, 371, 382
   deficiency 88
   dependent resistant rickets 91
Malabsorption 57, 79, 380
   diseases 239
   states 60, 101
   syndrome 51
Malaria 111, 180, 229, 232
Malnutrition 10, 70, 129, 189*f*, 224, 242, 243, 250, 251, 254, 256, 257, 261, 266
   acute 220, 228, 230*f*, 233
   causes of 380*t*
   childhood 261, 267
   chronic 235
   diarrhea-related 335
   ecology of 186
   edematous 200
   immunology of 242
   malignant 200
   micronutrient 180
   mild-moderate 214
   moderate acute 220, 228
   nonedematous 207
   on organs, adverse effect of 188*b*
   on systems, adverse effect of 188*b*
   pathogenesis of 344
   prevention of 224, 263, 265, 266
   secondary 187
   severe acute 37, 216, 218*f*, 219, 220, 227, 228, 230, 231, 242, 243, 254, 304
   uncomplicated severe acute 214
Malondialdehyde 24
Manganese 1, 11, 16, 16*f*, 18, 103, 272, 279
Manic depression 104
Mantoux test 37
Marasmus 32, 197, 198, 207, 208*f*, 209*f*, 211, 211*t*, 212, 235, 239, 243
   nutritional 188
Marfan sign 82
Massive edema 201*f*, 205*f*
   over feet and legs 205*f*
Mastitis 161
Maternal nutritional status, cause and effect 144*fc*
Maternal tissues, development of 135
Measles 206
Medical nutrition therapy 220
Megaloblastosis 51*f*
Meningocele 53*f*
Menkes kinky hair disease 101
Menstrual problems 292
Mental
   health 292
   impairment 224
   retardation 98
Mercaptopurine 416
Metabolic disorder 190, 402
Metabolic syndrome 286, 290
Microbia, interaction of 332
Micronutrient 1, 2, 8, 9, 9*t*, 12, 95, 96, 108, 137, 218, 233, 350, 374, 383, 396, 421
   deficiency 40, 41, 194, 223, 304, 306, 371, 381, 382
Mid-day Meal Program 263, 264
Migraines 402
Milk
   manual expression of 157*f*
   thiamine level 43
   types of 277
Minerals 2, 8, 9*t*, 95, 135, 139, 190, 206, 210, 350, 373
   daily requirement for 9*t*
   rich source of 17*f*
   supplementation 323
Minimal enteral nutrition 273

Mitogen 194
Molybdenum 103, 272
Monitoring therapy 76
Monoamine oxidases 416
Monosodium glutamate 403
Mood
   disorders 347
   stabilizers, conventional 292
Moon facies 204*f*
Morbilliform rashes 402
Muscle
   cramps 48, 105, 237
   mass 390
      reduced 390
   pains 50
   protein catabolism, enhancement of 196
   twitching 237
   wasting 202*f*, 211
   weakness 237
Myalgia 237
Myelin formation 117, 118

N

Nabarrow's thinners chart 34
N-acetyl cysteine 11, 25
Nails, atrophic 99*f*
National Family Health Survey 116, 133, 148, 184, 185
National Guideline and Calcium Supplementation 139
National Institute for Health and Care Excellence 332
National Iodine Deficiency Disorder Control Program 263
National Iron Plus Initiative 114
National Nutrition Monitoring Bureau 14
National Nutritional Anemia Control Program 263
National Nutritional Programs 178
National Vitamin A Prophylaxis Program 69
Nausea 237
Neomycin 51
Neonatal and childhood, integrated management of 216, 264
Neophobia 165
Neoplastic disorders, increased risk of 381
Nephrotic syndrome 128

Nervous system 254
Net protein utilization 5
Neural tube defect 53, 53*f*, 129
Neuropsychiatric dysfunctions 116
Neurotransmitter metabolism 117
Neutropenia 9
Niacin 8, 45, 137, 139, 143, 174, 257, 272, 397
Nickel 104
Nicotinamide 1, 8, 11, 18, 45, 47, 279
Nicotinic acid 8, 40, 41, 45, 46*f*
Night blindness 55, 65, 66, 263, 381
Nipple
   cracked 160
   flat 161
   inverted 161
   large 161
   retracted 161
   sore 160
Nitrites 403
Nitroblue tetrazolium 246
Non-nutritive sucking 271
Norepinephrine 289
North American Society for Pediatric Gastroenterology, Hepatology and Nutrition 375
Nucleotides 12, 13, 272
Nutrients 1
   calculation of range of 272
   in milk 150
   loss of 387
   parameter 397
   recommended daily amounts of 2
   reduced absorption of 194
   supplements in practice 427
Nutrition 133, 135, 136, 173, 181, 264, 303, 317, 330, 336, 342, 356, 386, 420, 426
   adequate 1
   antenatal 133
   assessment 292
   chart 397*t*
   during pregnancy 133, 143
   enteral 384
   history 304
   management 388
   promotion 180
   supplementary 264, 264*t*
   supplementation and food fortification 263
   therapeutic aspects of 374

Nutritional
 advice
  age-specific 324
  components of 336
 assessment 371, 381, 386
 complications 376
 deficiencies 300
 dwarfing 199, 212
 edema 104, 201f
 marasmus, Achar's grading 209t
 recovery syndrome 184, 221
 status 413
  assessment of 32, 33b, 34b, 38, 381
  evaluation of 282
  monitoring of 372
 stunting 212
 supplementation, oral 349
Nystagmus 129

O

Obesity 37, 47, 170, 243, 286, 288, 289, 295
 childhood 304, 313
 comorbidities of 289, 290b
 hormonal control of 289f
 hyperventilation syndrome 290
 hypothalamic 300
 maternal 136
 morbid 37
 pediatric 286
Oligodendrocytes 118
Oligodontia 89
Oligosaccharides 151
Oral allergy syndrome 402
Oral rehydration
 solution 336
 therapy 337
Oral therapy 112
Orthopedic disease 295
Osteodystrophy, renal 90
Osteomalacia 80, 237, 382
Osteopenia 371
Osteoporosis 9, 57, 105, 371
Otitis media, acute 219
Outpatient Therapeutic Program 220
Oxaloacetate 49
Oxygen radical absorption capacity 23
Oxytocin reflex 158

P

Pain
 abdominal 58, 237
 chest 292
 recurrent abdominal 292
Paladai feeding 276f
Palpitations 105
Pancreas 188
Pancreatic disease 65, 70
Pancreatic enzyme replacement therapy 342, 345, 348
Pancreatic insufficiency 347, 403
Pancreatitis 11
Panophthalmitis 67
Pantothenic acid 8, 41, 47, 272, 279, 397
Para-aminobenzoic acid 151
Para-aminosalicylic acid deficiency 51
Paralytic ileus 107, 237
Parasites 403
Parathormone 73
 release of 73
Parenteral nutrition 49, 350, 374, 384
 solutions 397
 total 100, 395
Paresthesia 222
Pectus
 carinatum 82, 83f
 excavatum 82, 83, 83f
Pediatric intensive care unit 388
Pediatrician
 responsibilities of 429b
 role of 429b
Pellagra 47f
Penicillamine therapy 48
Peptic disease 403
Pesticides 402, 403
Peyer's patches 247
Phagocytic function 194
Phenylalanine 119
Phenylketonuria 119
Phosphatase, high alkaline 74
Phosphate 236, 237, 272
 defective reabsorption of 92
 low levels of 74
Phospholipids 7
Phosphorus 10, 17, 17f, 140, 150, 191, 279, 397
 supplementation 280

Phosphorylation, oxidative 103, 106
Photophobia 99f, 129, 381
Phrynoderma 68
Phthisis bulbi 67, 68f
Physician
  responsibilities of 429b
  role of 429b
Phytohemagglutinin 248
Phytonutrients 16, 16f
Picky eaters 304, 311
Pigeon chest 83f
  deformity 81, 82f
Pink classification 265
Placenta, development of 135
Plasma calcium, low levels of 74
Pneumocystis
  carinii pneumonia 217
  jiroveci 242, 243
Pneumonia 217, 243
  signs of 229
Poisoning 9
Polycystic ovarian syndrome 286, 290, 292
Polydipsia 292, 361
Polytrauma 13
Polyuria 58, 292, 361
Pompe disease 43
Ponderal index 34, 37
Postdialysis weight 392
Pot belly 73
Potassium 9, 16, 16f, 17, 17f, 107, 190, 237, 272, 279, 397
Prader-Willi syndrome 288, 295
Prebiotics 12, 13
  role of 337
Prednisone 292
Pregnancy 143
Pre-kwashiorkor 197, 210
Probiotics 12, 13
Proctocolitis 402
Prolactin reflex 157
Propionyl-CoA carboxylase 49
Propranalol 416
Propyl gallate 12
Protein 1, 2, 4, 5, 106, 135, 143, 150, 174, 175, 191, 272, 279, 322, 383, 394, 395, 397, 421, 423
  biologically complete 4
  catabolic rate 391
  daily requirement for 5t
  derivative, purified 229
  dietary deficiency of 24
  energy
    malnutrition 11, 40, 41, 97f, 99, 184, 185, 188, 194, 199, 213, 261
    wasting 390, 390t, 393
  nutritional requirements of 18
  quality indices 5b
  reference 5
  requirement 5, 175, 175t
  serum 212
  synthesis, control of 40
  total serum 191
  visceral 392
  wasting, pathogenesis of 387
Provitamin A 23
Pseudohypoparathyroidism 288
Pseudotumor cerebri 68, 70, 118, 221, 300
Puberty, delayed 129, 371
Purpura 229
  fulminans 213f
Pyloric stenosis 403
Pyodermas 206
Pyridoxine 8, 40, 41, 48, 143, 174, 257, 272
  responsive convulsions 48
  sources of 48f
Pyruvate carboxylase 49

Q

Quaker upper arm circumference stick method 34, 35, 35b, 36f
Quetlet's index 34, 37
Quick anthropometric assessment 304

R

Rachitic rosary 73, 81, 82
Radiation therapy 239
Radio-allergo-sorbent test 406
Randomized controlled trial 352
Raptomycin, mammalian target of 249
Rasagiline 411
Red blood cells 52, 109
Refeeding syndrome 222, 222b, 235, 237, 237t, 239, 239t, 240fc, 258
  pathophysiology of 237, 238fc
Reflexes
  maternal 157
  swallowing 159
Refractory rickets, diagnosis of 92t
Rehabilitation 217
  nutritional 219b, 258

Relactation 160
Renal disease 57, 79, 88, 92
Renal failure 74, 237
   Rifle classification 389*t*
Renal replacement
   requirement 388
   therapy 386, 388, 390, 394
Respiration, types of 229
Respiratory failure 222, 237, 390
Respiratory tract infection, lower 217
Restless legs syndrome 118, 122
Reticular pigmentation 204
Retinal detachment 129
Retinol 54, 174, 381
Retinopathy of prematurity 11, 59
Retinyl stearate 12
Rhabdomyolysis 237
Rhesus disease 11
Rhinoconjunctivitis, acute 402
Riboflavin 1, 8, 11, 18, 41, 43, 45*f*, 139, 143, 174, 272, 397
   deficiency 45*f*
   sources of 44*f*
Ribonucleic acid 98
Rickets 10, 57, 83*f*, 86*f*, 88, 92, 223, 382
   acrobatic 84
   celiac 89
   clinical features of 74
   drug-induced 85, 89
   familial hypophosphatemic 85, 88, 91
   hepatic 85, 89
   malabsorptive 85, 89
   nutritional 79, 309*fc*
   oncogenic 91
   oncogenous 85, 88, 91
   pseudodeficiency 89
   radiological changes of 74
   refractory 90
   renal 85, 88, 90
   resistant 90
   tumor-related 91
   types of 88
Rifampicin 57, 79
Rifle classification 389*t*
Rooting reflex 159
Rotavirus 403
Roundworm 206
Roux-en-y gastric bypass 300

S

Salmonella 403
Sample diet chart 305*t*
Saxitoxin 402
Scaly skin 68
Schilling test 52
Sclerosis, multiple 47
Scombroid poisoning 402
Scotoma, central 104
Scurvy 85
Seborrhea 47
Sedentary behavior 288
   restriction of 315
Seizure 217, 222, 237
   febrile 118, 122
Selective serotonin reuptake inhibitors 292
Selenium 1, 11, 12, 18, 24, 137, 141, 194, 272, 371, 382, 396
Sensorium 222
Sensory stimulation 218
Sepsis 13, 390
   bacterial 232
Septicemia 243
Serotonin 119, 403
Serum tyrosine level, low 196
Sex maturity index 171*t*
Shakir tape method 34, 35
Shock 237
   anaphylactic 402
   treatment of 232
Short bowel syndrome 350
Short limb 84, 88
Short stature 84, 88, 129
Short trunk 84, 88
Sickle cell anemia 99
Skeletal
   deformities 88
   dysplasia 81
   maturation 300
   muscle 389
   radiographs 38
Skin 127, 294
   barrier function of 244
   changes 203
   fold thickness 291
   hyperkeratotic 50, 100
   infections 229
   pigmentation of 51*f*
   prick tests 403

Skinfold thickness 200
Sleep apnea 295, 300
  obstructive 290, 292
  pediatric 286
Sleep disturbances 48
Sleep problems 292
Slipped femoral epiphysis 88, 290, 292
Small bowel obstruction 300
Small for gestational age 111, 270
Sodium 5, 9, 106, 191, 237, 272, 279, 397
  metabisulfite 403
  versenate 58
Somatomedin 196
  levels, low 196
Soto's massive 93
Sparse light-colored hair 204f
Spine 82
Sports
  and games, classification of 423t
  nutrition 420
Staphylococcus aureus 402
Starch 2
  diet, low 339
Steatohepatitis, nonalcoholic 300
Steatorrhea 192, 195, 347
Stem cells 277
Sterols 7
Stillbirth 98
Stomatitis 45f
  angular 45, 45f
Stones, renal 10
Stool 229
Storage disorders 11
Street foods 180
Streptococcus mutans 103
Stress 128
  incontinence 290
  oxidative 20, 21, 25, 26
Stroke 118, 120b
  pediatric 120
Stunting 185, 197
Substantia nigra reticulate 117
Sucking reflex 159
Sucrose free diet 339
Sudden infant death syndrome 140, 213
Sunken eyes 229
Sunshine vitamin 56
Superoxide dismutase 11, 12, 103
  antioxidants like 18
Supplementary feeding
  program 220
  protocols 219
Sweating, excessive 99, 106

T

T cells 151
Tachycardia 104, 237
Tamoxifen 416
Tartrazine 403
Taurine 12, 13, 279
Teeth 81
Tetany 10, 84, 105
Theobromine 402
Theophyline 416
Therapeutic feeding protocols 219
Thiamine 8, 41, 143, 174, 272, 381, 397
  deficiency 237, 257
  sources of 42f
Thorax 81
Threadworm 206
Thrombocytopenia 222, 237
Thrombocytosis 120
Thromboembolism 300
Thymus atrophy 247
Thyroid
  clinical grading of 98t
  gland, enlargement of 98
  stimulating hormone 295
Thyroxin 197
Tissue growth, regulators of 40
T-lymphocytes
  lower levels of 248
  reduced number of 194
Tocopherol 1, 12, 18, 23
Tocotrienols 12, 23
Tongue, atrophy of 68
Toxins 402, 403
Trace elements 1, 8, 9, 9t, 108
Traffic light eating 299f
Transferrin 11, 12, 18
Triacylglycerols, medium-chain 272
Triceps skinfold thickness 34, 35
Triglycerides 7, 389
  long-chain 7
  medium-chain 7, 337, 383
  plasma levels of 388
Tropical sprue 64
Tryptamine 402, 403
Tuberculin test 37
Tuberculosis 37, 48, 206, 209f, 232
Tubular necrosis, acute 237
Tubules, renal 92
Tubulointerstitial disease 90
Tumor 57
  necrosis factor α 374

Index **449**

Turner syndromes 288
Tyramine 402, 403

U

Ulcer, peptic 111
Ulceration, corneal 55, 66
Undernutrition 185
   World Health Organization classification of 306t
Underweight 185
United Nations Children Emergency Fund 216
United States Institute of Medicine 136
Urate 12
Urea nitrogen appearance 391
Urinary tract infection 213, 219, 267
Urinary urea nitrogen 392
Urine
   culture 229
   nitrogen appearance 388t
   routine and culture sensitivity 218
   urea nitrogen 387, 388
Urticaria 401-403
   contact 402

V

Vanadium 104
Varicose veins 290
Vascular endothelial growth factor 151
Ventral pallidum 117
Very low birth weight 57, 79, 80, 274
Virus 403
Visceroptosis 84
Vision, maintenance of 54
Vital signs 293
Vitamin 2, 8, 17, 17f, 23, 40, 61, 135, 139, 237, 323, 350, 358
   A 7, 8, 12, 13, 21, 22, 26, 40, 41, 54, 64, 69, 70, 107, 137, 139, 141, 150, 177, 194, 272, 279, 371, 397
      prophylaxis program 263
      sources of 55f
   A deficiency 64, 65
      corneal lesions indicative of 229
      deficiency signs of 55
      extraocular manifestations of 68b
      primary 70
   antioxidant 23
   B 8
      complex 40, 41
      group 177
   B1 41, 42f, 137, 139, 143, 279, 396
      deficiency 257
   B12 8, 50, 137, 138, 257, 279, 371, 381, 397
      deficiency 51f, 350
      sources of 50f
   B2 8, 41, 43, 44f, 61, 137, 139, 143, 279
      deficiency 45
   B3 8, 41, 45, 257
   B5 41, 47
   B6 8, 16, 16f, 41, 48, 137, 139, 194, 279, 257
      deficiency 49, 104
   B7 8, 41, 49
   B9 8, 41, 52
   C 8, 11-13, 16, 16f, 17f, 18, 21-24, 40, 41, 53, 107, 137, 139, 141, 150, 194, 279, 396, 397
      deficiency 54, 55b
      rich foods 10
      sources of 54f
   D 7, 40, 41, 56, 76, 78, 137, 139, 140, 150, 266, 272, 279, 307, 358, 382
      levels, estimation of 73
      metabolism of 72, 73fc, 92
      sources of 57f
      status 75, 75t
   D deficiency 57, 72-74, 75t, 76, 78, 79, 92, 93, 140, 266, 281, 307, 315
      causes of 57b, 79b
      maternal 80
      rickets 78, 79, 86f, 88
      severity of 74
   D dependent rickets
      broad etiologic classification of 92b
      hereditary 88, 89
   D3 8
   daily requirement for 8t
   deficiency 41, 64, 68f, 97f, 194, 206, 210, 257, 373
   E 1, 7, 8, 12, 18, 23, 26, 40, 41, 58, 137, 139, 141, 194, 272, 279, 371, 396, 397
      sources of 59f
   K 7, 40, 41, 59, 150, 279, 382, 397
      dietary sources of 60f
   K deficiency 61
      bleeding, early-onset 61
   K1 272

recommended dietary allowance of 174t
requirements of 8
rich source of 17f
water-soluble 40, 41, 373
Vomiting 58, 106, 210, 237, 403
  persistent 217

W

Waist-to-hip ratio 291
Water 2, 190
  intoxication 106
  requirement 3
  soluble vitamins, deficiency of 381
Waterlow classification 199
Weakness 222, 237
Weight
  for age 33, 39
  for height 33, 34, 39, 199, 291, 306
  gain 136
    drugs causing 292b
    gestational 136
    goals 296t
  loss 361
    surgery 300
  range 4
Wellcome classification 198
Wernicke encephalopathy 381
Wernicke-Korsakoff syndrome 237
Wet beriberi 41, 42
White retinal lesions 55, 66
William syndrome 105
Wilson disease 11, 48, 101
World Health Organization 69, 169, 184, 199, 254, 289, 346
  growth charts 228

Wound healing 9, 128
  delayed 99
Wrist joint, widening of 73

X

Xanthurenic aciduria 48
Xerophthalmia 64, 65f, 66, 66f-68f, 263
  UNICEF treatment schedule of 56b, 69b
  World Health Organization
    classification of 55b, 66b
    treatment schedule of 56b, 69b
Xerophthalmic fundi 55, 66
Xerosis 66f
  conjunctival 55, 65, 66
  corneal 55, 66, 67f, 263
X-ray, chest 37, 218, 229

Y

Yellow classification 265
Yersinia infection 112

Z

Z score 306
Zinc 1, 9-12, 17, 17f, 18, 24, 98, 126-130, 137, 141, 174, 177, 191, 194, 272, 279, 358, 371, 382, 396, 397
  deficiency 11, 99, 100, 191, 249, 266, 281, 338, 371
    clinical features of 129, 129t
  fertilizer strategy 100
  functions 127f
  role of 126, 266
  supplementation 337

EU GSPR Authorised Reprsentative
Logos Europe, 9 rue Nicolas Poussin
1700, La Rochelle, France
Phone: +33 (0) 6 67 93 73 78
E-mail: contact@logoseurope.eu

www.ingramcontent.com/pod-product-compliance
Ingram Content Group UK Ltd.
Pitfield, Milton Keynes, MK11 3LW, UK
UKHW050454150426
5217IPUK00025B/1687